Clinical Gastroenterology

Series Editor:

George Y. Wu
Division of Gastroenterology-Hepatology
University of Connecticut School of Medicine
Farmington, CT, USA

More information about this series at http://www.springer.com/series/7672

Micheal Tadros • George Y. Wu

Editors

Management of Occult GI Bleeding

A Clinical Guide

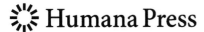 Humana Press

Editors
Micheal Tadros
Department of Gastroenterology
and Hepatology
Albany Medical Center
Albany, NY
USA

George Y. Wu
Department of Internal Medicine,
Division of Gastrenterology/Hepatology
University of Connecticut Health Center
Farmington, CT
USA

ISSN 2197-7399   ISSN 2197-7704   (electronic)
Clinical Gastroenterology
ISBN 978-3-030-71470-3   ISBN 978-3-030-71468-0   (eBook)
https://doi.org/10.1007/978-3-030-71468-0

This Humana imprint is published by the registered company Springer Nature Switzerland AG
The registered company address is: Gewerbestrasse 11, 6330 Cham, Switzerland

This book is dedicated to all our patients who have endured evaluations for obscure GI bleeding and to the physicians who so tirelessly have sought to determine and eliminate the causes, and to all the healthcare workers, who have persisted in being the guiding lights throughout the COVID-19 pandemic.

Preface

Occult gastrointestinal bleeding is a commonly encountered clinical problem in inpatient and outpatient practice. However, prompt delivery, accurate diagnoses, and effective therapy are often challenges. This textbook is designed to provide a comprehensive overview of the causes of occult GI bleeding, and an update on its management. The parts of the book are organized by organ and common causes of occult bleeding, prevalence, risk factors, typical presentations, diagnostic work up, advances on therapeutics, and pitfalls. Known genetic predispositions and special patient populations are discussed where data are available.

Occult GI bleeding is common indication of referral to a gastroenterologist. It usually presents as iron deficiency/microscopic anemia and/or microscopic detection of blood in stool in standard heme occult cards or by fecal immunohistochemical testing. The usual challenge is to determine the cause of the occult bleeding. It is imperative to develop a proper differential diagnosis to avoid delay in diagnosis and management. A major concern with occult GI bleeding is diagnosing or ruling out an underlying GI malignancy. Accordingly, the approach to elderly patients is different from young and middle aged ones due to increased prevalence of particular diseases with age. In addition, the expanding number of patients on non-steroidal anti-inflammatory agents as well as antiplatelet and anticoagulants medications increases the risk for occult bleeding.

The source of occult GI bleeding is usually identified with upper endoscopy and colonoscopy in 80–90% of patients. However, in the past, small bowel bleeding has been much more difficult to diagnose. However, advances in small bowel imaging and endoscopic modalities have led to enormous gains in diagnostic and therapeutic success rates in that organ.

This book provides a unique, comprehensive yet concise resource which contains detailed information for adult/pediatric gastroenterologists, primary care, internists, family doctors, and hospitalists. At the same time, the text is written to be comprehensible to other allied healthcare workers including nurse practitioners, nurses, physician assistants, and students in healthcare fields.

It is our hope that this volume will contribute to increasing awareness and prompt effective treatment that derives from understanding of the clinical problems and the modalities currently available to solve them.

Albany, NY, USA   Micheal Tadros
Farmington, CT, USA   George Y. Wu

Acknowledgments

Many thanks to those who worked exceptionally hard in the creation of this book. I would like to express my deepest appreciation to Dr. George Wu, the first physician I worked with pursuing a path in gastroenterology. His unwavering guidance and valuable advice still ring in my ears to this day. I could not have imagined a better advisor.

Special thanks to all my medical students, who present me with passion and enthusiasm for teaching in the field of medicine. Each of my students has shown the qualities required to become skilled physicians in the future, and I aspire towards working with them and assisting them in every aspect of the way.

I'm deeply appreciative to my division chief, Dr. James Litynski, for his continuous support, advice, and words of encouragement. Dr. Litynski is more of a friend and companion that leads with dedication and commitment. His guidance continues to help me in several aspects of my profession as a physician.

I would also like to extend my sincerest gratitude to Dr. Henry Pohl, Dr. John Birk, Dr. Michael Karsiak, Dr. Helen Swede, Dr. Scott Wetstone, and several others, who assisted in developing my clinical and academic career. I offer my sincere appreciation for the learning opportunities provided by these individuals who have encouraged me to dream for the best. Without these people, I would be lacking the skill that I hold today. Thank you.

Acknowledgments would be incomplete without offering recognition and gratitude to the souls of Dr. Cheryl Oncken, former chief of medicine at the University of Connecticut, and Dr. Thomas Devers, whose exceptional wisdom in the field of medicine continues to have an impact on me. These two prominent physicians have enabled me to become the physician I am today.

Lastly, I would like to acknowledge with gratitude the support and love of my entire family, as well as H.G. Cosman. I wouldn't be this successful without their inspiration and encouragement throughout my journey. They all kept me going, and their constant source of motivation is greatly appreciated (MT). The continued support of the Herman Lopata Chair in Hepatitis Research is gratefully acknowledged (GYW).

Contents

Contributors

Cassidy Alexandre, MD Department of Medicine, Division of Gastroenterology, Albany Medical Center, Albany, NY, USA

Nikki Allmendinger, MD Albany Medical Center, Albany, NY, USA

Ali Hani Al-Tarbsheh, MD Albany Medical College, Albany, NY, USA

Asra Batool, MD Albany Medical Center, Gastroenterology, Albany, NY, USA

Abbey Barnard, MD Veterans Affairs San Diego Healthcare System, San Diego, CA, USA

University of California-San Diego, Division of Gastroenterology, La Jolla, CA, USA

Victor N. Becerra, MD Albany Medical College Diagnostic Radiology, Albany, NY, USA

Kristina Bojanic, MD, PhD Department of Biophysics and Radiology, Faculty of Dental Medicine and Health Osijek, J. J. Strossmayer University of Osijek, Osijek, Croatia

Department of Biophysics and Radiology, Faculty of Medicine Osijek, J. J. Strossmayer University of Osijek, Osijek, Croatia

Department of Radiology, Health Center Osijek, Osijek, Croatia

Ethan Bortniker, MD Veterans Affairs San Diego Healthcare System, San Diego, CA, USA

University of California-San Diego, Division of Gastroenterology, La Jolla, CA, USA

Robert P.F. Brooks, MD Albany Medical College Diagnostic Radiology, Albany, NY, USA

Rosa T. Bui, MD Albany Medical Center, Gastroenterology, Albany, NY, USA

Deepika Devuni, MD Division of Gastroenterology, University of Massachusetts Medical School, Worcester, MA, USA

Katherine Donovan, MS Albany Medical Center, Albany, NY, USA

Peter Ells, MD Department of Medicine, Division of Gastroenterology, Albany Medical Center, Albany, NY, USA

Mark Hanscom, MD Division of Gastroenterology, University of Massachusetts Medical School, Worcester, MA, USA

Krishnakumar Hongalgi, MD Albany Medical Center, Albany, NY, USA

Jamie Horrigan, MD Department of Internal Medicine, Dartmouth-Hitchcock Medical Center, Lebanon, NH, USA

Jackcy Jacob, MD, FACP, FAAP Department of Internal Medicine, Albany Medical Center, Albany, NY, USA

Erik A. Jacobson, MD Albany Medical College Diagnostic Radiology, Albany, NY, USA

Neeha Kalakota, MD Division of Gastroenterology, Albany Medical Center, Albany, NY, USA

Katherine Kashinsky, MD Albany Medical Center, Albany, NY, USA

Peter E. Kim, MD Albany Medical College Diagnostic Radiology, Albany, NY, USA

Hwajeong Lee, MD Department of Pathology and Laboratory Medicine, Albany Medical Center, Albany, NY, USA

James Litynski, MD, FACG Division of Gastroenterology, Albany Medical Center, Albany, NY, USA

Craig A. McKinney, MD Division of Pediatric Gastroenterology, Hepatology and Nutrition, University of Virginia Children's Hospital, Charlottesville, VA, USA

Jeremy P. Middleton, MD Division of Pediatric Gastroenterology, Hepatology and Nutrition, University of Virginia Children's Hospital, Charlottesville, VA, USA

David Miller, MS Albany Medical Center, Albany, NY, USA

Sunil Narayan, MD Vascular and Interventional Radiology, Albany Medical College, Albany, NY, USA

Edgar R. Naut, MD, FACP, FHM Department of Medicine, Saint Francis Hospital and Medical Center, Hartford, CT, USA

Joseph M. Polito II, MD Albany Medical Center, Medicine, Albany, NY, USA

Caroline Polito, BS Stony Brook University Medical Center, Renaissance School of Medicine, Stony Brook, NY, USA

Perry K. Pratt, MD University of Connecticut Health, Division of Gastroenterology & Hepatology, Farmington, CT, USA

Julian Remouns, MD Albany Medical College, Albany, NY, USA

Enxhi Rrapi, BA Albany Medical College, Albany, NY, USA

Anthony K. Sayegh, MD Albany Medical College Diagnostic Radiology, Albany, NY, USA

Michael E. Schuster, MD Albany Medical College Diagnostic Radiology, Albany, NY, USA

Virali Shah, MBA Albany Medical College, Albany, NY, USA

Gagandeep Singh, MD, FHM Department of Medicine, Saint Francis Hospital and Medical Center, Hartford, CT, USA

Gary Siskin, MD Vascular and Interventional Radiology, Albany Medical College, Albany, NY, USA

Robert Smolic, MD, PhD Department of Pathophysiology, Physiology and Immunology, Faculty of Dental Medicine and Health Osijek, J. J. Strossmayer University of Osijek, Osijek, Croatia

Department of Pathophysiology, Faculty of Medicine Osijek, J. J. Strossmayer University of Osijek, Osijek, Croatia

Department of Medicine, Division of Gastroenterology/Hepatology, University Hospital Osijek, Osijek, Croatia

Martina Smolić, MD, PhD Department of Pharmacology and Biochemistry, Faculty of Dental Medicine and Health Osijek, J. J. Strossmayer University of Osijek, Osijek, Croatia

Department of Pharmacology, Faculty of Medicine Osijek, J. J. Strossmayer University of Osijek, Osijek, Croatia

Steven C. Stain, MD Department of Surgery, Albany Medical College, Albany, NY, USA

Rebecca J. Stetzer, MD Albany Medical College, Albany, NY, USA

Micheal Tadros, MD, MPH, FACG Department of Gastroenterology and Hepatology, Albany Medical Center, Albany, NY, USA

Marcel Tafen, MD Division of Trauma and Surgical Critical Care, Albany Medical College, Albany, NY, USA

Omar Tageldin, MD Department of Internal Medicine, Albany Medical Center, Albany, NY, USA

Haleh Vaziri, MD University of Connecticut Health, Division of Gastroenterology & Hepatology, Farmington, CT, USA

Alicia Wiczulis, MD Albany Medical Center, Albany, NY, USA

George Y. Wu, MD, PhD Department of Internal Medicine, Division of Gastrenterology/Hepatology, University of Connecticut Health Center, Farmington, CT, USA

Part I
Introduction

Chapter 1
An Introduction to the Clinical Approach and Management of Occult Gastrointestinal Bleeding

Jamie Horrigan, Micheal Tadros, and Jackcy Jacob

Introduction and Definitions

The clinical presentation GI blood loss depends on the location of the bleeding as well as the volume and rate of the bleeding. Minuscule blood loss of 0.5–1.5 mL per day in the GI tract is normal and not visualized, whereas larger blood volumes of 100–200 mL or greater produce visible blood in the stool [3]. Visible bleeding is defined as overt GI bleeding which most commonly presents in one of the following ways: (1) hematemesis – coffee-ground colored emesis typically from an upper GI source, (2) hematochezia – bright red blood or clots typically from a location in the distal GI tract or less commonly a briskly bleeding upper GI source, or (3) melena – tarry, black or maroon colored stool typically from an upper GI source or from degradation of blood in slow transit from the proximal colon [4]. *Occult* GI bleeding is not visible to the naked eye and is defined by a positive fecal occult blood test (FOBT) with or without iron deficiency anemia (IDA) [2]. When enough blood is lost over time and not adequately replaced by the body, iron deficiency can develop and eventually manifests as IDA. Chronic GI blood loss as little as 5–10 ml/day can lead to IDA [5].

In most instances, the cause of overt or occult bleeding is readily identified by esophagogastroduodenoscopy (EGD) and/or colonoscopy. However, when EGD

J. Horrigan
Department of Internal Medicine, Dartmouth-Hitchcock Medical Center, Lebanon, NH, USA
e-mail: jamie.m.horrigan@hitchcock.org

M. Tadros (✉)
Department of Gastroenterology and Hepatology, Albany Medical Center, Albany, NY, USA
e-mail: tadrosm1@amc.edu

J. Jacob
Department of Internal Medicine, Albany Medical Center, Albany, NY, USA
e-mail: jacobj@amc.edu

© The Author(s), under exclusive license to Springer Nature
Switzerland AG 2021
M. Tadros, G. Y. Wu (eds.), *Management of Occult GI Bleeding*, Clinical
Gastroenterology, https://doi.org/10.1007/978-3-030-71468-0_1

Table 1.1 Definitions of gastrointestinal bleeding

Gastrointestinal bleeding	Typical manifestation	Definition
Overt[a]: Bleeding is visible	Hematemesis	Vomiting of bright red blood or dark colored "coffee-grounds"
	Melena	Black, tarry, foul smelling stool
	Hematochezia	Bright red or maroon, bloody stool
Occult: Bleeding is invisible	Iron deficiency anemia (IDA) and/or	Hemoglobin <13 g/dL in men and < 12 g/dL in women. Often with low mean corpuscular volume MCV < 90 (early IDA may present with a normal MCV).
	Positive fecal occult blood test (FOBT)	Absence of overt bleeding with presence of blood in stool by guaiac or immunohistochemical testing
Obscure: Bleeding is visible or invisible		Recurrent or persistent bleeding that is overt or occult as above but with no source found after comprehensive testing of the upper, mid, and lower GI tract[b]

[a] Patients with overt bleeding may have iron deficiency anemia and will have a positive FOBT
[b]Raju et al. [31]

and colonoscopy fail to identify the source of the bleeding, the term *potential small bowel bleeding* is used. Anatomically, small bowel bleeding includes sources distal to the ampulla of Vater and proximal to the ileocecal valve, much of which is beyond the reach of a traditional enteroscope or colonoscope. If additional testing of the small bowel by video capsule endoscopy (VCE), enteroscopy, or radiographic studies such as angiography are also unable to find the source, the bleeding is termed *obscure*. Of note, prior to technological advancements over the last several decades, the term *obscure* bleeding was used to describe occult or overt bleeding following a normal EGD and colonoscopy and essentially became synonymous with small bowel bleeding. However, with the ability to visualize the small bowel with VCE, since 2001, and deep enteroscopy, since 2004, a small bowel source of GI bleeding is found in >70% of cases that were previously classified as obscure bleeding [2, 6]. Table 1.1 clarifies the often misused definitions.

Findings in Occult GI Bleeding

Iron Deficiency Anemia

Iron is essential for hemoglobin production. Thus the inadequate uptake and storage or excessive loss of iron will eventually lead to anemia, defined as a hemoglobin <13 g/dL in men and < 12 g/dL in women. While iron deficiency anemia (IDA) is most often caused by blood loss, other causes such as hemolysis, malabsorption, or increased demand for iron (such as in neonates and pregnant women) need to be excluded. IDA is most common in neonates and young children, followed by menstruating and pregnant women, and is least common in male adults. Consequently, when iron deficiency anemia is seen in groups other than premenopausal women, it is often assumed to be due to gastrointestinal loss [5].

Occult GI bleeding typically causes a slow and indolent drop in the hemoglobin along with other lab markers of iron deficiency including low serum iron, high iron-binding capacity, and low serum ferritin levels in early stages. Microcytosis is often not present until later stages of iron deficiency. It is important to note, however, that about 40% of the time, the anemia remains normocytic [1]. Serum ferritin levels are a marker of iron stores. Ferritin levels below 15 ng/mL are consistent with IDA, although, using 30 ng/mL as a cutoff may improve sensitivity [7]. Additionally, since ferritin is an acute phase reactant and often quite elevated in patients with chronic inflammatory conditions, a higher threshold is used to reflect IDA i.e. ferritin levels below 50 or 100 ng/mL in these patients. In patients with quiescent inflammatory bowel disease (IBD), for example, iron deficiency is defined as ferritin <30 ng/mL or transferrin saturation < 16%, whereas in IBD patients with active disease the serum ferritin cut off is 100 ng/mL [1, 8, 9].

Fecal Occult Blood Testing (FOBT)

As noted earlier, melena or hematochezia may be seen when a patient passes large volumes of blood (100 mL or more) from the GI tract. However, when less than 100 ml is passed, stool may be dark or appear normal. This is when fecal occult blood testing (FOBT) may be useful to identify suspected GI bleeding. Fecal occult blood tests start to become positive at a level of about 2 mL per day or higher, but the sensitivity increases considerably as the volume of fecal blood increases [8]. Testing for occult blood is often performed through guaiac-based stool tests, fecal immunochemical tests (FIT), and heme-porphyrin based tests.

Guaiac is a brown resin from the guaiacum tree that turns a blue color when it oxidized by the pseudoperoxidase activity of hemoglobin. Guaiac tests preferentially detect lower GI tract bleeding due to degradation of the hemoglobin that occurs in the upper GI tract. Nevertheless, there are a number of upper GI lesions that can be detected on guaiac based testing if enough blood loss is present [9].

Similarly, immunochemical testing is also sensitive and specific for lower GI tract bleeding, but not upper GI tract bleeding due to hemoglobin degradation. Immunochemical tests work by detecting human globin epitopes and thus, do not require dietary restriction and is less affected by concomitant medication use. Discontinuation of aspirin/NSAIDs is not needed as in other forms of testing. Additionally, only one stool sample is required as opposed to the three samples required for guaiac based FOBT. The heme-porphyrin assay which accurately measures the total stool hemoglobin by the porphyrin derived from heme through spectrofuorometric method, can be confounded by myoglobin, which is also found in red meats, making dietary restriction necessary. On the contrary, ingestion of vitamin C, such as in fruits, fruit juices, or supplements, may cause false-negative results as vitamin C inhibits oxidation [10, 11].

Historically, the goal of FOBT was to detect microscopic bleeding in the GI tract and aid in the detection of colorectal neoplasia. Overuse of FOBT, especially in the inpatient setting, where it is inappropriately used for any anemia, has led to increased false positive tests [12]. Additionally, inadequate sampling (one instead of three) has led to inappropriate use in the outpatient setting with premature referral to invasive testing [13]. As noted earlier, in patients with IDA, a negative FOBT does not necessarily rule out GI bleeding, especially if located in the upper GI tract. The FOBT was falsely negative in 42% of patients with IDA who had lesions on upper endoscopy that were the likely the source of the bleed [14].

More information about FOBT is provided in Chap. 2.

Sources of Occult GI Bleeding

Occult GI bleeding can occur anywhere in the GI tract from the oropharynx to the anus and a source is found in approximately 60% of cases. The majority of patients (30–55%) end up having an upper GI source while 20–30% have a colorectal source. About 10% of patients have synchronous lesions in which there are both upper and lower GI lesions. In those patients in which the lesion is not found on EGD or colonoscopy, a thorough small bowel evaluation reveals the source in 30–50% of these patients [15, 16].

As summarized above, the causes of occult GI bleeding are commonly categorized by their location within the GI tract and usually divided into endoscopic areas: upper GI tract, small bowel, or lower GI tract. They can also be further classified by the different pathologic categories: neoplastic, vascular, inflammatory, genetic, or other as shown in Table 1.2 [5].

Non-Gastrointestinal Causes of Bleeding

The GI work up for iron deficiency anemia sometimes returns negative. Though this is a textbook on occult GI bleeding, it warrants special warning to the clinician that the source of the anemia still needs to be aggressively sought and may ultimately be an area anatomically close to the GI tract. Unseen bleeding from epistaxis, hemangiomas, or occult trauma to the nasal or oropharyngeal passage, for example, may result in ingestion of blood unbeknownst to the patient. As such, a thorough physical exam or referral to otolaryngology may end up finding the source. Rarely, history of blood from the oropharynx can be confused as hematemesis when in fact, it is from bleeding from the respiratory tract (hemoptysis) that the patient could be ingesting [17].

Table 1.2 Sources of occult GI bleeding

Neoplastic	Vascular	Inflammatory	Genetic	Other
Carcinoma – esophageal, gastric, small bowel, colon Adenoma Polyposis syndromes Gastrointestinal stromal cell tumor (GIST) Kaposi sarcoma Lynphona Leiomyoma or leiomyosarcoma Carclnoic Lipoma	Vascular ectasias (at any site) Post-surgical (biopsy site, polypectomy, anastomotic bleeding) Anorectal disease (hemorrhoid, fissure) Diverticular bleed Gastric aAntral vascular ectasia (GAVE) Ischemia (i.e. ischemic colitis) Dieulafoy's lesion Cameron lesion Meckel's diverticulum Amyloidosis Gastrointestinal hemangioma Vasculitis	Aorto-enteric fistulas Inflammatory bowel disease (IBD) Erosive esophagitis Erosive gastritis Cameron lesion Colitis (including medication-induced) Ulcerative jejunitis from celiac disease Endometriosis Portal hypertensive gastropathy or enteropathy Varices (esophageal, gastric, small bowel) Ulcer (any site, including medication-induced)	Osler-Weber-Rendu sydrome Blue rubber bleb nevus syndrom Neurofibromatosis type I or II Gardner's syndrome Klippel-Trenaunay-Weber syndrome Ehlers-Danlos syndrome Hermans ky-Pudlak syndrome	**Infectious diseases:** Clostridioides difficile Cytomegalovirus Parasitic infection Helicobacter pylori Tuberculosis **Non-GI causes that can mimic GI bleeding:** Long-distance running Hemoptysis Oropharyngeal bleeding (i.e epistaxis) Gynecologic bleeding Factitious bleeding (self-induced)

[a]Lee and Laberge [42]
[a]Rockey [43]

Management

The Role of Thorough History and Physical

The differential diagnosis of GI bleeding is broad. Thus, a targeted approach based on the patient's symptoms, past medical history, family history, and physical exam may result in a swift and more efficient investigation.

Many patients with occult GI bleeding present with moderate to severe anemia on labs, but can be surprisingly asymptomatic due to the chronicity of the bleeding with adequate compensation. Thus, these patients may not present with the typical signs or symptoms of anemia, such as fatigue, weakness, and reduced exercise capacity. More subtle symptoms of chronic iron deficiency anemia include hair loss, hand and feet paresthesias, restless leg syndrome (often seen even in iron deficiency alone prior to the anemia), and in men, impotence. It may not be until severe anemia with hemoglobin <7 mg/dl that the patient will finally begin to display more disconcerting symptoms such as pallor, headache or dizziness from hypoxia, tinnitus from the increased circulatory response, or dyspnea from high output cardiac failure [1].

A detailed history of gastrointestinal symptoms such as heartburn, dysphagia, odynophagia, recurrent nausea, vomiting, or prolonged anorexia should direct the clinician to an upper GI source. A history of severe reflux symptoms or difficulty swallowing may suggest esophagitis. Epigastric abdominal pain, burning in the epigastrium after eating, or intolerance of foods may suggest gastritis or gastric ulcers, especially in patients who have a history smoking, of overusing NSAIDs, or having a diet known to be associated with gastritis or ulcers. A history of alcoholism, especially with cirrhosis, could also be suggestive of peptic ulcer disease as well as premalignant colonic neoplasia [18]. Symptoms consistent with a lower GI source include a change in the stool caliber, diarrhea, constipation, lower abdominal pain. Parasitic infections can cause a constellation of non-specific symptoms including abdominal pain, flatulence, nausea, diarrhea, and signs of iron deficiency anemia. Exposure to typical water sources and foods prone to parasite ingestion or inoculation will be important.

Furthermore, a chronic overt GI bleed, such as recurrent variceal bleeding, may present as occult GI bleeding. These patients may have chronic melena that goes unnoticed or is ignored. The delayed presentation of an overt GI bleed will likely result in IDA. Patients with chronic liver disease may develop chronic GI bleeding and IDA from portal hypertensive gastropathy and gastric antral vascular ectasia (GAVE). Angiodysplasias may present as chronic GI bleeding due to frequent rebleeding and the presence of multiple lesions [19, 20].

Patients with red flag signs such as a history of unintentional weight loss or family history of malignancy may have a mass lesion, typically of the lower GI tract. It is important to remember that these patients may not have GI symptoms at all and, if they are above the age of 45–50 years old, colorectal cancer is at the top of the differential, especially if they have never had colorectal screening in the past. Additionally, a history of radiation or malignancy related treatment to an area of the GI tract might suggest mucosal injury as the source of bleeding, such as radiation proctitis.

Concurrent diagnosis of aortic stenosis and occult GI bleeding may suggest bleeding from acquired coagulopathy, known as Heyde's syndrome, in which the patient develops angiodysplasias [21]. Patients with end stage renal disease (ESRD) are also at risk of gastric vascular ectasias and colonic angiodysplasias, though the pathophysiology is not well understood [22]. The implantation of left ventricular assistive devices (LVAD) have an increased association with angiodysplasias as well [23]. A history of liver disease or portal hypertension might suggest varices or portal hypertensive gastropathy. Sometimes the diagnosis is not yet made, and the clinician must be vigilant for physical exam findings such as caput medusa, spider angiomas, or abdominal distention due to ascites, which will be the key to diagnosis.

A history of severe epistaxis may suggest a vascular lesion, especially when associated with telangiectasias of the lips, tongue, or palms. Multiple vascular lesions might also indicate hereditary hemorrhagic telangiectasias, and a careful family history must be elicited. Blue or colored papules on the skin, in the right setting, may suggest blue rubber bleb nevus syndrome, which is a rare, severe, sporadically occurring disorder characterized by multiple venous malformations.

Special Populations

Special populations warrant a mention here to make sure that key sources of occult bleeding are not missed. Specifically, pre-menopausal women, patients less than 40 years old, particularly pediatric patients, and patients on anticoagulants.

Anticoagulant Use

Positive FOBT in patients on chronic antiplatelets, NSAIDs, or anticoagulation should not be attributed to medication use unless endoscopy is unrevealing. There are mixed data on whether antiplatelet, anticoagulants, and NSAIDs increase or decrease the positive predictive value or sensitivity of detecting colorectal neoplasms [24]. Ultimately, positive fecal occult blood tests, in patients taking either low-dose aspirin or warfarin, should be managed in the same fashion as patients not taking these medications [25].

Pediatric Patients

Many times, simple demographic data may help drive the work up. For example, in patients less than 40 years of age, small bowel tumors, inflammatory bowel disease, Dieulafoy's lesion, or Meckel's diverticulum (especially in the pediatric population) may be the likely etiology [26]. Bleeding in older patients tend to be from neoplasia or medication-induced GI complications, such as mucosal ulcers or gastropathy due to NSAIDs. Younger patients tend to have inflammatory lesions and are more prone to have bleeding from ulceration of a Meckel's diverticulum in the small bowel. The ulceration occurs in the distal mucosa and occurs due to acid secretion by ectopic gastric mucosa within the diverticulum [27]. Dieulafoy's lesions were named in 1898 by a French surgeon, and are submucosal arterial malformations that are difficult to diagnose as they are most commonly located in the small bowel [28]. In neonates, small bowel lesions would also include necrotizing enterocolitis. In infants, milk-protein allergy would also be of consideration. Other causes of small bowel bleeding in patients less than age 40 are seen in Table 1.3.

Table 1.3 Common occult GI bleeding in the small bowel based on age

Under age 40 years	Over age 40 years
Neoplasia (typically of small bowel)	Vascular ectasia
Inflammatory bowel disease (IBD)	Dieulafoy's lesions
Dieulafoy's lesions	Neoplasia
Meckel's diverticulum	NSAID-induced ulcers
Polyposis syndromes	Aorto-enteric fistula (if history of prior surgery)
	Small bowel varices
	Portal hypertensive enteropathy

Table adapted from Welli et al. [44]

Pre-Menopausal Women

IDA in pre-menopausal women is often due to heavy menses. As such, gynecologic sources of bleeding should be excluded before a full GI workup. However, women with GI symptoms and a positive FOBT or IDA warrant evaluation with EGD and colonoscopy for an occult GI bleeding source. In a study of 186 premenopausal women with a positive FOBT who underwent endoscopy, 23% had a clinically important lesion. These lesions were often in the upper GI tract and related to peptic ulcer disease (3%) or gastric cancer (3%). In these women, hemoglobin <10 g/dl, positive FOBT, and GI symptoms predicted clinically significant findings on endoscopy [29].

Clinical Approach to Occult GI Bleeding

The clinical approach to a patient with occult GI bleeding. or suspected occult GI bleeding will depend on the patient's age, clinical history, and whether the patient has a positive FOBT or IDA. It is important to assess the patient's stability, and formulate an effective diagnostic and treatment plan. We will go through the management of several patient populations based on their clinical presentations using the American College of Gastroenterology (ACG) clinical guidelines on small bowel bleeding from 2015, the American Gastroenterological Association (AGA) medical position on obscure GI bleeding from 2007, and the AGA Clinical Practice Guidelines on the Gastrointestinal Evaluation of Iron Deficiency Anemia from 2020 [2, 30].

The Patient with a Positive FOBT, But Without Iron Deficiency Anemia

If an asymptomatic patient has suspected GI bleeding with a positive FOBT and no IDA, then colonoscopy is recommended, especially if the patient is over 50 years [31]. The reason colonoscopy is preferred as a first step is because of the high risk of colonic carcinoma, the fact that upper GI sources of bleeding typically cause symptoms, and the high prevalence of false-positive FOBT and FIT. If the patient

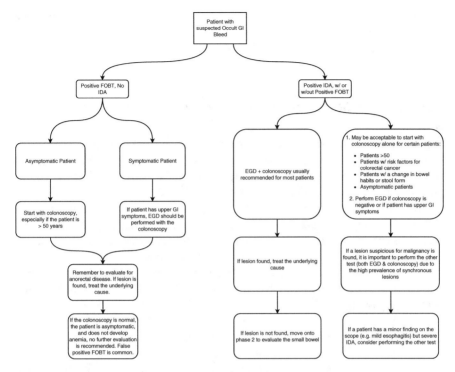

Fig. 1.1 Diagnostic algorithm for patients with suspected occult gastrointestinal (GI) bleeding with positive fecal occult blood test (FOBT) and/or positive iron deficiency anemia (IDA). EGD = esophagogastroduodenoscopy.

has upper GI symptoms, EGD should be performed along with the colonoscopy. If the colonoscopy is normal, the patient is asymptomatic, and does not develop anemia, then no further evaluation is recommended [Fig. 1.1] [2, 4, 31].

Since false positive FOBT is common, particularly with guaiac-based tests, testing error must be considered if the clinical scenario is inconsistent with bleeding. As guaiac-based tests rely on the pseudoperoxidase activity of hemoglobin, consumption of trace blood in red meats may cause a false-positive test. Similarly, foods that contain peroxidase, such as cruciferous vegetables (i.e. broccoli, cauliflower) can also cause a false positive. Swallowing blood from epistaxis or gingival bleeding may also produce a positive FOBT. Lastly, a positive FOBT may also be due to anorectal disease, including hemorrhoidal bleeding or the presence of a fissure [1, 12, 32]. A large study of asymptomatic patients found that the presence of hemorrhoids was an independent risk factor for false positive FIT results. Some studies have supported this finding, while others have shown no association [33, 34]. Hemorrhoids are rarely a cause of IDA, unless there is an overt bleed [35]. Given the disparities between studies, we recommend a colonoscopy in older patients with positive FOBT results to rule out more serious colorectal pathology even if the patient has known hemorrhoids. If the patient has hemorrhoids and a persistently positive FOBT after normal colonoscopy, then no further evaluation is warranted. If a younger patient has a positive FOBT, is asymptomatic, and does not have IDA or risk factors for colorectal cancer, it is reasonable to observe the patient. Lastly, if the patient has hemorrhoids, positive FOBT, and IDA, then evaluation of the upper and lower GI tract is warranted per the algorithm below.

The Patient with Iron Deficiency Anemia +/− Positive FOBT

Patients with iron deficiency anemia not attributed to hematologic or malabsorption causes, particularly men and post-menopausal women warrant evaluation regardless of whether FOBT is positive or negative to rule out serious pathology. The most common etiologies of occult GI bleeding and resulting IDA in these patients include colonic carcinoma, mucosal injury from long term aspirin (or other nonsteroidal anti-inflammatory drug use), angiodysplasia, gastric carcinoma, peptic ulcer disease, esophagitis, H. pylori infection, GAVE, gastrectomy, and small bowel tumors [1]. Thus, patients with IDA and a positive FOBT often require both EGD and colonoscopy as an initial workup. In particular, IDA in men and postmenopausal women must be assumed due to GI blood loss and warrants evaluation with both EGD and colonoscopy [2, 31]. Additionally, premenopausal women without a history of menorrhagia and incidental finding of IDA or patients with IDA and concurrent GI symptoms should undergo both EGD and colonoscopy.

For certain patient populations, it is acceptable to start with either colonoscopy or endoscopy as the initial diagnostic test. Consider colonoscopy as the initial diagnostic test in a patient with IDA over 50 years old without any GI symptoms if they have risk factors for colorectal cancer such as a family history or a change in stool form or frequency. Consider EGD as the initial diagnostic test in a patient with upper GI symptoms, a history of NSAID use or abuse, heavy alcohol use or cirrhosis, or those with a history of developmental disability, or inability to express GERD symptoms. If one test is normal, it is reasonable to perform the other for a complete evaluation. EGD and colonoscopy may be performed in succession during on the same day for patient convenience, decreased sedation use, and cost reduction. Some physicians prefer to give the patient a bowel prep for a colonoscopy, and if the colonoscopy is normal, then perform the EGD next. The decision of whether to perform the second scope should be individualized based on patient findings. For example, if the severity of the IDA is not fully explained by the severity of the lesion (i.e. mild esophagitis seen with significant IDA), then a colonoscopy is reasonable to evaluate for a significant lower GI lesion since on average, 10% of patients will have synchronous lesions [2, 15, 31].

During the EGD, duodenal biopsies should be performed to rule out celiac disease. Of note, according to the ACG small bowel bleeding guidelines, celiac disease is no longer considered a cause of GI bleeding. Instead, the thought is that celiac disease causes iron deficiency anemia from malabsorption, not occult GI bleeding. However, in rare cases, ulcerative jejunitis, lymphoma, and adenocarcinoma can occur from celiac disease complications and result in small bowel bleeding [2]. Biopsies should also be performed in the colon, particularly in patients with diarrhea, as 50% of microscopic colitis have mild anemia [36].

Small Bowel Evaluation

If EGD and colonoscopy are normal, and the patient has severe IDA, persistent symptoms of small bowel lesions (diarrhea), or failure of IDA to correct with adequate replacement therapy, then an evaluation of the small bowel or second-look endoscopy is warranted [2, 31]. The most commonly used diagnostic tool for small bowel evaluation is a video capsule endoscopy (VCE), whereby a wireless camera in capsular form is ingested by the patient to help visualize portions of the small bowel inaccessible by EGD and colonoscopy. The diagnostic yield of VCE is 38–83% in patients with suspected small bowel bleeding [37]. Not every patient can undergo VCE, particularly those with stricturing Crohn's disease, clinical signs of obstruction, a history of radiation to the small bowel, certain motility disorders, and pregnant patients [38]. In these patients with contraindications to VCE, radiographic tests, such as computed tomographic enterography (CTE) can also be used [Fig. 1.2] [2]. Another drawback of VCE is its poor ability to localize a lesion in terms of guiding deep enteroscopy for intervention [2].

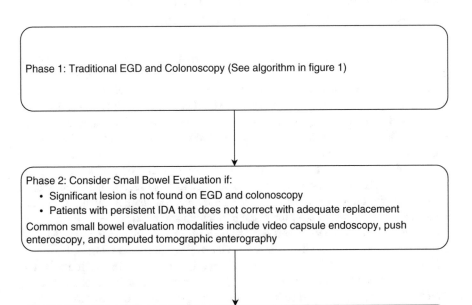

Fig. 1.2 Phases of diagnostic evaluation of patients with occult gastrointestinal (GI) bleeding EGD = esophagogastroduodenoscopy; IDA = iron deficiency anemia

Another commonly used diagnostic tool for the small bowel is push enteroscopy which has the benefits of intervention as well as better visualization of the proximal small bowel 45–90 cm distal to the ligament of Treitz. Push endoscopy has a diagnostic yield of 3–70% in cases of suspected small bowel bleeding [2]. However, most of the lesions found on push endoscopy are actually within reach of a traditional endoscope, which reiterates the importance of a careful first inspection of the upper GI tract with EGD and the importance of second-look endoscopy [39, 40]. Disadvantages of push enteroscopy include patient discomfort as compared to a traditional EGD and looping of the enteroscope in the stomach. Of note however, it actually offers a better view of the duodenum and proximal jejunum compared to the VCE. However, if push enteroscopy is normal, it is reasonable to move onto VCE for visualization of the more distal small bowel. With the advances in technology, there is now also single balloon, double balloon, and spiral enteroscopy which allow for examination of the full length of the small bowel. More details are discussed in the endoscopy chapter.

The Patient Who Warrants Second-Look Endoscopy/ Colonoscopy Due to Potential Missed Lesions

As noted earlier, second-look endoscopy is warranted to patients with refractory anemia for whom a comprehensive initial exam did not uncover the bleeding source. Endoscopy is an invaluable tool, but lesions are often missed. Studies have shown that 3.5% to greater than 30% of clinically significant non-small bowel lesions are missed on EGD, push enteroscopy, and colonoscopy that are incidentally detected by VCE. This means that these lesions were within reach of the traditional EGD and colonoscopes, but were missed.

Second-look entails repeating the EGD or colonoscopy or performing a push enteroscopy. The latter can be considered another form of second-look endoscopy, as it allows for direct visualization of the upper gastrointestinal much beyond the ligament of Treitz, particularly the distal duodenum and proximal jejunum which is challenging to see with VCE and out of reach of a traditional endoscope. Missed lesions occur more commonly in the lower GI tract than the upper GI tract. However, when the missed lesion is in the upper GI tract, it is most commonly found in the antrum. Cameron lesions can be missed in patients with a large hiatal hernia. Colorectal cancer can be missed in patients with a poor prep. Arteriovenous malformations or Dieulafoy's lesions can be missed if they are present in the gastro-duodenum and may require a side view scope. Anal cancer can be missed if a rectal exam was not done or during rapid colonoscope insertion. Varices can be missed if they are deflated (as in under-resuscitated patients). Due to the high prevalence of these missed lesions, it may be worthwhile to repeat EGD and colonoscopy in a

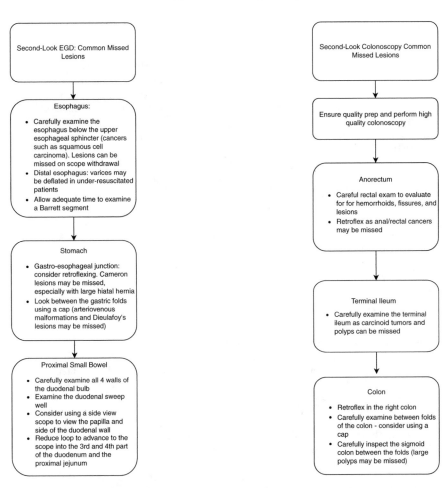

Fig. 1.3 Recommendations evaluation of missed lesions during second-look endoscopy. EGD = esophagogastroduodenoscopy

patient with persistent IDA that does not correct with adequate replacement and a positive FOBT, especially when the first examination was done at a different healthcare center [41], [Fig. 1.3].

Subsequent chapters will delve into the specifics of screening tests, endoscopic evaluation, imaging, differential based on the sites of the lesion, management, and special populations.

Acknowledgments The authors thank Ms. Elizabeth Irish and the Albany Medical College Library for their contribution to this chapter.

Appendix 1

		Gastrointestinal bleeding	
		Occult – unseen by the patient and clinician	Overt – seen by the patient and clinician
SOURCE OF BLEED or PATHOLOGY	**Obvious**-positive EGD or colonoscopy (or small bowel testing*)	**Occult/obvious source**	Overt/obvious source
	Obscure-negative EGD, colonoscopy (or small bowel evaluation*) but patient continues to bleed (5% of all bleeds)	**Occult/obscure source**	Overt/obscure source

*Small bowel evaluation may include video capsule endoscopy and enteroscopy.
EGD: Esophagogastroduodenoscopy.

Bibliography

1. Short MW, Domagalski JE, Am Fam Physician. 87. 2013;98–104.
2. Gerson LB, Fidler JL, Cave DR, Leighton JA, Am J Gastroenterol. 2015;110:1265–87. https://www.gastrojournal.org/article/S0016-5085(20)34847-2/fulltext#articleInformation.
3. Dybdahl JH, Daae LN, Larsen S. Occult faecal blood loss determined by chemical tests and a 51 Cr method. Scand J Gastroenterol. 1981;16(2):245–52. https://doi.org/10.3109/00365528109181963.
4. Luke RG, Lees W, Rudick J. Appearances of the stools after the introduction of blood into the caecum. Gut. 1964;5:77–9. https://doi.org/10.1136/gut.5.1.77.
5. Rockey DC. Occult gastrointestinal bleeding. N Engl J Med. 1999;341(1):38–46. https://doi.org/10.1056/nejm199907013410107.
6. Pasha SF, Leighton JA, Das A, Harrison ME, Decker GA, Fleischer DE, et al. Double-balloon enteroscopy and capsule endoscopy have comparable diagnostic yield in small-bowel disease: a meta-analysis. Clin Gastroenterol Hepatol. 2008;6(6):671–6. https://doi.org/10.1016/j.cgh.2008.01.005.
7. Kaitha S, Bashir M, Ali T. Iron deficiency anemia in inflammatory bowel disease. World J Gastrointest Pathophysiol. 2015;6(3):62–72. https://doi.org/10.4291/wjgp.v6.i3.62.
8. Rockey DC. Occult gastrointestinal bleeding. Gastroenterol Clin N Am. 2005;34(4):699–718. https://doi.org/10.1016/j.gtc.2005.08.010.
9. Rockey DC, Koch J, Cello JP, Sanders LL, McQuaid K. Relative frequency of upper gastrointestinal and colonic lesions in patients with positive fecal occult-blood tests. N Engl J Med. 1998;339(3):153–9. https://doi.org/10.1056/nejm199807163390303.
10. Nicholson BD, Thompson M, Price CP, Heneghan C, Pluddemann A. Home-use faecal immunochemical testing: primary care diagnostic technology update. Br J Gen Pract. 2015;65(632):156–8. https://doi.org/10.3399/bjgp15X684229.
11. Brenner H, Tao S, Haug U. Low-dose aspirin use and performance of immunochemical fecal occult blood tests. JAMA. 2010;304(22):2513–20. https://doi.org/10.1001/jama.2010.1773.
12. Mathews B, Ratcliffe T, Sehgal R, Abraham J, Monash B. Fecal occult blood testing in hospitalized patients with upper gastrointestinal bleeding. J Hosp Med. 2017;12(7):567–9. https://doi.org/10.12788/jhm.2773.

13. Nadel MR, Berkowitz Z, Klabunde CN, Smith RA, Coughlin SS, White MC. Fecal occult blood testing beliefs and practices of U.S. primary care physicians: serious deviations from evidence-based recommendations. J Gen Intern Med. 2010;25(8):833–9. https://doi.org/10.1007/s11606-010-1328-7.
14. Lee MW, Pourmorady JS, Laine L. Use of fecal occult blood testing as a diagnostic tool for clinical indications: a systematic review and meta-analysis. Am J Gastroenterol. 2020; https://doi.org/10.14309/ajg.0000000000000495.
15. Zuckerman GR, Prakash C, Askin MP, Lewis BS. AGA technical review on the evaluation and management of occult and obscure gastrointestinal bleeding. Gastroenterology. 2000;118(1):201–21. https://doi.org/10.1016/s0016-5085(00)70430-6.
16. Murphy B, Winter DC, Kavanagh DO. Small bowel gastrointestinal bleeding diagnosis and management – a narrative review. Front Surg. 2019.;6:25; https://doi.org/10.3389/fsurg.2019.00025.
17. Dahlerup JF, Eivindson M, Jacobsen BA, Jensen NM, Jorgensen SP, Laursen SB, et al. Diagnosis and treatment of unexplained anemia with iron deficiency without overt bleeding. Dan Med J. 2015;62(4):C5072.
18. Zwas FR, Lyon DT. Occult GI bleeding in the alcoholic. Am J Gastroenterol. 1996;91(3):551–3.
19. Gkamprela E, Deutsch M, Pectasides D. Iron deficiency anemia in chronic liver disease: etiopathogenesis, diagnosis and treatment. Ann Gastroenterol. 2017;30(4):405–13. https://doi.org/10.20524/aog.2017.0152.
20. Stein J, Connor S, Virgin G, Ong DE, Pereyra L. Anemia and iron deficiency in gastrointestinal and liver conditions. World J Gastroenterol. 2016;22(35):7908–25. https://doi.org/10.3748/wjg.v22.i35.7908.
21. Islam S, Cevik C, Islam E, Attaya H, Nugent K. Heyde's syndrome: a critical review of the literature. J Heart Valve Dis. 2011;20(4):366–75.
22. Trivedi H, Yang J, Szabo A. Gastrointestinal bleeding in patients on long-term dialysis. J Nephrol. 2015;28(2):235–43. https://doi.org/10.1007/s40620-014-0132-6.
23. Singh G, Albeldawi M, Kalra SS, Mehta PP, Lopez R, Vargo JJ. Features of patients with gastrointestinal bleeding after implantation of ventricular assist devices. Clin Gastroenterol Hepatol. 2015;13(1).:107–14.e1 https://doi.org/10.1016/j.cgh.2014.05.012.
24. Sawhney MS, McDougall H, Nelson DB, Bond JH. Fecal occult blood test in patients on low-dose aspirin, warfarin, clopidogrel, or non-steroidal anti-inflammatory drugs. Dig Dis Sci. 2010;55(6):1637–42. https://doi.org/10.1007/s10620-010-1150-4.
25. Greenberg PD, Cello JP, Rockey DC. Asymptomatic chronic gastrointestinal blood loss in patients taking aspirin or warfarin for cardiovascular disease. Am J Med. 1996;100(6):598–604. https://doi.org/10.1016/s0002-9343(96)00009-5.
26. Bresci G. Occult and obscure gastrointestinal bleeding: causes and diagnostic approach in 2009. World J Gastrointest Endosc. 2009;1(1):3–6. https://doi.org/10.4253/wjge.v1.i1.3.
27. Sagar J, Kumar V, Shah DK. Meckel's diverticulum: a systematic review. J R Soc Med. 2006;99(10):501–5. https://doi.org/10.1258/jrsm.99.10.501.
28. Lee YT, Walmsley RS, Leong RW, Sung JJ. Dieulafoy's lesion. Gastrointest Endosc. 2003;58(2):236–43. https://doi.org/10.1067/mge.2003.328.
29. Vannella L, Aloe Spiriti MA, Cozza G, Tardella L, Monarca B, Cuteri A, et al. Benefit of concomitant gastrointestinal and gynaecological evaluation in premenopausal women with iron deficiency anaemia. Aliment Pharmacol Ther. 2008;28(4):422–30. https://doi.org/10.1111/j.1365-2036.2008.03741.x.
30. https://www.gastrojournal.org/article/S0016-5085(20)34847-2/fulltext#articleInformation.
31. Raju GS, Gerson L, Das A, Lewis B, American Gastroenterological A. American Gastroenterological Association (AGA) institute medical position statement on obscure gastrointestinal bleeding. Gastroenterology. 2007;133(5):1694–6. https://doi.org/10.1053/j.gastro.2007.06.008.
32. Robertson DJ, Lee JK, Boland CR, Dominitz JA, Giardiello FM, Johnson DA et al. Recommendations on fecal immunochemical testing to screen for colorectal neoplasia: a con-

sensus statement by the US multi-society task force on colorectal cancer. Gastroenterology. 2017;152(5):1217–37 e3. https://doi.org/10.1053/j.gastro.2016.08.053.

33. Kim NH, Park JH, Park DI, Sohn CI, Choi K, Jung YS. Are hemorrhoids associated with false-positive Fecal immunochemical test results? Yonsei Med J. 2017;58(1):150–7. https://doi.org/10.3349/ymj.2017.58.1.150.

34. Chiang TH, Lee YC, Tu CH, Chiu HM, Wu MS. Performance of the immunochemical fecal occult blood test in predicting lesions in the lower gastrointestinal tract. CMAJ. 2011;183(13):1474–81. https://doi.org/10.1503/cmaj.101248.

35. Clinical Practice Committee AGA. American Gastroenterological Association medical position statement: diagnosis and treatment of hemorrhoids. Gastroenterology. 2004;126(5):1461–2. https://doi.org/10.1053/j.gastro.2004.03.001.

36. Boland K, Nguyen GC. Microscopic colitis: a review of collagenous and lymphocytic colitis. Gastroenterol Hepatol (N Y). 2017;13(11):671–7.

37. Rondonotti E, Villa F, Mulder CJ, Jacobs MA, de Franchis R. Small bowel capsule endoscopy in 2007: indications, risks and limitations. World J Gastroenterol 2007;13(46):6140–6149. https://doi.org/10.3748/wjg.v13.i46.6140.

38. Bandorski D, Kurniawan N, Baltes P, Hoeltgen R, Hecker M, Stunder D, et al. Contraindications for video capsule endoscopy. World J Gastroenterol. 2016;22(45):9898–908. https://doi.org/10.3748/wjg.v22.i45.9898.

39. Linder J, Cheruvattath R, Truss C, Wilcox CM. Diagnostic yield and clinical implications of push enteroscopy: results from a nonspecialized center. J Clin Gastroenterol. 2002;35(5):383–6. https://doi.org/10.1097/00004836-200211000-00005.

40. Zaman A, Katon RM. Push enteroscopy for obscure gastrointestinal bleeding yields a high incidence of proximal lesions within reach of a standard endoscope. Gastrointest Endosc. 1998;47(5):372–6. https://doi.org/10.1016/s0016-5107(98)70221-4.

41. Koffas A, Laskaratos FM, Epstein O. Non-small bowel lesion detection at small bowel capsule endoscopy: a comprehensive literature review. World J Clin Cases. 2018;6(15):901–7. https://doi.org/10.12998/wjcc.v6.i15.901.

42. Lee EW, Laberge JM. Differential diagnosis of gastrointestinal bleeding. Tech Vase Interv Radiol. 2004;7(3):112–22. https://doi.org/10.1053/j.tvir.2004.12.001.

43. Rockey DC. Occult and obscure gastrointestinal bleeding: causes and clinical management. Nat Rev. Gastroenterol Hepatol. 2010;7(5):265–79. https://doi.org/10.1038/nrgastro.2010.42.

44. Welli ML, Hansel SL, Bruining DM, Fletcher JG, Froemming AT, Barlow JM, et al. CT for evaluation of acute gastrointestinal bleeding. Radiographies. 2018;38((4]):1089–107. https://doi.org/10.1148/rg.2018170138.

Chapter 2
Non-Invasive Office Screening Methods

Edgar R. Naut and Gagandeep Singh

Office Base Screening

Small intestinal bleeding accounts for 5–10% of patients who present with gastro-intestinal bleeding and remains a relatively uncommon cause [1]. As has previously been defined occult gastrointestinal bleeding is not visible to either the patient or the physician and is detected by either by fecal occult blood testing (FOBT), or iron deficiency anemia with or without a positive FOBT [1–3]. Unfortunately there are no guidelines or recommendations on screening this population. As a result non-invasive office base screening is based on the recommendations for accessing iron deficiency anemia as well as colorectal cancer screening. This is in addition to obtaining a thorough history and physical.

Anemia

The World Health Organization (WHO) defines anemia, as a condition in which the number of red cells or their oxygen carrying capacity is not sufficient to meet physi-ologic needs [4]. The WHO estimates the global burden of disease for anemia is about 30% of the world population [5–7]. The diagnosis is often made on laboratory full blood count testing for screening or the evaluation of another condition [4]. Anemia is associated with significant morbidity and mortality. A decrease in quality of life, cognitive function and work productivity have been reported [5, 7, 8].

The most common anemia is iron deficiency anemia (IDA) representing about 50% of all anemias' worldwide. Total body iron ranges from three to four grams

E. R. Naut (✉) · G. Singh
Department of Medicine, Saint Francis Hospital and Medical Center, Hartford, CT, USA
e-mail: gsingh@TrinityHealthOfNE.org

© The Author(s), under exclusive license to Springer Nature
Switzerland AG 2021
M. Tadros, G. Y. Wu (eds.), *Management of Occult GI Bleeding*, Clinical
Gastroenterology, https://doi.org/10.1007/978-3-030-71468-0_2

with a net daily loss of one to two milligrams [9]. This is usually balanced through dietary iron. Iron deficiency anemia has a high prevalence in women [8]. The WHO reported in 1992 that 37% of all women were anemic and in the United States 12% of reproductive age women had iron deficiency. In addition 4% of women 20–49 years of age and 3% of women 50–69 years of age had iron deficiency anemia [5, 8, 9]. In addition iron deficiency is the most common nutritional deficiency worldwide. Despite this and IDA being so prevalent there are no consistent guidelines on the screening for IDA.

Guidelines

In the United States the Center for Disease Control and Prevention (CDC) recommends screening females of childbearing age every five to ten years and more frequently if clinically indicated [10]. In addition they recommend screening pregnant women at the first prenatal visit [10]. This contrasts the United States preventive Services Task Force (USPSTF) who finding insufficient evidence to recommend routine screening [11].

Making the Diagnosis of Iron Deficiency Anemia

Commonly the evaluation for anemia is initiated from findings picked up on history and physical. The diagnosis can be difficult to make in some cases where there are co-contaminant inflammatory states. Some findings have been associated with all anemias such as conjunctival pallor, nail-bed pallor, absence of nail bed blanching and palmar crease pallor [7, 12]. Other findings are specific for IDA (see Table 2.1). For example some of the symptoms associated with IDA include paleness, fatigue (in iron deficiency with or without anemia), dyspnea, headache, restless leg syndrome, and pica symptoms [5, 7, 8]. Physical findings commonly seen include alopecia, atrophic glossitis, dry skin [7]. In addition IDA anemia should be suspected in patients who are undergoing hemodialysis, middle age obese individuals, and obesity at any age [6]. Certain medications have also been associated with IDA such as Antacids, H2 blockers, Proton pump inhibitors, Nonsteroidal anti-inflammatory drugs (NSAIDs), aspirin, Zinc, and manganese supplements [8].

Once IDA is suspected and a complete blood count (CBC) confirms the presence of anemia several red blood cells indices help suggest IDA. A mean corpuscular volume (MCV) below 80 fL has a reported sensitivity of 97.6% for IDA; however IDA can present with normocytic anemia 40% of the time [8]. In addition the MCV may be low in other conditions such as thalassemia. The Mentzer index, which is the ratio of MCV to red blood cell count, can be used to help distinguish between IDA and Thalassemia trait [13]. A value greater than 13 suggests IDA. The red

Table 2.1 Signs and Symptoms of Iron Deficiency Anemia

Signs	Symptoms
Pallor	Fatigue
Alopecia	Dyspnea
Atrophic glossitis	Restless leg syndrome
Angular stomatitis	Headache
Defects of the nail bed (koilonchia and Mees lines)	Pica symptoms
Dry skin	Neurocognitive dysfunction
Dry and damaged hair	Angina pectoris
Cardiac murmur	Vertigo
Tachycardia	Tinnitus
Syncope	Taste disturbance
Hemodynamic instability	
Plummer-Vinson syndrome	

Table 2.2 Test for the diagnosis of iron deficiency anemia

Test	Limitations
Serum Iron/TIBC	Diurnal variations
Percent transferrin saturation	Not diagnostic by itself
Ferritin	Increased during inflammatory states independently of iron studies
Reticulocyte count	Not diagnostic
Soluble transferrin receptor (sTFRC)	Lacks standardization among different immune assays
Serum hepcidin	Not readily available in many laboratories
Reticulocyte hemoglobin concentration	Iron availability can be influenced by multiple factors

blood cell distribution width (RDW) may be elevated in patients with IDA and normal in patients with thalassemia [8].

Bone marrow aspiration and Perl's staining is the gold standard for the diagnosis of iron deficiency (ID), as it shows an absence of stainable iron in the bone marrow [6]. However other test are available which can reliably diagnose IDA. These test include serum iron, total iron binding capacity (TIBC), percent transferrin saturation (TSAT), serum ferritin, reticulocyte count, soluble (serum) transferrin receptor levels, serum hepcidin, and reticulocyte hemoglobin concentration (CHr) (see Table 2.2) [5, 6]. A peripheral blood smears can also give valuable infomation in diagnosing ID (Fig. 2.1).

Serum Iron/TIBC

Serum iron represents the amount of iron bound to transferrin. This allows iron to be incorporated into hemoglobin in developing erythroblast. The transferrin bound iron pool has a high turnover that can be up to six times a day. This in conjunction

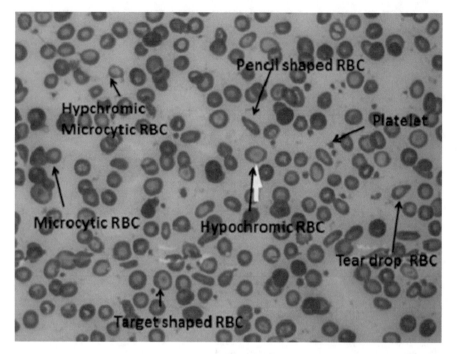

Fig. 2.1 Peripheral blood film with changes attributed to iron deficiency anemia [32]. (Copyright © 2012, Springer Nature)

with diurnal variation, and external factors make serum iron unreliable in diagnosing ID [5]. TIBC (expressed in micrograms/deciliter) is a functional measure of the level of transferrin circulating; an elevated TIBC is consistent with IDA [5, 8, 14].

Percent Transferrin Saturation

The TSAT is calculated by using the formula (Iron × 100)/TIBC and is expressed as a percent [8]. A very low TSAT usually less than 10–15% is consistent with IDA however it is not diagnostic by itself [5, 8].

Ferritin

In the absence of inflammation, ferritin (microgram/Liter) correlates with total body iron stores. A ferritin level of less than 15 microgram/L in patients older than five years old is diagnostic for ID and has a sensitivity of 59% and a specificity of 99% [7, 9]. The American Gastroenterology Association (AGA) gastrointestinal evaluation of iron deficiency anemia recommend using a ferritin threshold of less than 45 microgram/L to diagnose iron deficiency [9]. At this level the sensitivity of ferritin is 85% and the specificity is 92%. Unfortunately ferritin levels increase during inflammatory states independently of iron stores [5, 7]. In acute and chronic inflammatory disorders such as malignant disease, liver or kidney disease ferritin levels of 50 micrograms/L or higher may still have ID. As such cut off of 100 micrograms/L and 200 micrograms/L have been suggested in patients with chronic kidney disease and hemodialysis respectively [7]. The AGA suggest using adjuvant testing to help establish the diagnosis of iron deficiency such as serum iron, transferrin saturation, or C-reactive protein [9].

Reticulocyte Count

A corrected reticulocyte count expressed as a percent of red blood cells can provide an estimate of appropriate bone marrow production compared to normal with an index greater than two being incompatible with IDA [5].

Soluble Transferrin Receptor (sTFRC)

Soluble transferrin receptor is cleaved by the membrane protease in the erythroid cells when not stabilized by diferric transferrin. In the presence of iron the TFRC mRNA is destabilized. In the absence of iron the mRNA becomes stable resulting in an up regulation of the TFRC [5, 6]. TRFC levels are not affected by inflammation and it has been suggested as a tool in differentiating IDA and anemia of chronic disease (ACD) [6]. It can also be used in identifying ID in patients with inflammatory conditions [5, 6]. Although it is not as sensitive and specific as a ferritin level of less the 30 microgram/L it does have a sensitivity and specificity of 86 and 75% respectively [6]. Unfortunately there is a lack of standardization among different immune assays. This results in difficulty comparing studies and translating into routing clinical practice.

Serum Hepcidin

Is a biomarker that is decreased in ID and are undetectable in severe IDA. As with TRFC there are different test available and it is not readily available in many laboratory. However studies have shown promise and this may be available in the future [6].

Reticulocyte Hemoglobin Concentration

The CHr measures recent iron availability and it has not been widely adopted due to the fact that iron availability can be influenced by a number of factors [5].

Stool Testing for Occult Blood

Occult gastrointestinal bleeding should be suspected in patients with positive stool testing for blood [1, 2]. In most cases these patients would have had testing done as an alternative for colorectal cancer screening (CRS). Colorectal cancer is the second leading cause of cancer death in the United States and the third leading cancer diagnosis [15, 16]. Colorectal cancer screening is recommended for average risk patients from the age of 50 to 75 by most society guidelines and expert groups [17–20]. The preferred modality is colonoscopy however fecal occult blood testing (FOBT) has been shown to be an effective screening tool and is an alternative for patients who do not wish to have a colonoscopy as the initial test. In some studies guaiac based or immunochemical have been shown to decreases colorectal cancer mortality by about 30% [21]. Screening can be done with sensitive guaiac-based fecal occult blood testing, fecal immunochemical testing (FIT), or multi-target stool DNA testing [18, 22]. These test detect blood or shredded debris by polyps, adenomas or cancers [21]. Guidelines recommend high sensitivity guaiac based FOBT annually or biennially and, FIT annually (see Table 2.3) [21].

Sensitive Guaiac-Based Fecal Occult Blood Testing

Guiac-based screening test (Hemoccult SENSA, Beckman Coulter) have been shown to reduce CRC death [18, 23]. However they are less sensitive then FIT test. The reported sensitivity and specificity of this two test are 62–70% and 87–96% respectively [18, 23]. In addition there has been concerns about dietary restrictions when using guaiac based testing. Certain foods, vitamins, or medications can produce false positive and false negative so in general dietary restrictions are recommended [24]. The current recommendation is to obtain six stool samples from three bowel movements on three separate days. The sample should be returned to the lab within 14 days [25]. A single digital rectal exam sample is not sensitive for CRS

Table 2.3 Stool testing for occult blood

Test	Sensitivity	Specificity
Guiac-based screening test (Hemoccult SENSA, Beckman coulter)	62–70%	87–96%
Fecal immunochemical testing (FIT)		
OC-light test using a cutoff of 10 microgram hemoglobin per gram of feces	79–88%	91–93%
OC FIT-CHEK family of tests using a cutoff of 20 microgram hemoglobin per gram of feces	73–75%	91–95%
Multi-target stool DNA testing (FIT-DNA)	92% (95% CI 84–97%)	84% (95% CI 84–85%)

Bibbins-Domingo et al. [33]

however a positive result would warrant further investigation. Another limitation of the test has been its low ability to detect polyps and its inability to determine clinically significant disease [24].

Fecal Immunochemical Testing (FIT)

In the United States there are multiple FITs from different manufacturers with different test methods and performance characteristics [23]. The OC FIT-CHEK family of FITs has the highest sensitivity and specificity. The OC-Light test using a cutoff of 10 microgram hemoglobin per gram of feces to detect CRC has sensitivity and specificity of 79–88% and 91–93%, respectively; For the OC FIT-CHEK family of tests using a cutoff of 20 microgram hemoglobin per gram of feces it ranges from 73% to 75% and 91% to 95%, respectively as reported by Lin et al. [23]. Dickerson et al. reported a sensitivity of 79% and specificity of 94% for available FIT test for the detection of CRC [25]. A study performed by Goede et al. comparing guaiac fecal occult blood to FIT testing in Ontario, Canada showed that switching to FIT testing at a high cut-off increased health benefits without increasing colonoscopy demands [26]. The test provides several advantages including only requiring one sample and does not require dietary modifications [18].

Multi-Target Stool DNA Testing (FIT-DNA)

Multi-target stool DNA testing has increased single test sensitivity however it is less specific then FIT alone. The test characteristics of the only FIT-DNA test available in the United States (Cologuard; Exact Sciences) were studied and the sensitivity and specificity to detect colorectal cancer was 92% and 84% respectively. Its sensitivity to detect advanced precancerous lesions was 42%, and its specificity to detect "all non-advanced findings" was 87% [18, 27]. Although sensitivity is the most important aspect of cancer screening test, specificity is also important as it limits the amount of false positive results and hence unnecessary interventions [27].

Other Considerations

Celiac Disease

Celiac disease, which is also known as gluten-sensitivity enteropathy, is a systemic disorder that affects about 1% of Americans [28]. Celiac disease results in a T-Cell-mediated immune response to gluten. This immune response in people whom have the genetic predisposition results in the malabsorption of nutrients due to damage to the small intestine [28]. Celiac disease is often under diagnosed and in the United States estimates 10–15% of persons with this condition are diagnosed [28]. Undiagnosed celiac disease is a significant cause of IDA and in general screening for it is recommended in patients presenting with IDA [4]. Screening usually involves serum IgA antibodies to tissue transglutaminase (tTG) or Transglutaminase 2 (TG2) [28]. In addition four biopsies from the second part of the duodenum are recommended during endoscopy have been recommended [4]. However the AGA recommends against routine small bowel biopsy unless serologic testing is positive [9]. Other indications for celiac disease screening as well as genetic modalities are beyond the scope of this chapter.

Infectious Diseases

Infectious diseases, particularly parasitic diseases lead to extracorporeal iron losses and anemia of inflammation [29]. The World Health Organization has classified a severe health problem in over 60 developing countries for children under five as well as pregnant women. One of the main reasons is extracorporeal iron loss [29]. Hookworm is the most important parasitic disease in humans and the burden is mainly due to extra-corporeal blood loss [29]. Other parasites include Schistosomiasis and less commonly Trichuris. In the right setting such as in returning travelers or recent immigrants from high-risk areas testing stool examination for ova and parasite can be performed. More advanced testing such as polymerase chain reaction (PCR), serology or antigen testing is beyond the scope of this chapter.

Helicobacter pylori (H. pylori) is a common chronic bacterial infection which has been associated with peptic ulcer disease and gastric cancer which can result in iron deficiency in addition plays a role in unexplained IDA. Both the American College of Gastroenterology (ACG) and the AGA recommend screening patients with unexplained ID for *H. Pylori* [9, 30]. The AGA goes further and recommends noninvasive testing for *H. Pylori* with treatment if positive over no testing [9]. This is preferred over routine gastric biopsy in patients with unremarkable endoscopies. An approach of urea breath testing after a negative endoscopy was noted to have significant cost savings when compared with routine gastric biopsy at the time of the endoscopy [9]. This resulted in minimal harm from the short term delay in diagnosis from false-negative noninvasive testing. Other available noninvasive test for *H. Pylori* include stool antigen testing and serology. However a recent Cochrane database review found that for most people urea breath tests had a high diagnostic accuracy when compared to serology and stool antigen testing in the diagnosis of *H. Pylori* [31].

Conclusion

There are no guidelines regarding non-invasive office screening methods for occult gastrointestinal bleeding. The findings of occult gastrointestinal bleeding in the office are often incidental and found as a result of recommended screening for other conditions such as iron deficiency anemia and colorectal cancer screening. In addition if symptoms of anemia develop the search for the etiology may lead to the diagnosis of occult gastrointestinal bleeding. Once the diagnosis of IDA is made screening for celiac disease and when appropriate infectious etiology should be undertaken.

Acknowledgement The author thanks the Saint Francis Hospital and Medical Center library for their contribution to this chapter.

References

1. Gerson LB, Fidler JL, Cave DR, Leighton JA. ACG clinical guideline: diagnosis and Management of Small Bowel Bleeding. Am J Gastroenterol. 2015;110(9):1265–87. quiz 88
2. Naut ER. The approach to occult gastrointestinal bleed. Med Clin North Am. 2016;100(5):1047–56.
3. Bull-Henry K, Al-Kawas FH. Evaluation of occult gastrointestinal bleeding. Am Fam Physician. 2013;87(6):430–6.
4. Banerjee AK, Celentano V, Khan J, Longcroft-Wheaton G, Quine A, Bhandari P. Practical gastrointestinal investigation of iron deficiency anaemia. Expert Rev Gastroenterol Hepatol. 2018;12(3):249–56.
5. Auerbach M, Adamson JW. How we diagnose and treat iron deficiency anemia. Am J Hematol. 2016;91(1):31–8.
6. Camaschella C. New insights into iron deficiency and iron deficiency anemia. Blood Rev. 2017;31(4):225–33.
7. Lopez A, Cacoub P, Macdougall IC, Peyrin-Biroulet L. Iron deficiency anaemia. Lancet. 2016;387(10021):907–16.
8. Hempel EV, Bollard ER. The evidence-based evaluation of iron deficiency Anemia. Med Clin North Am. 2016;100(5):1065–75.
9. Ko CW, Siddique SM, Patel A, Harris A, Sultan S, Altayar O, et al. AGA clinical practice guidelines on the gastrointestinal evaluation of iron deficiency anemia. Gastroenterology. 2020;159:1085–94.
10. Recommendations to prevent and control iron deficiency in the United States. Centers for Disease Control and Prevention. MMWR Recomm Rep. 1998;47(RR-3):1–29.
11. Available from: https://www.uspreventiveservicestaskforce.org/Page/Document/RecommendationStatementFinal/iron-deficiency-anemia-screening. Accessed 29 Nov 2016.
12. Strobach RS, Anderson SK, Doll DC, Ringenberg QS. The value of the physical examination in the diagnosis of anemia. Correlation of the physical findings and the hemoglobin concentration. Arch Intern Med. 1988;148(4):831–2.
13. Mentzer WC. Differentiation of iron deficiency from thalassaemia trait. Lancet. 1973;1(7808):882.
14. Bouri S, Martin J. Investigation of iron deficiency anaemia. Clin Med (Lond). 2018;18(3):242–4.

15. Selby K, Baumgartner C, Levin TR, Doubeni CA, Zauber AG, Schottinger J, et al. Interventions to improve follow-up of positive results on fecal blood tests: a systematic review. Ann Intern Med. 2017;167(8):565–75.
16. Hillyer GC, Jensen CD, Zhao WK, Neugut AI, Lebwohl B, Tiro JA, et al. Primary care visit use after positive fecal immunochemical test for colorectal cancer screening. Cancer. 2017;123(19):3744–53.
17. Wilt TJ, Harris RP, Qaseem A, Physicians HVCTFotACo. Screening for cancer: advice for high-value care from the American College of Physicians. Ann Intern Med. 2015;162(10):718–25.
18. Bibbins-Domingo K, Grossman DC, Curry SJ, Davidson KW, Epling JW, García FAR, et al. Screening for colorectal cancer: US preventive services task force recommendation statement. JAMA. 2016;315(23):2564–75.
19. Care CTFoPH. Recommendations on screening for colorectal cancer in primary care. CMAJ: Can Med Assoc J = journal de l'Association medicale canadienne. 2016;188(5):340–8.
20. Lansdorp-Vogelaar I, von Karsa L. Cancer IAfRo. European guidelines for quality assurance in colorectal cancer screening and diagnosis. First Edition – Introduction. Endoscopy. 2012;44(Suppl 3):SE15–30.
21. Sur D, Colceriu M, Sur G, Floca E, Dascal L, Irimie A. Colorectal cancer: evolution of screening strategies. Med Pharm Rep. 2019;92(1):21–4.
22. Knudsen AB, Zauber AG, Rutter CM, Naber SK, Doria-Rose VP, Pabiniak C, et al. Estimation of benefits, burden, and harms of colorectal cancer screening strategies: modeling study for the US preventive services task force. JAMA. 2016;315(23):2595–609.
23. Lin JS, Piper MA, Perdue LA, Rutter CM, Webber EM, O'Connor E, et al. Screening for colorectal cancer: updated evidence report and systematic review for the US preventive services task force. JAMA. 2016;315(23):2576–94.
24. Shapiro JA, Bobo JK, Church TR, Rex DK, Chovnick G, Thompson TD, et al. A comparison of fecal immunochemical and high-sensitivity guaiac tests for colorectal cancer screening. Am J Gastroenterol. 2017;112(11):1728–35.
25. Dickerson L, Varcak SC. Colorectal cancer screening: the role of the noninvasive options. JAAPA. 2016;29(9):1–3.
26. Goede SL, Rabeneck L, van Ballegooijen M, Zauber AG, Paszat LF, Hoch JS, et al. Harms, benefits and costs of fecal immunochemical testing versus guaiac fecal occult blood testing for colorectal cancer screening. PLoS One. 2017;12(3):e0172864.
27. Imperiale TF, Ransohoff DF, Itzkowitz SH, Levin TR, Lavin P, Lidgard GP, et al. Multitarget stool DNA testing for colorectal-cancer screening. N Engl J Med. 2014;370(14):1287–97.
28. Crowe SE. In the clinic. Celiac disease. Ann Intern Med. 2011;154(9):ITC5-1-ITC5-15; quiz ITC5–6.
29. Shaw JG, Friedman JF. Iron deficiency anemia: focus on infectious diseases in lesser developed countries. Anemia. 2011;2011:260380.
30. Chey WD, Leontiadis GI, Howden CW, Moss SF. ACG clinical guideline: treatment of helicobacter pylori infection. Am J Gastroenterol. 2017;112(2):212–39.
31. Best LM, Takwoingi Y, Siddique S, Selladurai A, Gandhi A, Low B, et al. Non-invasive diagnostic tests for helicobacter pylori infection. Cochrane Database Syst Rev. 2018;3:CD012080.
32. Abdelrahman EG, Gasim GI, Musa IR, Elbashir LM, Adam I. Red blood cell distribution width and iron deficiency anemia among pregnant Sudanese women. Diagn Pathol. 2012;7:168.
33. Bibbins-Domingo K, Grossman DC, Curry SJ, Davidson KW, Epling JW, García FAR, et al. Screening for colorectal cancer: US preventive services task force recommendation statement. JAMA. 2016;315(23):2564–75.

Chapter 3
Endoscopic Detection

Joseph M. Polito II and Caroline Polito

Introduction

Occult gastrointestinal (GI) bleeding refers to the presentation of a positive fecal occult blood test without an obvious cause for the blood loss [1]. Once a patient presents with occult GI bleeding, it is important to determine if iron deficiency anemia is present. In patients with a positive fecal occult blood test but no evidence of anemia, a colonoscopy should be considered. In patients with upper GI symptoms, an upper endoscopy should be performed as well [2, 3]. Upper GI symptoms include heartburn, difficulty swallowing, stomach pain, nausea, and vomiting [4]. For patients who have a positive fecal occult blood test and an iron deficiency anemia, both an upper endoscopy and colonoscopy are recommended [2, 3]. If upper endoscopy and colonoscopy do not indicate the source of the bleeding, the next step is to evaluate the small bowel [5]. The majority of these patients will undergo a wireless capsule endoscopy [6].

Upper Endoscopy

Upper endoscopy allows for the visualization of the esophagus, stomach, and proximal duodenum. It can also be used to sample tissue [7]. Typically upper endoscopies are performed using a high-definition white light endoscope [8]. Patients with

J. M. Polito II (✉)
Albany Medical Center, Medicine, Albany, NY, USA
e-mail: JPolito@AlbanyGI.com

C. Polito
Stony Brook University Medical Center, Renaissance School of Medicine,
Stony Brook, NY, USA
e-mail: Caroline.polito@Stonybrookmedicine.edu

© The Author(s), under exclusive license to Springer Nature
Switzerland AG 2021
M. Tadros, G. Y. Wu (eds.), *Management of Occult GI Bleeding*, Clinical
Gastroenterology, https://doi.org/10.1007/978-3-030-71468-0_3

29

upper GI symptoms, especially symptoms indicative of gastroesophageal reflux disease (GERD), often receive upper endoscopies [9]. In addition, if imaging of the upper GI tract shows suspected neoplasms, ulcers, strictures, mucosal abnormalities, or obstructions, an upper endoscopy may be performed [7]. Lesions in the upper digestive tract are often detected in those who test positive for fecal occult blood or have an iron deficiency anemia [10–13]. Upper GI symptoms are also associated with the detection of lesions in the upper digestive tract. However, the prevalence of lesions in the upper GI tract is greater than or equal to that of colonic lesions even in those without symptoms [10–13]. Upper GI sources of bleeding are found in 36–56% of patients with an iron deficiency anemia [14–16] and in 29% of patients who test positive for fecal occult blood and do not have an iron deficiency anemia. Approximately 50% of these patients will be symptomatic [14]. In addition, 5–17% of patients have both upper and lower GI lesions [14–16]. Upper endoscopy can employ a number of therapeutic interventions including biopsy, polypectomy, dilation of strictures, stent placement, removal of foreign bodies, percutaneous gastrostomy tube placement, treatment of GI bleeding with injection, banding, coagulation, sclerotherapy, and endoscopic therapy for esophageal intestinal metaplasia [7].

Colonoscopy

Colonoscopy is the preferred approach for evaluation of the colon, rectum, and the distal portion of the terminal ileum and can detect a wide range of lesions, including polyps, diverticula, cancers, and angiodysplasias. It allows for the visualization of the entire colonic mucosa as well as the ability to obtain tissue biopsies [17]. While colonoscopy is effective in reducing colon cancer rates overall, it is more effective in reducing the risk of rectal and left sided colon cancer than right sided colon cancer [18]. One technique to improve visualization is retroflexion, which is when the colonoscope is bent into a U-shape to allow the viewing lens to look backwards. Reflexion is often used in the right colon to improve the effectiveness of colonoscopy given the fact that right sided colon polyps can be located on the backs of haustral folds in the cecum and ascending colon [19]. Retroflexion in the right colon is successful in over 90% of cases with very low complication rates while yielding a significant improvement in the adenoma detection rate [20]. Good bowel preparation is important for all colonoscopies and is necessary for proper visualization. An excellent bowel prep will allow for 95% of the mucosal surface to be seen allowing for a high adenoma detection rate while a poor bowel prep will result in fecal matter blocking visualization and require a repeat bowel preparation [21]. Diagnostic indications include screening or surveillance for colon cancer, evaluating signs and symptoms suggestive of colonic or distal small bowel disease such as gastrointestinal bleeding or diarrhea, assessing a response to treatment for patients with colonic diseases like inflammatory bowel disease, and evaluating abnormalities found on imaging studies [17] including barium enema [22], abdominal computed tomography (CT) [23], positron emission tomography (PET) [24], and magnetic resonance imaging (MRI) [25]. Some radiographic findings that are considered abnormal and may warrant performing a colonoscopy include thickening of the wall of the colon or terminal ileum [26], mass lesions [27], and strictures [28]. It also can be used for therapeutic interventions, such as stricture dilation, stent placement, colonic decompression, and foreign body removal [17]. Colonoscopies are generally considered the gold standard for colon cancer screening and surveillance. If polyps are found during the colonoscopy, they are usually removed endoscopically if possible [29].

Small Bowel Evaluation

If a complete endoscopy and colonoscopy with adequate visualization do not reveal the source of occult gastrointestinal bleeding, evaluation of the small bowel is recommended [1]. Wireless capsule endoscopy is the preferred initial approach for evaluating the small bowel [1]. Other endoscopic options include push enteroscopy [30], single balloon endoscopy, double balloon endoscopy [31] and spiral enteroscopy.

Wireless Capsule Endoscopy

Wireless capsule endoscopy is generally the first choice for evaluating suspected small bowel bleeding. Wireless video endoscopy, also referred to as video capsule endoscopy (VCE), is a noninvasive technology designed to provide diagnostic imaging of the small intestine. It can also provide limited visualization of the esophagus, stomach, and cecum. The images acquired from wireless capsule endoscopy are of high resolution and have a 1:8 magnification, which is greater than that of a conventional endoscope. This allows for visualization of individual villi. The capsule moves passively, does not inflate the bowel, and images the mucosa in a collapsed state [31]. The main advantages of wireless capsule endoscopy are that it is relatively noninvasive and permits examination of the entire length of the small bowl most of the time. Its main disadvantage is that it cannot be guided nor steered and it does not allow for tissue sampling or therapeutic intervention. In addition, not all of the small bowel mucosa is visualized as the capsule passes through the small intestine while being pushed along by peristalsis [31]. The diagnostic yield of capsule endoscopy is highest when it is performed as close as possible to the bleeding episode [32–35]. Double-ended wireless video capsules, which can capture images from both ends of the video capsule, have also been developed for the examination of the colon [36].

Wireless video endoscopy identifies causes of small bowel bleeding more often than push enteroscopy in most reports [37–45]. Studies have suggested that wireless capsule endoscopy is equal to or more sensitive than other methods for the diagnosis of small bowel sources of blood loss. A meta-analysis of 14 observational studies compared wireless capsule endoscopy with other procedures for suspected small bowel bleeding and estimated that the overall yield of wireless capsule endoscopy was 63%, which is significantly higher than push enteroscopy with a yield of 26% and barium studies with a yield of 8% [37]. Overall, the yield of wireless video endoscopy for occult small bowel bleeding has been reported to be in the range of 30–70% [6, 32, 33, 37–40, 42, 46–52]. One trial of 89 patients with suspected small bowel bleeding that compared capsule endoscopy with push enteroscopy found that performing capsule endoscopy before push enteroscopy was a more effective strategy than beginning with push enteroscopy. The capsule endoscopy first strategy significantly reduced the percentage of patients needing a second procedure from 79% to 25% [53]. In another randomized trial of 136 patients with suspected small bowel bleeding who had undergone upper endoscopy, colonoscopy, and push enteroscopy, patients were assigned to either capsule endoscopy or radiographic evaluation. The diagnostic yield for capsule endoscopy was 30% in comparison to radiographic evaluation with a 7% yield, but the rate of recurrent bleeding between the two groups was the same [48]. Another study involving 305 patients undergoing capsule endoscopy for suspected small bowel bleeding did not find a significant difference between those with a positive and negative video capsule endoscopy. It also did not find a difference in rebleeding rates between those who underwent treatment and those who did not [54]. Repeat capsule endoscopy is recommended for patients whose initial capsule endoscopy is negative given that the entire small bowel mucosa may not be visualized with a single pass and could miss the source of GI bleeding. The capsule does not follow an axial path but rather tumbles and is unable to see behind all of the folds of the small intestine [55].

Push Enteroscopy

Push enteroscopy is an alternative means of visualization of the small bowel. It involves oral passage of a push enteroscope or a pediatric colonoscope past the ligament of Treitz. In the case of the enteroscope, the instrument is 200–250 cm long but the depth of insertion can be limited by looping within the stomach or small bowel or by patient discomfort. About 25–80 cm of the jejunum distal to the ligament of Treitz can be evaluated [56]. The amount of jejunum that can be viewed can be increased when an overtube designed to reduce looping in the stomach is used. However, it has not been conclusively determined whether or not this improves the diagnostic and therapeutic ability of push enteroscopy [57, 58].

Multiple studies have determined that the diagnostic yield of push enteroscopy in identifying bleeding lesions is estimated to be between 3% and 70% [2] with angioectasia being the most common diagnosis [59–61]. One benefit of push enteroscopy in comparison to wireless capsule endoscopy is that it can sample tissue and perform therapeutic maneuvers which include clipping of bleeding lesions or ablation and hemostasis of bleeding using bipolar cautery.

In a study of 95 patients with suspected small bowel bleeding who underwent push enteroscopy, it was concluded that many lesions detected during enteroscopy were within reach of a standard endoscope. This indicates that a careful repeat standard upper endoscopy may be appropriate prior to push enteroscopy or other diagnostic procedures [59].

Single Balloon

Single balloon enteroscopy allows for both evaluation and therapeutic intervention in the small bowel. Single balloon enteroscopy consists of a long, 1400 mm enteroscope, an overtube with a distal inflatable balloon, and a control unit to inflate and deflate the balloon. The overtube is designed to minimize looping of the small bowel while pleating it back over the overtube and the enteroscope [62]. It can be used anterograde via the mouth or retrograde via the rectum with intubation and advancement proximal to the ileocecal valve. Single balloon enteroscopy is typically performed with fluoroscopic assistance and the use of CO_2 instead of air for insufflation of the bowel as CO_2 is absorbed more quickly across the bowel mucosa (Fig. 3.1). Using air for the insufflation of the bowel can prolong the procedure time and single balloon enteroscopy requires higher volumes of gas insufflation, which can cause discomfort and limit advancement of the enteroscope [62]. Bowel prep is not required for enteroscopy. The enteroscope is initially advanced as far as possible using the same technique as a standard endoscope. The tip of the enteroscope is hooked on a fold in the bowel to stabilize it and the

Fig. 3.1 Fluoroscopic image of single balloon enteroscopy

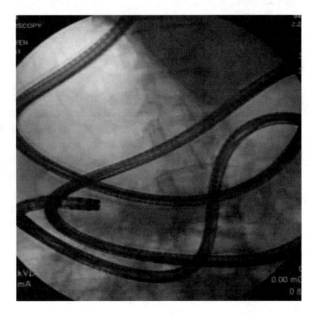

overtube is then advanced over the enteroscope. The balloon is inflated and both the enteroscope and overtube are withdrawn together. The balloon is deflated and the enteroscope is then advanced as far as possible at which point the process is repeated [62]. This results in pleating of the bowel over the overtube and subsequent shortening of the bowel. The combination of anterograde and retrograde enteroscopy can potentially allow for complete evaluation of the small bowel. Single balloon enteroscopy is a safe procedure with <1% risk of perforation during diagnostic procedures [62].

Double Balloon

Double balloon enteroscopy is similar to single balloon enteroscopy. The primary difference is that the enteroscope has a distal balloon in addition to the overtube balloon. The enteroscope is advanced as far as possible and the balloon is inflated to anchor its position [56]. The overtube is then advanced towards the end of the enteroscope at which point the overtube balloon is inflated and both enteroscope and overtube are withdrawn together pleating the bowel in an accordion like fashion over the overtube. The enteroscope balloon is deflated and the process is repeated. Double balloon enteroscopy allows for complete evaluation of the jejunum and ileum [56]. It is typically done in an antegrade fashion but can be done retrograde via the rectum. Diagnostic yields for obscure GI bleeding range from 40% to 80% [56]. Perforation is rare but is more common in patients who have had prior bowel surgery. Pancreatitis has been reported as a complication of double balloon enteroscopy as well [56].

Spiral Enteroscopy

Spiral enteroscopy allows for antegrade evaluation of the small bowel. It involves an overtube with a soft raised helix at its distal end. The enteroscope is manually turned in a clockwise manner to cause pleating of the small bowel on the enteroscope [63]. It has a shorter examination time in comparison to double-balloon and single-balloon enteroscopy as well as more stability during withdrawal but it requires two operators [64]. Motorized spiral enteroscopy have recently been developed that would allow for single operator use [65]. The drive motor is located in the endoscope handle and is activated by foot pedals, which controls the direction and speed of rotation of a coupler located in the middle of the endoscope's insertion tube [66]. Studies have shown that motorized spiral enteroscopy have short procedural durations and high depth of maximum insertion while maintaining a high diagnostic and therapeutic efficacy [67].

Type	Overtube	Depth of Insertion	Procedure time	Completion Rate*	Diagnostic Yield
Capsule	No	Reaches cecum 85% of the time [68]	480 min [68]	51.2–94.2% [69–71]	48–60.9% [69, 72]
Push	Can be with or without [73]	46–80 cm beyond the ligament of Treitz with overtube [44, 57, 60, 74–80]	30 min [60, 74, 75]	0%	15–80% [81, 82]
Single balloon	Yes	Antegrade: 133–270 cm Retrograde: 73–199 cm [83–87]	53–69 min [86, 88]	0–24% [83, 89–91]	41–65% [83–87, 89–93]
Double balloon	Yes	Antegrade: 220–360 cm Retrograde: 124–183 [94–98]	73–123 min [94–98]	92% [95, 97–103]	40–80% [88–92, 104]
Spiral	Yes	175–262 cm (anterograde or retrograde) [105–107]	34–37 min [105–107]	8–92.6% [103, 108]	12–75% [64, 83–87, 89–93, 105–107]

*Total small bowel visualization

Intraoperative Enteroscopy

Intraoperative enteroscopy involves the insertion of an endoscope through an enterotomy site, orally, or rectally during surgery [109, 110]. The surgeon telescopes the bowel over the endoscope, allowing for visualization of the entire length of the small bowel in more than 90% of patients. The diagnostic yield has been reported to be between 60% and 88% with rates of recurrent bleeding of 13–60% [2]. There can, however, be associated morbidity and mortality. Complications from intraoperative enteroscopy including serosal tears, avulsion of the superior mesenteric vein, congestive heart failure, azotemia, and prolonged ileus have been reported [110]. A large, multidisciplinary study looking at intraoperative enteroscopy for patients who had bleeding or anemia had a diagnostic yield of 69%. Segmental resection was performed in 90% of these patients with a symptom recurrence rate of 20%. There were no serious complications reported [111].

Technical Aspects

Endoscope technology has seen significant advances in recent years. Available endoscopes in the United States have been designed with improved resolution and magnification compared to earlier models, thus allowing for the ability to distinguish submillimeter closely approximated lesions. Upper endoscopes generally have outer diameters of 9.2–10.8 mm with slimmer 5.8 mm diameter endoscopes

Fig. 3.2 Olympus GIF
190 upper endoscope

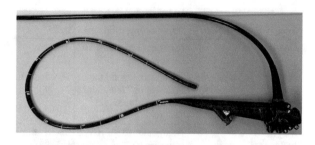

Fig. 3.3 Olympus CF 190
colonoscope

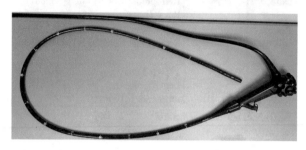

available for specific clinical situations such as esophageal strictures. Working
lengths range from 1030 mm to 1100 mm allowing for intubation of the third portion of the duodenum (Fig. 3.2).

Available colonoscopes have outer diameters ranging from 9.5 mm for pediatric
colonoscopes to 13.2 mm for adult colonoscopes depending on the manufacturer.
Field of vision is generally 140 degrees up to 170 degrees for some colonoscopes
[112] (Fig. 3.3).

A pixel is defined as a tiny area of illumination on a display screen. Standard
Resolution (SD) is defined as a 4:3 (width: height) aspect ratio with a 640 × 480
pixel lines resulting in over 300,000 pixels to produce the image. Modern endoscopes allow for high definition (HD) imaging which produces increased image
detail and thus the ability to discern more subtle mucosal lesions. HD endoscope
systems allow for 1080 × 1024 up to 1920 × 1080 pixel format. In addition to high
definition, many endoscopes have variable degrees of magnification as well as a
near focus mode to improve detection of subtle lesions [112].

Endoscopes have left/right and up/down controls which allow for angulation of
the tip (Fig. 3.4). A working channel allows for the use of various instruments such
as biopsy forceps, snares, and coagulation devices to be passed through the endoscope (Fig. 3.5). Water irrigation and suction are also available to help clear visual
fields of fecal residue or blood (Fig. 3.6). Variable stiffness colonoscopes allow for
adjustment of the stiffness of the colonoscope to reduce looping [113] (Fig. 3.7).

Looping during colonoscopy most commonly occurs in the sigmoid colon and
transverse colon, which results in paradoxical retrograde or static movement of the
colonoscope relative to the bowel during antegrade intubation of the bowel. Looping
is often associated with "redundant" colons and can reduce cecal intubation rates.
Cecal intubation rates for endoscopists are a quality measure and should be at least
90–95% [114]. Risk factors for failure to reach the cecum include poor bowel

Fig. 3.4 Colonoscope
control knobs

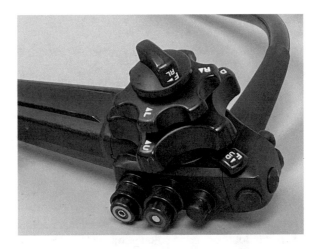

Fig. 3.5 Working
channel cap

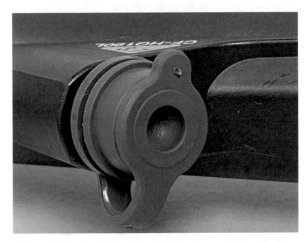

Fig. 3.6 Colonoscope tip
with suction, irrigation,
and biopsy channels

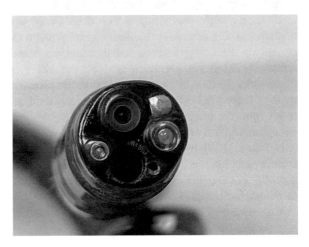

Fig. 3.7 Variable stiffness control

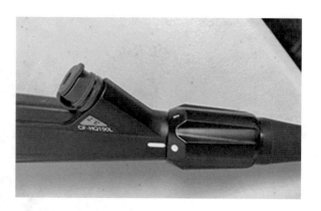

preparation and female sex. Women have longer colons relative to men, increasing the risk of looping during colonoscopy [115]. Once the cecum has been reached, the colonoscope is slowly withdrawn using maneuvers that allow for careful inspection of the mucosa and haustral folds. The colonoscope is retroflexed in the rectum by bending backwards on itself to inspect the distal rectum. A similar maneuver is used in upper endoscopy to look back up at the cardia of the stomach, which is not well seen upon entering the stomach from the esophagus if only a forward view is utilized [116].

Endoscopic technology that enhances visualization of the mucosa and microvasculature compared to white light endoscopy has also been developed. Narrow Band Imaging utilizes an electronically activated filter allowing only blue and green light [117], which is absorbed by hemoglobin thus making blood and vascular structures dark and enhancing differences between the mucosa and the surrounding vasculature [118]. This technology has improved the detection of flat or carpet-like polyps and the ability to differentiate neoplastic from non-neoplastic tissue [119].

Endoscopies are not without risks. Preprocedural complications that arise from preparation for an endoscopy include respiratory distress or arrest from sedation, possibly with oxygen saturation dropping below 80% [120] as well as potential medication allergic reactions and side effects, such as cardiorespiratory complications from using diazepam (Valium) and midazolam (Versed) [121]. Midazolam is commonly used for conscious sedation and has been known to cause grand mal seizures [122]. Bowel preparations also come with a variety of potential complications, which include hypoglycemia in diabetic patients since the patient is required to be NPO for 6–8 hrs before the procedure and fluid and electrolyte imbalances can result from the preparations. Examples of electrolyte imbalances include hyperphosphatemia following a phosphate bowel preparation, especially in patients with renal failure [123], hypocalcemia [124], and hypovolemia. The use of topical anesthetic agents run the risk of disruption in pharyngeal motor function [125], angioneurotic edema, and in the case of using topical benzocaine, acute toxic methemoglobinemia [126].

Colonoscopies have a number of potential procedural complications. Perforation is estimated to occur in approximately 0.2% of diagnostic colonoscopies. One retrospective review found that 64% of perforations are rectosigmoid and 13% are cecal [127]. Perforation may be due to direct mechanical trauma from force at the tip of the endoscope or pneumatic distension when intraluminal pressure exceeds 210 mmHg [128]. In therapeutic colonoscopy, there is deliberate mucosal injury when performing a polypectomy or biopsy, which may directly cause perforation. As a result, the site of perforation in a polypectomy is most commonly the site of the polyp. Hemorrhage, endocarditis [129], bacteremia [130], splenic injury [131], and vasovagal reactions are other risks of colonoscopies.

The most serious complications involving upper endoscopies are perforation and hemorrhage. Perforations during upper endoscopies occur at a rate of 0.02–0.2% [125]. The most common site for perforation is the distal third of the esophagus [132]. Angulation of the posterior wall of the stomach may make it difficult to navigate and the distal third of the esophagus is most likely to be inflamed or have a tumor. Other risks include infection, aspiration, Mallory-Weis tears [133], and cardiac dysrhythmia [134].

References

1. Gerson LB, Fidler JL, Cave DR, Leighton JA. ACG clinical guideline: diagnosis and management of small bowel bleeding. Am J Gastroenterol. 2015 Sep;110(9):1265.
2. Raju GS, Gerson L, Das A, Lewis B. American Gastroenterological Association (AGA) institute medical position statement on obscure gastrointestinal bleeding. Gastroenterology. 2007 Nov 1;133(5):1694–6.
3. Bull-Henry K, Al-Kawas FH. Evaluation of occult gastrointestinal bleeding. Am Fam Physician. 2013 Mar 15;87(6):430–6.
4. Hunt R, Quigley E, Abbas Z, et al. Coping with common gastrointestinal symptoms in the community: a global perspective on heartburn, constipation, bloating, and abdominal pain/discomfort May 2013. J Clin Gastroenterol. 2014 Aug 1;48(7):567–78.
5. Pasha SF, Leighton JA, Das A, et al. Double-balloon enteroscopy and capsule endoscopy have comparable diagnostic yield in small-bowel disease: a meta-analysis. Clin Gastroenterol Hepatol. 2008 Jun 1;6(6):671–6.
6. Liao Z, Gao R, Xu C, Li ZS. Indications and detection, completion, and retention rates of small-bowel capsule endoscopy: a systematic review. Gastrointest Endosc. 2010 Feb 1;71(2):280–6.
7. Early DS, Ben-Menachem T, Decker GA, Evans JA, Fanelli RD, Fisher DA, Fukami N, Hwang JH, Jain R, Jue TL, Khan KM. Appropriate use of GI endoscopy. Gastrointest Endosc. 2012 Jun 1;75(6):1127–31.
8. Ezoe Y, Muto M, Horimatsu T, et al. Magnifying narrow-band imaging versus magnifying white-light imaging for the differential diagnosis of gastric small depressive lesions: a prospective study. Gastrointest Endosc. 2010 Mar 1;71(3):477–84.
9. Lichtenstein DR, Cash BD, Davila R, et al. Role of endoscopy in the management of GERD. Gastrointest Endosc. 2007 Aug 1;66(2):219–24.
10. Levin B, Lieberman DA, McFarland B, Smith RA, Brooks D, Andrews KS, Dash C, Giardiello FM, Glick S, Levin TR, Pickhardt P. Screening and surveillance for the early detection of colorectal cancer and adenomatous polyps, 2008: a joint guideline from the American Cancer Society, the US multi-society task force on colorectal cancer, and the American College of Radiology. CA Cancer J Clin. 2008 May;58(3):130–60.

11. Chen YK, Gladden DR, Kestenbaum DJ, Collen MJ. Is there a role for upper gastrointestinal endoscopy in the evaluation of patients with occult blood-positive stool and negative colonoscopy? Am J Gastroenterol. 1993 Dec;1:88(12).

12. Geller AJ, Kolts BE, Achem SR, Wears R. The high frequency of upper gastrointestinal pathology in patients with fecal occult blood and colon polyps. Am J Gastroenterol. 1993 Aug;1:88(8).

13. Hsia PC, Al-Kawas FH. Yield of upper endoscopy in the evaluation of asymptomatic patients with Hemoccult--positive stool after a negative colonoscopy. Am J Gastroenterol. 1992 Nov;1:87(11).

14. Rockey DC, Cello JP. Evaluation of the gastrointestinal tract in patients with iron-deficiency anemia. N Engl J Med. 1993 Dec 2;329(23):1691–5.

15. Till SH, Grundman MJ. Lesson of the week: prevalence of concomitant disease in patients with iron deficiency anaemia. BMJ. 1997 Jan 18;314(7075):206.

16. Kepczyk MT, Kadakia CS. Prospective evaluation of gastrointestinal tract in patients with iron-deficiency anemia. Dig Dis Sci. 1995 Jun 1;40(6):1283–9.

17. Rex DK, Petrini JL, Baron TH, et al. Quality indicators for colonoscopy. Am J Gastroenterol. 2006 Apr;101(4):873.

18. Doubeni CA, Corley DA, Quinn VP, et al. Effectiveness of screening colonoscopy in reducing the risk of death from right and left colon cancer: a large community-based study. Gut. 2018 Feb 1;67(2):291–8.

19. Miyamoto H, Naoe H, Oda Y, et al. Impact of retroflexion in the right colon after repeated forward-view examinations. JGH Open. 2018 Dec;2(6):282–7.

20. Cohen J, Grunwald D, Grossberg LB, Sawhney MS. The effect of right colon retroflexion on adenoma detection: a systematic review and meta-analysis. J Clin Gastroenterol. 2017 Oct;51(9):818.

21. Clark BT, Rustagi T, Laine L. What level of bowel prep quality requires early repeat colonoscopy: systematic review and meta-analysis of the impact of preparation quality on adenoma detection rate. Am J Gastroenterol. 2014 Nov;109(11):1714.

22. Rex DK, Rahmani EY, Haseman JH, et al. Relative sensitivity of colonoscopy and barium enema for detection of colorectal cancer in clinical practice. Gastroenterology. 1997 Jan 1;112(1):17–23.

23. Freeny PC, Marks WM, Ryan JA, Bolen JW. Colorectal carcinoma evaluation with CT: preoperative staging and detection of postoperative recurrence. Radiology. 1986 Feb;158(2):347–53.

24. Ogunbiyi OA, Flanagan FL, Dehdashti F, et al. Detection of recurrent and metastatic colorectal cancer: comparison of positron emission tomography and computed tomography. Ann Surg Oncol. 1997 Dec 1;4(8):613–20.

25. Sun L, Wu H, Guan YS. Colonography by CT, MRI and PET/CT combined with conventional colonoscopy in colorectal cancer screening and staging. World J Gastroenterol: WJG. 2008 Feb 14;14(6):853.

26. Schreyer AG, Rath HC, Kikinis R, et al. Comparison of magnetic resonance imaging colonography with conventional colonoscopy for the assessment of intestinal inflammation in patients with inflammatory bowel disease: a feasibility study. Gut. 2005 Feb 1;54(2):250–6.

27. Tedesco FJ, Waye JD, Avella JR, Villalobos MM. Diagnostic implications of the spatial distribution of colonic mass lesions (polyps and cancers): a prospective colonoscopic study. Gastrointest Endosc. 1980 Aug 1;26(3):95–7.

28. Gumaste V, Sachar DB, Greenstein AJ. Benign and malignant colorectal strictures in ulcerative colitis. Gut. 1992 Jul 1;33(7):938–41.

29. Regula J, Rupinski M, Kraszewska E, et al. Colonoscopy in colorectal-cancer screening for detection of advanced neoplasia. N Engl J Med. 2006 Nov 2;355(18):1863–72.

30. Appleyard M, Fireman Z, Glukhovsky A, et al. A randomized trial comparing wireless capsule endoscopy with push enteroscopy for the detection of small-bowel lesions. Gastroenterology. 2000 Dec 1;119(6):1431–8.

31. Wang A, Banerjee S, Barth BA, et al. Wireless capsule endoscopy. Gastrointest Endosc. 2013 Dec 1;78(6):805–15.

32. Hartmann D, Schmidt H, Bolz G, et al. A prospective two-center study comparing wireless capsule endoscopy with intraoperative enteroscopy in patients with obscure GI bleeding. Gastrointest Endosc. 2005 Jun 1;61(7):826–32.

33. Pennazio M, Santucci R, Rondonotti E, et al. Outcome of patients with obscure gastrointestinal bleeding after capsule endoscopy: report of 100 consecutive cases. Gastroenterology. 2004 Mar 1;126(3):643–53.

34. Goenka MK, Majumder S, Kumar S, et al. Single center experience of capsule endoscopy in patients with obscure gastrointestinal bleeding. World J Gastroenterol: WJG. 2011 Feb 14;17(6):774.

35. Yamada A, Watabe H, Kobayashi Y, et al. Timing of capsule endoscopy influences the diagnosis and outcome in obscure-overt gastrointestinal bleeding. Hepato-Gastroenterology. 2012 May;59(115):676–9.

36. Hong SN, Kang SH, Jang HJ, Wallace MB. Recent advance in colon capsule endoscopy: What's new? Clin Endosc. 2018 Jul;51(4):334.

37. Triester SL, Leighton JA, Leontiadis GI, et al. A meta-analysis of the yield of capsule endoscopy compared to other diagnostic modalities in patients with obscure gastrointestinal bleeding. Am J Gastroenterol. 2005 Nov;100(11):2407.

38. Lewis BS, Swain P. Capsule endoscopy in the evaluation of patients with suspected small intestinal bleeding: results of a pilot study. Gastrointest Endosc. 2002 Sep 1;56(3):349–53.

39. Delvaux MM, Saurin JC, Gaudin JL, et al. Comparison of wireless endoscopic capsule and push-enteroscopy in patients with obscure occult/overt digestive bleeding: results of a prospective, blinded, multicenter trial. Gastrointest Endosc. 2002;55:5.

40. Van Gossum A. A prospective comparative study between push enteroscopy and wireless video capsule in patients with obscure digestive bleeding. Gastrointest Endosc. 2002;97:AB-88

41. Beejay UA, Haber GB, Rasul I, et al. A pilot trial comparing the diagnostic utility and reproduceability of given (R) diagnostic imaging system to conventional enteroscopy in the evaluation of chronic obscure gastrointestinal bleeding. Am J Gastroenterol. 2002;97(9S):S299.

42. Ell C, Remke S, May A, et al. The first prospective controlled trial comparing wireless capsule endoscopy with push enteroscopy in chronic gastrointestinal bleeding. Endoscopy. 2002 Sep;34(09):685–9.

43. Mylonaki M, Fritscher-Ravens A, Swain P. Wireless capsule endoscopy: a comparison with push enteroscopy in patients with gastroscopy and colonoscopy negative gastrointestinal bleeding. Gut. 2003 Aug 1;52(8):1122–6.

44. Adler DG, Knipschield M, Gostout C. A prospective comparison of capsule endoscopy and push enteroscopy in patients with GI bleeding of obscure origin. Gastrointest Endosc. 2004 Apr 1;59(4):492–8.

45. Mata A, Bordas JM, Feu F, et al. Wireless capsule endoscopy in patients with obscure gastrointestinal bleeding: a comparative study with push enteroscopy. Aliment Pharmacol Ther. 2004 Jul;20(2):189–94.

46. Mergener K, Schembre DB, Brandabur JJ, et al. Clinical utility of capsule endoscopy-a single center experience. Am J Gastroenterol. 2002;9(97):S299–300.

47. Scapa E, Jacob H, Lewkowicz S, et al. Initial experience of wireless-capsule endoscopy for evaluating occult gastrointestinal bleeding and suspected small bowel pathology. Am J Gastroenterol. 2002 Nov;97(11):2776.

48. Laine LA, Sahota A, Shah A. Does capsule endoscopy improve outcomes in obscure GI bleeding: randomized controlled trial of capsule endoscopy vs. dedicated small bowel radiography. Gastro Endosc. 2009 Apr 1;69(5):AB99.

49. Park JJ, Cheon JH, Kim HM, et al. Negative capsule endoscopy without subsequent enteros-copy does not predict lower long-term rebleeding rates in patients with obscure GI bleeding. Gastrointest Endosc. 2010 May 1;71(6):990–7.
50. Koulaouzidis A, Yung DE, Lam JH, et al. The use of small-bowel capsule endoscopy in iron-deficiency anemia alone; be aware of the young anemic patient. Scand J Gastroenterol. 2012 Sep 1;47(8–9):1094–100.
51. Lepileur L, Dray X, Antonietti M, et al. Factors associated with diagnosis of obscure gas-trointestinal bleeding by video capsule enteroscopy. Clin Gastroenterol Hepatol. 2012 Dec 1;10(12):1376–80.
52. Koulaouzidis A, Rondonotti E, Giannakou A, Plevris JN. Diagnostic yield of small-bowel capsule endoscopy in patients with iron-deficiency anemia: a systematic review. Gastrointest Endosc. 2012 Nov 1;76(5):983–92.
53. De Leusse A, Vahedi K, Edery J, et al. Capsule endoscopy or push enteroscopy for first-line exploration of obscure gastrointestinal bleeding? Gastroenterology. 2007 Mar 1;132(3):855–62.
54. Min YW, Kim JS, Jeon SW, et al. Long-term outcome of capsule endoscopy in obscure gas-trointestinal bleeding: a nationwide analysis. Endoscopy. 2014 Jan;46(01):59–65.
55. Cave DR, Fleischer DE, Leighton JA, et al. A multicenter randomized comparison of the Endocapsule and the Pillcam SB. Gastrointest Endosc. 2008 Sep 1;68(3):487–94.
56. Chauhan SS, Manfredi MA, Dayyeh BK, et al. Enteroscopy. Gastrointest Endosc. 2015 Dec 1;82(6):975–90.
57. Benz C, Jakobs R, Riemann JF. Do we need the overtube for push-enteroscopy? Endoscopy. 2001 Aug;33(08):658–61.
58. Taylor AC, Chen RY, Desmond PV. Use of an overtube for enteroscopy-does it increase depth of insertion? A prospective study of enteroscopy with and without an overtube. Endoscopy. 2001 Mar;33(03):227–30.
59. Zaman A, Katon R. Push enteroscopy for obscure GI bleeding yields a high incidence of proxi-mal lesions within the reach of standard endoscopy. Gastrointest Endosc. 1997;45(4):AB103.
60. Foutch PG, Sawyer R, Sanowski RA. Push-enteroscopy for diagnosis of patients with gastro-intestinal bleeding of obscure origin. Gastrointest Endosc. 1990 Jul 1;36(4):337–41.
61. Lewis BS, Wenger JS, Waye JD. Small bowel enteroscopy and intraoperative enteroscopy for obscure gastrointestinal bleeding. Am J Gastroenterol. 1991 Feb 1;86(2)
62. Manno M, Barbera C, Bertani H, et al. Single balloon enteroscopy: technical aspects and clinical applications. World J Gastrointest Endosc. 2012 Feb 16;4(2):28.
63. Akerman PA. Spiral enteroscopy versus double-balloon enteroscopy: choosing the right tool for the job. Gastrointest Endosc. 2013 Feb 1;77(2):252–4.
64. Baniya R, Upadhaya S, Subedi SC, Khan J, Sharma P, Mohammed TS, Bachuwa G, Jamil LH. Balloon enteroscopy versus spiral enteroscopy for small-bowel disorders: a systematic review and meta-analysis. Gastrointest Endosc. 2017 Dec 1;86(6):997–1005.
65. Mans L, Arvanitakis M, Neuhaus H, Devière J. Motorized spiral enteroscopy for occult bleeding. Dig Dis. 2018;36:325–7.
66. Neuhaus H, Beyna T, Schneider M, Devière J. Novel motorized spiral enteroscopy: first clini-cal case. Gastrointest Endosc. 2016 May 1;83(5):AB637.
67. Beyna T, Arvanitakis M, Schneider M, Gerges C, Böing D, Devière J, Neuhaus H. Motorised spiral enteroscopy: first prospective clinical feasibility study. Gut. 2021;70(2):261–7.
68. Swain P, Fritscher-Ravens A. Role of video endoscopy in managing small bowel disease. Gut. 2004 Dec 1;53(12):1866–75.
69. He C, Lai H, Huang J, Li A, Xue Q, Liu S, Ren Y. Su1274 comparing diagnostic yield of preoperative capsule endoscopy with double balloon Enteroscopy in patients with overt small intestinal bleeding. Gastrointest Endosc. 2018 Jun 1;87(6):AB307.
70. Vuik FE, Moen S, Nieuwenburg SA, Kuipers EJ, Spaander MC. Applicability of colon cap-sule endoscopy as pan-endoscopy: from bowel preparation, transit times, and completion rate to rating times and patient acceptance. Endoscopy. 2020 Apr;52(S 01):OP69.

71. Luo YY, Pan J, Chen YZ, Jiang X, Zou WB, Qian YY, Zhou W, Liu X, Li ZS, Liao Z. Magnetic steering of capsule endoscopy improves small bowel capsule endoscopy completion rate. Dig Dis Sci. 2019 Jul 15;64(7):1908–15.

72. Cavallaro F, Tontini GE, Bozzi R. Feasibility, safety and diagnostic yield of Omom CE, a new capsule endoscopy system: the first experience in Caucasian patients. Gastroenterol Pancreatol Liver Disord. 2017;4(7):1–4.

73. Chauhan SS, Manfredi MA, Dayyeh BK, Enestvedt BK, Fujii-Lau LL, Komanduri S, Konda V, Maple JT, Murad FM, Pannala R, Thosani NC. Enteroscopy. Gastrointestinal endoscopy. 2015;82(6):975–90.

74. Benz C, Jakobs R, Riemann JF. Does the insertion depth in push enteroscopy depend on the working length of the enteroscope? Endoscopy. 2002 Jul;34(07):543–5.

75. Sharma BC, Bhasin DK, Makharia G, Chhabra M, Vaiphei K, Bhatti HS, Singh K. Diagnostic value of push-type enteroscopy: a report from India. Am J Gastroenterol. 2000 Jan 1;95(1):137–40.

76. Taylor AC, Buttigieg RJ, McDonald IG, Desmond PV. Prospective assessment of the diagnostic and therapeutic impact of small-bowel push enteroscopy. Endoscopy. 2003 Nov;35(11):951–6.

77. Ell C, Remke S, May A, Helou L, Henrich R, Mayer G. The first prospective controlled trial comparing wireless capsule endoscopy with push enteroscopy in chronic gastrointestinal bleeding. Endoscopy. 2002 Sep;34(09):685–9.

78. Mata A, Bordas JM, Feu F, Gines A, Pellise M, Fernández-Esparrach G, Balaguer F, Pique JM, Llach J. Wireless capsule endoscopy in patients with obscure gastrointestinal bleeding: a comparative study with push enteroscopy. Aliment Pharmacol Ther. 2004 Jul;20(2):189–94.

79. Chong J, Tagle M, Barkin JS, Reiner DK. Small bowel push-type fiberoptic enteroscopy for patients with occult gastrointestinal bleeding or suspected small bowel pathology. Am J Gastroenterol (Springer Nature). 1994 Dec 1;89(12).

80. May A, Nachbar L, Schneider M, Ell C. Prospective comparison of push enteroscopy and push-and-pull enteroscopy in patients with suspected small-bowel bleeding. Am J Gastroenterol. 2006 Sep 1;101(9):2016–24.

81. Nakamura M, Niwa Y, Ohmiya N, Miyahara R, Ohashi A, Itoh A, Hirooka Y, Goto H. Preliminary comparison of capsule endoscopy and double-balloon enteroscopy in patients with suspected small-bowel bleeding. Endoscopy. 2006 Jan;38(01):59–66.

82. Hayat M, Axon AT, O'Mahony S. Diagnostic yield and effect on clinical outcomes of push enteroscopy in suspected small-bowel bleeding. Endoscopy. 2000 May;32(05):369–72.

83. Tsujikawa T, Saitoh Y, Andoh A, Imaeda H, Hata K, Minematsu H, Senoh K, Hayafuji K, Ogawa A, Nakahara T, Sasaki M. Novel single-balloon enteroscopy for diagnosis and treatment of the small intestine: preliminary experiences. Endoscopy. 2008 Jan;40(01):11–5.

84. Upchurch BR, Sanaka MR, Lopez AR, Vargo JJ. The clinical utility of single-balloon enteroscopy: a single-center experience of 172 procedures. Gastrointest Endosc. 2010 Jun 1;71(7):1218–23.

85. Ramchandani M, Reddy DN, Gupta R, Lakhtakia S, Tandan M, Rao GV, Darisetty S. Diagnostic yield and therapeutic impact of single-balloon enteroscopy: series of 106 cases. J Gastroenterol Hepatol. 2009 Oct;24(10):1631–8.

86. Khashab MA, Lennon AM, Dunbar KB, Singh VK, Chandrasekhara V, Giday S, Canto MI, Buscaglia JM, Kapoor S, Shin EJ, Kalloo AN. A comparative evaluation of single-balloon enteroscopy and spiral enteroscopy for patients with mid-gut disorders. Gastrointest Endosc. 2010 Oct 1;72(4):766–72.

87. Domagk D, Mensink P, Aktas H, Lenz P, Meister T, Luegering A, Ullerich H, Aabakken L, Heinecke A, Domschke W, Kuipers E. Single-vs. double-balloon enteroscopy in small-bowel diagnostics: a randomized multicenter trial. Endoscopy. 2011 Jun;43(06):472–6.

88. Lenz P, Domagk D. Double-vs. single-balloon vs. spiral enteroscopy. Best Pract Res Clin Gastroenterol. 2012 Jun 1;26(3):303–13.

89. May A, Färber M, Aschmoneit I, Pohl J, Manner H, Lotterer E, Möschler O, Kunz J, Gossner L, Mönkemüller K, Ell C. Prospective multicenter trial comparing push-and-pull enteroscopy with the single-and double-balloon techniques in patients with small-bowel disorders. Am J Gastroenterol. 2010 Mar 1;105(3):575–81.

90. Kawamura T, Yasuda K, Tanaka K, Uno K, Ueda M, Sanada K, Nakajima M. Clinical evaluation of a newly developed single-balloon enteroscope. Gastrointest Endosc. 2008 Dec 1;68(6):1112–6.

91. Takano N, Yamada A, Watabe H, Togo G, Yamaji Y, Yoshida H, Kawabe T, Omata M, Koike K. Single-balloon versus double-balloon endoscopy for achieving total enteroscopy: a randomized, controlled trial. Gastrointest Endosc. 2011 Apr 1;73(4):734–9.

92. Aktas H, de Ridder L, Haringsma J, Kuipers EJ, Mensink PB. Complications of single-balloon enteroscopy: a prospective evaluation of 166 procedures. Endoscopy. 2010 May;42(05):365–8.

93. Frantz DJ, Dellon ES, Grimm IS, Morgan DR. Single-balloon enteroscopy: results from an initial experience at a US tertiary-care center. Gastrointest Endosc. 2010 Aug 1;72(2):422–6.

94. Heine GD, Hadithi M, Groenen MJ, Kuipers EJ, Jacobs MA, Mulder CJ. Double-balloon enteroscopy: indications, diagnostic yield, and complications in a series of 275 patients with suspected small-bowel disease. Endoscopy. 2006 Jan;38(01):42–8.

95. Yamamoto H, Kita H, Sunada K, Hayashi Y, Sato H, Yano T, Iwamoto M, Sekine Y, Miyata T, Kuno A, Ajibe H. Clinical outcomes of double-balloon endoscopy for the diagnosis and treatment of small-intestinal diseases. Clin Gastroenterol Hepatol. 2004 Nov 1;2(11):1010–6.

96. Di Caro S, May A, Heine DG, Fini L, Landi B, Petruzziello L, Cellier C, Mulder CJ, Costamagna G, Ell C, Gasbarrini A. The European experience with double-balloon enteroscopy: indications, methodology, safety, and clinical impact. Gastrointest Endosc. 2005 Oct 1;62(4):545–50.

97. Gross SA, Stark ME. Initial experience with double-balloon enteroscopy at a US center. Gastrointest Endosc. 2008 May 1;67(6):890–7.

98. Mehdizadeh S, Ross A, Gerson L, Leighton J, Chen A, Schembre D, Chen G, Semrad C, Kamal A, Harrison EM, Binmoeller K. What is the learning curve associated with double-balloon enteroscopy? Technical details and early experience in 6 US tertiary care centers. Gastrointest Endosc. 2006 Nov 1;64(5):740–50.

99. Yamamoto H, Sekine Y, Sato Y, Higashizawa T, Miyata T, Iino S, Ido K, Sugano K. Total enteroscopy with a nonsurgical steerable double-balloon method. Gastrointest Endosc. 2001 Feb 1;53(2):216–20.

100. Nakase H, Matsuura M, Mikami S, Chiba T. Diagnosis and treatment of obscure GI bleeding with double balloon endoscopy. Gastrointest Endosc. 2007 Sep 1;66(3):S78–81.

101. May A, Nachbar L, Schneider M, Neumann M, Ell C. Push-and-pull enteroscopy using the double-balloon technique: method of assessing depth of insertion and training of the enteroscopy technique using the Erlangen Endo-trainer. Endoscopy. 2005 Jan;37(01):66–70.

102. Möschler O, May A, Müller MK, Ell C. Null for the German DBE study group. Complications in and performance of double-balloon enteroscopy (DBE): results from a large prospective DBE database in Germany. Endoscopy. 2011 Jun;43(06):484–9.

103. Messer I, May A, Manner H, Ell C. Prospective, randomized, single-center trial comparing double-balloon enteroscopy and spiral enteroscopy in patients with suspected small-bowel disorders. Gastrointest Endosc. 2013 Feb 1;77(2):241–9.

104. Sanaka MR, Navaneethan U, Kosuru B, Yerneni H, Lopez R, Vargo JJ. Antegrade is more effective than retrograde enteroscopy for evaluation and management of suspected small-bowel disease. Clin Gastroenterol Hepatol. 2012 Aug 1;10(8):910–6.

105. Akerman PA, Agrawal D, Chen W, Cantero D, Avila J, Pangtay J. Spiral enteroscopy: a novel method of enteroscopy by using the endo-ease discovery SB overtube and a pediatric colonoscope. Gastrointest Endosc. 2009 Feb 1;69(2):327–32.

106. Buscaglia JM, Dunbar KB, Okolo PI, Judah J, Akerman PA, Cantero D, Draganov PV. The spiral enteroscopy training initiative: results of a prospective study evaluating the discovery SB overtube device during small bowel enteroscopy (with video). Endoscopy. 2009 Mar;41(03):194–9.
107. Judah JR, Draganov PV, Lam Y, Hou W, Buscaglia JM. Spiral enteroscopy is safe and effective for an elderly United States population of patients with numerous comorbidities. Clin Gastroenterol Hepatol. 2010 Jul 1;8(7):572–6.
108. Judah JR, Collins D, Gaidos JK, Hou W, Forsmark CE, Draganov PV. Prospective evaluation of gastroenterologist-guided, nurse-administered standard sedation for spiral deep small bowel enteroscopy. Dig Dis Sci. 2010 Sep 1;55(9):2584–91.
109. Zaman A, Sheppard B, Katon RM. Total peroral intraoperative enteroscopy for obscure GI bleeding using a dedicated push enteroscope: diagnostic yield and patient outcome. Gastrointest Endosc. 1999 Oct 1;50(4):506–10.
110. Ress AM, Benacci JC, Sarr MG. Efficacy of intraoperative enteroscopy in diagnosis and prevention of recurrent, occult gastrointestinal bleeding. Am J Surg. 1992 Jan 1;163(1):94–9.
111. Green J, Schlieve CR, Friedrich AK, et al. Approach to the diagnostic workup and management of small bowel lesions at a tertiary care center. J Gastrointest Surg. 2018 Jun 1;22(6):1034–42.
112. Bhat YM, Dayyeh BK, Chauhan SS, et al. High-definition and high-magnification endoscopes. Gastrointest Endosc. 2014 Dec 1;80(6):919–27.
113. Xie Q, Chen B, Liu L, Gan H. Does the variable-stiffness colonoscope makes colonoscopy easier? A meta-analysis of the efficacy of the variable stiffness colonoscope compared with the standard adult colonoscope. BMC Gastroenterol. 2012 Dec;12(1):151.
114. Hoff G, Holme Ø, Bretthauer M, et al. Cecum intubation rate as quality indicator in clinical versus screening colonoscopy. Endosc Int Open. 2017 Jun;5(06):E489–95.
115. Witte TN, Enns R. The difficult colonoscopy. Can J Gastroenterol Hepatol. 2007;21(8):487–90.
116. Ahlawat R, Ross AB. Esophagogastroduodenoscopy. StatPearls [Internet] 2018 Oct 27. StatPearls Publishing.
117. Gono K, Obi T, Yamaguchi M, et al. Appearance of enhanced tissue features in narrow-band endoscopic imaging. J Biomed Opt. 2004 May;9(3):568–78.
118. Singh R, Mei SC, Sethi S. Advanced endoscopic imaging in Barrett's oesophagus: a review on current practice. World J Gastroenterol: WJG. 2011 Oct 14;17(38):4271.
119. Chiu HM, Chang CY, Chen CC, et al. A prospective comparative study of narrow-band imaging, chromoendoscopy, and conventional colonoscopy in the diagnosis of colorectal neoplasia. Gut. 2007 Mar 1;56(3):373–9.
120. Hart R, Classen M. Complications of diagnostic gastrointestinal endoscopy. Endoscopy. 1990 Sep;22(05):229–33.
121. Arrowsmith JB, Gerstman BB, Fleischer DE, Benjamin SB. Results from the American Society for Gastrointestinal Endoscopy/US Food and Drug Administration collaborative study on complication rates and drug use during gastrointestinal endoscopy. Gastrointest Endosc. 1991 Jul 1;37(4):421–7.
122. Alexander JA, Smith BJ. Midazolam sedation for percutaneous liver biopsy. Dig Dis Sci. 1993 Dec 1;38(12):2209–11.
123. Fine A, Patterson J. Severe hyperphosphatemia following phosphate administration for bowel preparation in patients with renal failure: two cases and a review of the literature. Am J Kidney Dis. 1997 Jan 1;29(1):103–5.
124. Oliveira L, Wexner SD, Daniel N, DeMarta D, Weiss EG, Nogueras JJ, Bernstein M. Mechanical bowel preparation for elective colorectal surgery. Dis Colon Rectum. 1997 May 1;40(5):585–91.
125. Zubarik R, Eisen G, Mastropietro C, Lopez J, Carroll J, Benjamin S, Fleischer DE. Prospective analysis of complications 30 days after outpatient upper endoscopy. Am J Gastroenterol. 1999;94(6):1539–45.

126. Brown CM, Levy SA, Susann PW. Methemoglobinemia: life-threatening complication of endoscopy premedication. Am J Gastroenterol. 1994;89(7):1108–9.
127. Gedebou TM, Wong RA, Rappaport WD, Jaffe P, Kahsai D, Hunter GC. Clinical presentation and management of iatrogenic colon perforations. Am J Surg. 1996 Nov 1;172(5):454–8.
128. BURT AV. Pneumatic rupture of the intestinal canal: with experimental data showing the mechanism of perforation and the pressure required. Arch Surg. 1931 Jun 1;22(6):875–902.
129. Hall C, Dorricott NJ, Donovan IA, Neoptolemos JP. Colon perforation during colonoscopy: surgical versus conservative management. Br J Surg. 1991 May;78(5):542–4.
130. Low DE, Shoenut JP, Kennedy JK, Sharma GP, Harding GK, Den Boer B, Micflikier AB. Prospective assessment of risk of bacteremia with colonoscopy and polypectomy. Dig Dis Sci. 1987 Nov 1;32(11):1239–43.
131. Taylor FC, Frankl HD, Riemer KD. Late presentation of splenic trauma after routine colonoscopy. Am J Gastroenterol. 1989 Apr;1:84(4).
132. Berry BE, Ochsner JL. Perforation of the esophagus: a 30 year review. J Thorac Cardiovasc Surg. 1973 Jan 1;65(1):1–7.
133. Penston JG, Boyd EJ, Wormsley KG. Mallory-Weiss tears occurring during endoscopy: a report of seven cases. Endoscopy. 1992 May;24(04):262–5.
134. Levy N, Abinader E. Continuous electrocardiographic monitoring with Holter electrocardiocorder throughout all stages of gastroscopy. Am J Dig Dis. 1977 Dec 1;22(12):1091–6.

Chapter 4
Radiologic Detection

Michael E. Schuster, Erik A. Jacobson, Anthony K. Sayegh, Victor N. Becerra, Robert P.F. Brooks, and Peter E. Kim

CT

CT is a valuable radiologic modality in the workup of occult GI bleeding. CT scans use X-rays, which produce ionizing radiation, to build cross-sectional images of the body. The images, or "slices," are created based on the differential densities of the internal structures [1]. Densities can be measured directly on the image, utilizing the Hounsfield Units (HU) scale. CT has high patient throughput and, other than CTC, requires no patient preparation [2, 3].

Non-contrast CT has limited diagnostic utility in the workup of OGIB due to the poor contrast resolution of the image. Hemorrhage may be visualized as circumferential thickening of the bowel wall [4]. Intraluminal hemorrhage may be seen based on its density (30–45 HU for unclotted blood and 45–70 HU for clotted blood) [5, 6].

Techniques which use oral and/or IV contrast can significantly improve the diagnostic utility of CT. Imaging can be timed for assessment of the arteries (CTA), for identifying sources of active bleeding. CT enterography (CTE) is performed in an enteric phase (about 50 s after contrast administration) or portal venous phase (60–70 s after contrast administration) to accentuate bowel wall enhancement. These techniques can be performed in conjunction with a delayed phase (typically 90 s or longer after contrast administration) to improve conspicuity of bleeding sites. Standard CT scans with IV contrast can show sources of occult GI bleeding such as gastric ulcers (Fig. 4.1) and sigmoid adenocarcinoma (Fig. 4.2).

M. E. Schuster (✉) · E. A. Jacobson · A. K. Sayegh · V. N. Becerra · R. P.F. Brooks · P. E. Kim
Albany Medical College Diagnostic Radiology, Albany, NY, USA
e-mail: schustm@amc.edu; jacobse3@amc.edu; sayegha@amc.edu; becerrv@amc.edu; brooksr2@amc.edu; kimp@amc.edu

M. Tadros, G. Y. Wu (eds.), *Management of Occult GI Bleeding*, Clinical Gastroenterology, https://doi.org/10.1007/978-3-030-71468-0_4

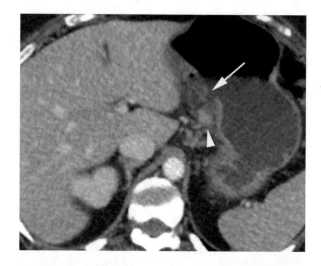

Fig. 4.1 There is a focal discontinuity in the gastric antrum (arrow), relating to a gastric ulcer. Arrowhead relates to an adjacent focus of hemorrhage. Endoscopy one day later showed a gastric ulcer with blood clot and no perforation, NSAID induced

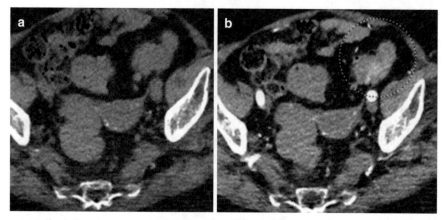

Fig. 4.2 Precontrast (**a**) and postcontrast (**b**) CT shows high attenuation in the lumen of the sigmoid colon (encircled on **b**), representing the site of bleeding. Invasive adenocarcinoma was found on pathology

CT Enterography (CTE)

CT enterography (CTE) allows excellent visualization of the entire bowel wall, as well as evaluation of extraenteric structures [7]. In this technique, improved visualization of the bowel mucosa is obtained with fluid distention. Standard technique includes bowel distention with an orally ingested neutral oral contrast (such as Volumen, a 0.1% weight/volume barium suspension). Routine protocol typically involves ingestion of a volume of 1.35 liters Volumen in the 45–60 min prior to CT, with an additional volume of 500 mL water in the last 15 min prior to scanning [7, 8]. Optimal bowel distention is achieved by drinking the oral contrast material slowly, rather than rapidly.

Intravenous contrast administration is a required component of CTE. A routine CTE is performed with a single scan after the administration of IV contrast. Optimal small bowel wall enhancement corresponds to an "enteric phase", about 50 s after the administration of IV contrast [8, 9]. Most institutions perform a single contrast CTE with a delay of 50 –70 s (portal venous phase).

While a single phase study is typically sufficient in the workup of patients with Crohn's disease (Fig. 4.3), a multiphase CTE is often helpful in the workup of patients with occult GI bleeding [10, 11]. The multiple phases increase sensitivity for bleeding sites by showing the accumulation of intravenous contrast on more delayed phases. A non-contrast series is probably not necessary, though some centers will perform non-contrast imaging to avoid potential confusion from high density objects such as ingested tablets. Double contrast (arterial and portal venous or more delayed) and triple contrast (arterial, enteric, and delayed) techniques have been described [10]. Angiodysplasia can be identified as an avidly enhancing plaque in the enteric phase [7]. Hara showed a sensitivity of 33% and specificity of 85% in occult GI bleeding.

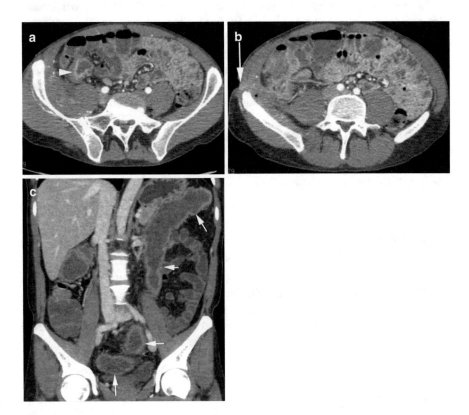

Fig. 4.3 CTE demonstrates complications of Crohn's disease, with ascending colitis (arrowhead in **a**) and inflammation related to enterocutaneous fistula (arrow in **b**). Note the adjacent iliacus myositis in **a**. Note the mucosal enhancement and wall thickening (arrows in **c**) in Crohn's colitis

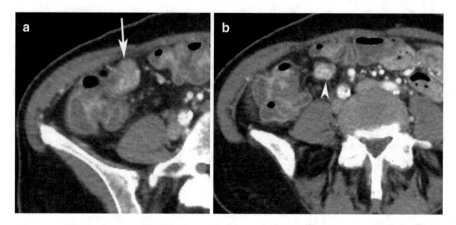

Fig. 4.4 CT enterography shows enhancing lesion of the terminal ileum (arrow in **a**), representing neuroendocrine tumor. Adjacent mesenteric metastasis is noted (arrowhead in **b**)

There are good data that video capsule endoscopy (VCE) and CTE provide complementary information [11–17]. While VCE is more sensitive than CTE for mucosal lesions, CTE is more sensitive for mural lesions [11, 18, 19]. CTE is more sensitive for small bowel neoplasms, a more common source of bleeding in younger patients (see Fig. 4.4). CTE could be considered as a first line of evaluation in younger patients and those with Crohn's disease. There are also data that CTE is a very effective triage tool in determining who may benefit from double balloon enteroscopy [20].

Disadvantages of CTE include ionizing radiation exposure, potential allergic reaction to IV contrast, and contrast induced nephropathy. Patients with GI bleeding are more likely to have compromised renal function, which may preclude the administration of IV contrast. Disadvantages of VCE include retained capsule.

CT Enteroclysis

In this technique, a neutral contrast is instilled through a fluoroscopically placed nasojejunal tube. The invasive and labor-intensive nature make enteroclysis a much less common option, and diagnostic yields have not been shown to be increased [3, 19]. Nevertheless, this option could be considered in patients who cannot tolerate the large volume of orally ingested contrast required for CTE.

CT Colonography

CT Colonography (CTC) is a non-invasive screening technique for colorectal cancer. After a complete bowel preparation, the patient is scanned in supine and prone

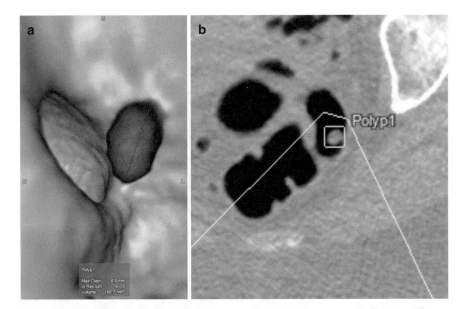

Fig. 4.5 3D-reformatted "fly through" image shows an 8 mm polyp in the sigmoid colon, color coded red by polyp selecting tool in Vitrea postprocessing software package (**a**).The polyp is demonstrated on the axial source image through the pelvis (**b**)

positions, utilizing a low-dose technique [21]. Supine and prone imaging is performed to better detect polyps and move any residual fluid in the colon between the two positions. 3-dimensional "fly-through" images are created to aid detection, in addition to the standard 2-dimensional slices (Fig. 4.5).

CT colonography may be considered in patients who cannot tolerate colonoscopy. After incomplete colonoscopy, CT colonography may have findings 19% of the time [22]. CT colonography can be obtained the same day after incomplete colonoscopy. If the patient wishes to have CT colonography instead of colonoscopy, a full bowel preparation is still required. Several studies have shown a high sensitivity and specificity for CTC for detecting polyps 6 mm or larger [23, 24].

CT Angiography

CT Angiography (CTA) has greater utility in the workup of patients with acute GI bleeding [25]. The arterial timing of contrast can be helpful in identifying sites of active hemorrhage by showing pooling of contrast at sites of active hemorrhage [26, 27]. In patients with intermittent episodes of gastrointestinal bleeding, CTA or multiphase CT that includes arterial phase is useful for identifying sites of hemorrhage [28]. See Fig. 4.6, with conventional angiography correlate.

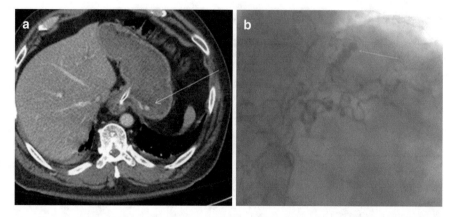

Fig. 4.6 There is active bleeding from a gastric vascular malformation (arrow in **a**). Bleeding site is confirmed at conventional angiography (arrow in **b**)

Fig. 4.7 Image from a dual energy CT in a patient with metastatic renal cell carcinoma to the small bowel. Fused image with iodine map accentuates the site of contrast accumulation (arrow), representing a site of active hemorrhage

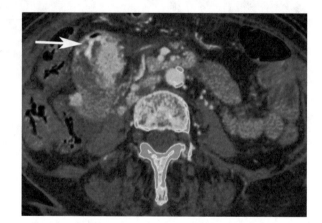

Dual Energy CT

Dual energy CT is a relatively new technology that uses X-rays of different energies to provide more information than a conventional CT. There is evidence that dual energy may aid in identifying sites of GI bleeding [29]. Iodine-based CT contrast can be made more apparent with low energy reconstructions of the CT data, as well as with iodine maps (Fig. 4.7). There is also potential for radiation dose reduction, as virtual non-contrast images can be created from the dual energy data.

MR Enterography

MR Enterography (MRE) is a technique to evaluate the small bowel. The oral preparation for MR enterography (MRE) is identical to that of CTE. Intravenous contrast is required, as it is with CTE. Advantages over CTE include lack of ionizing

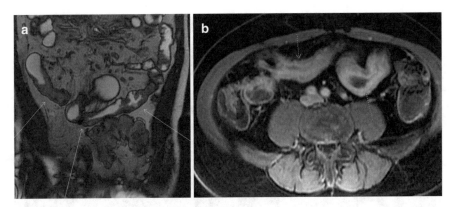

Fig. 4.8 Coronal T2 weighted image (**a**) and axial post contrast T1-weighted image (**b**) show skip areas of small bowel wall thickening (arrows in **a** and **b**), as well as wall hyperenhancement in **b**. Findings are compatible with areas of active Crohn's disease

radiation, reduced risk of contrast allergy, greater contrast resolution, and lack of contrast induced nephropathy. There is a risk of nephrogenic systemic fibrosis (NSF), a debilitating multisystem process that affects the skin, with some contrast agents [30]. MRE has poorer spatial resolution compared to CTE, and artifact related to bowel peristalsis is greater due to the longer scan times. This can be minimized by giving glucagon by intramuscular injection or slow IV push [31].

MR Enterography is an excellent option in patients who have history of inflammatory bowel disease. Complications of Crohn's Disease are well demonstrated with MRE (Fig. 4.8), and the cumulative radiation dose from repeated CT exams can be mitigated with MRE. MRE is also a good option for patients with allergy to contrast given for CT. A disadvantage of MRE compared to CT is a higher likelihood of poor or non-diagnostic studies in patients who are unable to tolerate the oral preparation or to remain motionless for the (longer) duration exam. Studies have shown that MRE is as or more accurate than CTE in the detection of small-bowel diseases, particularly in detecting neoplastic diseases [32]. See Figs. 4.9 and 4.10. Both CTE and MRE have been shown to be effective in evaluating small bowel vascular lesions which may be missed by endoscopy [33, 34], See Fig. 4.11.

Barium Studies

Barium studies can be useful in the workup of GI bleeding, particularly in patients who have contraindications for endoscopy. While no longer generally considered a first line modality, many important findings can be seen with double contrast barium studies, though diagnostic yields are low compared to endoscopy [35–37]. Barium studies have no role in the evaluation of patients with active GI bleeding. Double contrast upper GI exams may show causes of occult GI bleeding such as ulcers and

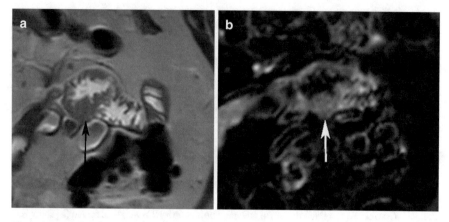

Fig. 4.9 Coronal images from MR enterography demonstrate metastatic melanoma (arrows) to the jejunum. Coronal T2 weighted image (**a**) and Coronal post contrast image (**b**)

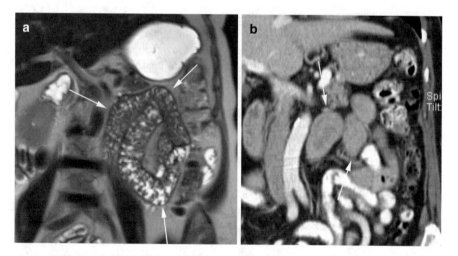

Fig. 4.10 Coronal T2 weighted image from MR enterography shows nodular thickening of the jejunum (arrows in **a**) in a patient with celiac disease. Note the excellent bowel contrast compared to the patient's conventional CT with oral contrast (**b**), which shows bowel wall thickening in this same region (arrows in **b**)

cancers (see Figs. 4.12 and 4.13). Barium enema may occasionally be useful to find neoplastic causes of occult bleeding (see Fig. 4.14), though CTC has higher diagnostic yield for detecting colonic neoplasia [38].

Nuclear Medicine

Technetium (Tc) 99 m sulfur colloid and Tc99m pertechnetate-labeled autologous red blood cells (RBCs) are two nuclear techniques for evaluating occult GI bleeding (Figs. 4.15-4.16) [39–42]. Tc99m sulfur colloid has a short circulating half-life of

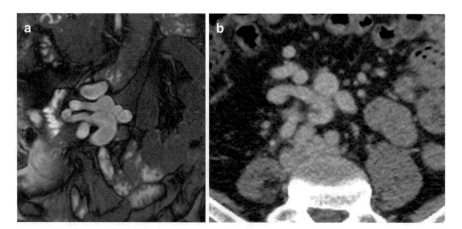

Fig. 4.11 Small bowel varices are well seen on MRI (Coronal FIESTA image, **a**) and axial contrast enhanced CT (**b**)

Fig. 4.12 There are three gastric ulcers on double contrast upper GI (arrows), which demonstrate pooling of contrast

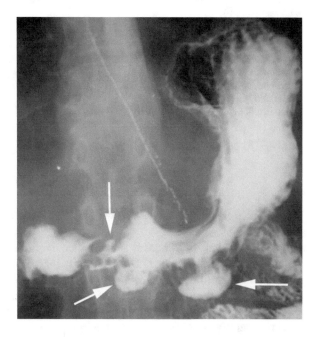

3 min and rapid uptake by the reticuloendothelial system (liver, spleen, and bone marrow) [42]. Imaging is generally performed for only 20–30 min, decreasing the opportunity to identify intermittent lower GI bleed. High background counts in the liver and spleen can obscure upper GI bleeds. For these reasons, 99mTc-erythrocytes are generally superior [43, 44].

Scintigraphy is indicated for overt gastrointestinal bleeding. Per the SNMMI guidelines for gastrointestinal bleeding scintigraphy (GIBS), the goal is to

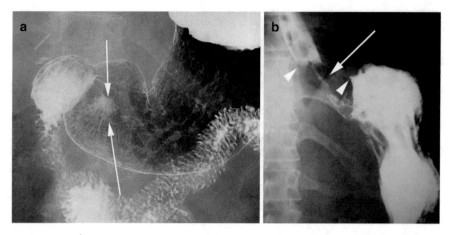

Fig. 4.13 Two examples of gastric adenocarcinoma. Pooling of contrast with radiating folds (arrows in **a**) are seen in this gastric adenocarcinoma. Irregular stricture (arrow in **b**) related to gastric adenocarcinoma, invading the lower esophagus. Note the irregular overhanging edges (arrowheads in **b**)

Fig. 4.14 Irregular stricture (arrow) on barium enema with overhanging edges corresponds to a site of sigmoid adenocarcinoma

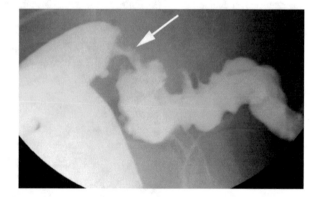

determine whether the patient is actively bleeding, to localize the bleeding bowel segment, and to estimate the rate of blood loss [45]. This allows for treatment planning and risk stratification [16, 46–48]. GIBS is best for evaluation of the mid- to lower GI tract. Selected patients can then be sent to angiography (Fig. 4.16).

A Tc99m pertechnetate study, otherwise known as a Meckel's scan, is typically used for identifying a Meckel's diverticulum in the pediatric population [49]. This is due to its affinity for gastric mucosa, as evidenced by its sensitivity of up to 97% in children but only up to 60% in adults [50]. Its specificity remains high at 95% for both adult and pediatric populations.

If a Meckel's scan (see Fig. 4.17) is employed for the workup of lower GI bleeding in an adult, images are typically taken at short intervals from 30 to 90 minutes and, in the event of a possible intermittent bleed, less frequent image captures can be performed over a 24 h period [49]. Diagnostic utility can be improved in adults

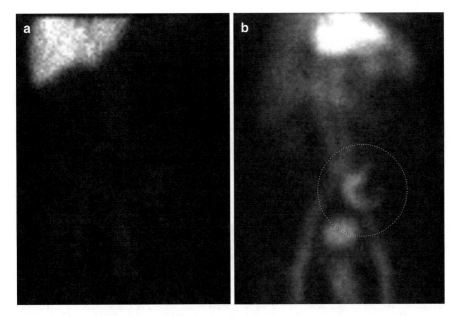

Fig. 4.15 Patient underwent a GI bleeding scan performed with 10 mCi Tc-99 m sulfur colloid which did not show signs of gastrointestinal bleeding (**a**). Two days later, 25 mCi Tc-99 m labeled autologous red blood cells were injected intravenously (**b**). Active gastrointestinal bleeding is seen in the left lower abdomen (site is encircled)

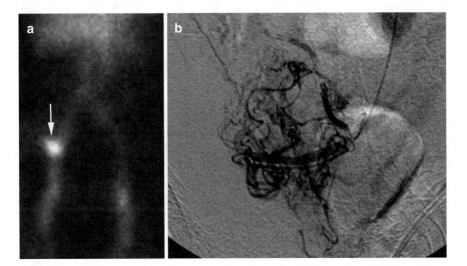

Fig. 4.16 GI bleeding scan demonstrates pooling of radiotracer in the right lower quadrant (arrow in **a**). Subsequent angiography shows a tangle of vessels (**b**) relating to a cecal arteriovenous malformation

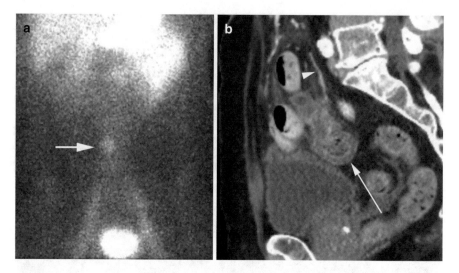

Fig. 4.17 Meckel's scan demonstrates radiotracer uptake in the midline lower abdomen (arrow in **a**), corresponding to ectopic gastric mucosa in a Meckel's diverticulum. Sagittal (**b**) reformatted images from contrast-enhanced CT shows peripheral enhancement of the Meckel's diverticulum (arrow). Note the primary Meckel's vessel arising directly from the SMA (arrowhead), well demonstrated on CT

with premedication with a histamine receptor antagonist with or without pentagastin, employment of bladder lavage with saline, or nasogastric suctioning [51, 52]. CT may be useful in identifying the Meckel's diverticulum and Meckel's vessel arising from the SMA (Fig. 4.17b) [53, 54].

Conclusions

There are multiple radiologic modalities that are useful in the workup patients with obscure GI bleeding. There are good data that CT and VCE provide complementary information. MRE is very useful, particularly for Crohn's disease. Nuclear medicine RBC scans and Meckel's scans are useful in selected patients, and angiography is helpful both for diagnosis and treatment. Fluoroscopy and CT colonography can be helpful particularly in patients who cannot tolerate endoscopy. Advanced techniques such as dual energy CT will likely become more ubiquitous and aid in the diagnosis of patients with GI bleeding.

References

1. Herman GT. Fundamentals of computerized tomography: image reconstruction from projection. 2nd ed: Springer; 2009.
2. Geoffroy Y, Rodallec MH, Boulay-Coletta I, Julies MC, Ridereau-Zins C, Zins M. Multidetector CT angiography in acute gastrointestinal bleeding: why, when, and how. Radiographics. 2011;31(3):E35–46.

3. He B, Yang J, Xiao J, Gu J, Chen F, Wang L, et al. Accuracy of computed tomographic enterography for obscure gastrointestinal bleeding. Acad Radiol. 2018;25:196–201.
4. Sugi MD, Menias CO, Lubner MG, Bhalia S, Mellnick VM, Kwon MH, Katz DS. CT findings of acute small-bowel entities. Radiographics. 2018;38(5):1352–69.
5. Hamilton JD, Kumaravel M, Censullo ML, Cohen AM, Kievlan DS, West OC. Multidetector CT evaluation of active extravasation in blunt abdominal and pelvic trauma patients. Radiographics. 2008;28(6):1603–16.
6. Lubner M, Menias C, Rucker C, et al. Blood in the belly: CT findings of hemoperitoneum. Radiographics. 2007;27(1):109–25.
7. Elsayes KM, Al-Hawary MM, Jagdish J, Ganesh HS, Platt JF. CT enterography: principles, trends, and interpretation of findings. Radiographics. 2010;30:1955–70.
8. Sheedy SP, Kolbe AB, Fletcher JG, Fidler JL. Computed tomography enterography. Radiol Clin N Am. 2018;56:649–70.
9. Schindera ST, Nelson RC, DeLong DM, et al. Multi-detector row CT of the small bowel: peak enhancement temporal window – initial experience. Radiology. 2007;243(2):438–44.
10. Hara AK, Walker FB, Silva AC, Leighton JA. Preliminary estimate of triphasic CT enterography performance in hemodynamically stable patients with suspected gastrointestinal bleeding. Am J Roentgenol. 2009;193:1252–60.
11. Huprich JE, Fletcher JG, Fidler JL, Alexander JA, Guimarães LS, Siddiki HA, et al. Prospective blinded comparison of wireless capsule endoscopy and multiphase CT enterography in obscure gastrointestinal bleeding. Radiology. 2011;260:744–51.
12. Agrawal JR, Travis AC, Mortele KJ, Silverman SG, Maurer R, Reddy SI, et al. Diagnostic yield of dual-phase computed tomography enterography in patients with obscure gastrointestinal bleeding and a non-diagnostic capsule endoscopy. J Gastroenterol Hepatol. 2012;27:751–9.
13. Boriskin HS, Devito BS, Hines JJ, Scarmato VJ, Friedman B. CT enterography vs. capsule endoscopy. Abdom Imaging. 2008;34:149–55.
14. Chu Y, Wu S, Qian Y, et al. Complimentary imaging modalities for investigating obscure gastrointestinal bleeding: capsule endoscopy, double-balloon enteroscopy, and computed tomographic enterography. Gastroenterol Res Pract. 2016;2016:1–8.
15. Haghighi D, Zuccaro G, Vargo J, Conwell D, Dumot J, Santisi J, et al. Comparison of capsule endoscopy (CE) findings of healthy subjects (HS) to an obscure gastrointestinal bleeding (OGIB) patient population. Gastrointest Endosc. 2005;61:AB104.
16. Kim BSM, Li BT, Engel A, et al. Diagnosis of gastrointestinal bleeding: a practical guide for clinicians. World J Gastrointest Pathophysiol. 2014;5:467–78.
17. Singh-Bhinder N, Kim DH, Holly BP, et al. ACR appropriateness criteria ® nonvariceal upper gastrointestinal bleeding. J Am Coll Radiol. 2017;14(5S):S177–S188.
18. Limsrivilai J, Srisajjakul S, Pongprasobchai S, Leelakusolvong S, Tanwandee T. A prospective blinded comparison of video capsule endoscopy versus computed tomography enterography in potential small bowel bleeding. J Clin Gastroenterol. 2017;51:611–8.
19. Wang Z, Chen J-Q, Liu J-L, Qin X-G, Huang Y. CT enterography in obscure gastrointestinal bleeding: a systematic review and meta-analysis. J Med Imag Radiat Oncol. 2013;57:263–73.
20. Yen H-H. Clinical impact of multidetector computed tomography before double-balloon enteroscopy for obscure gastrointestinal bleeding. World J Gastroenterol. 2012;18:692.
21. Chen SC, Lu DS, Hecht JR, et al. CT colonography: value of scanning in both the supine and prone positions. AJR Am J Roentgenol. 1999;172(3):595–9.
22. Hendrikus JM, van Leeuwen MS, Laheij RJ, Vleggaar FP. CT-colonography after incomplete colonoscopy. Dis Colon Rectum. 56(5):593–9.
23. Pickhardt PJ, Hassan C, Halligan S, Marmo R. Colorectal cancer: CT colonography and colonoscopy for detection – systematic review and meta-analysis. Radiology. 2011;259(2):393–405.
24. Plumb AA, Halligan S, Pendse DA, Taylor SA, Malett S. Sensitivity and specificity of CT colonography for the detection of colonic neoplasia after positive faecal occult blood testing: systematic review and meta-analysis. Eur Radiol. 2014 May;24(5):1049–58.
25. Wu L-M. Usefulness of CT angiography in diagnosing acute gastrointestinal bleeding: a meta-analysis. World J Gastroenterol. 2010;16:3957.
26. Kuhle WG, Sheiman RG. Detection of active colonic hemorrhage with use of helical CT: findings in a swine model. Radiology. 2003;228:743–52.

27. Wells ML, Hansel SL, Bruining DH, Fletcher JG, Froemming AT, Barlow JM, Fidler JL. CT for evaluation of acute gastrointestinal bleeding. Radiographics. 2018;38(4):1089–107.
28. Tseng C-M, Lin I-C, Chang C-Y, et al. Role of computed tomography angiography on the management of overt obscure gastrointestinal bleeding. PLoS One. 2017;12(3):1–9 OR e0172754. https://doi.org/10.1371/journal.pone.0172754.
29. Sun H, Xue HD, Wang YN, et al. Dual-source dual-energy computed tomography angiography for active gastrointestinal bleeding: a preliminary study. Clin Radiol. 2013 Feb;68(2):139–47.
30. Thomsen HS. Nephrogenic systemic fibrosis: a serious late adverse reaction to gadodiamide. Eur Radiol. 2006;16:2619–21.
31. Dillman JR, Smith EA, Khalatbari S, Strouse PJ. IV glucagon use in pediatric MR enterography: effect on image quality, length of examination, and patient tolerance. AJR Am J Roentgenol. 2013;201(1):185–9.
32. Masselli G, Di Tola M, Casciani E, Polettini E, Laghi F, Monti R, Giulia Bernieri M, Gualdi G. Diagnosis of small-bowel diseases: prospective comparison of multi-detector row CT Enterography with MR enterography. Radiology. 2015;279(2):420–31.
33. Huprich JE, Barlow JM, Hansel SL, Alexander JA, Fidler JL. Multiphase CT enterography evaluation of small-bowel vascular lesions. AJR Am J Roentgenol. 2013;201(1):65–72.
34. Amzallag-Bellenger E, Oudjit A, Ruiz A, Cadiot G, Soyer PA, Hoeffel CC. Effectiveness of MR enterography for the assessment of small-bowel diseases beyond crohn disease. Radiographics. 2012;32(5):1423–44.
35. Gerson LB, Fidler JL, Cave DR, Leighton JA. ACG clinical guideline: diagnosis and management of small bowel bleeding. Am J Gastroenterol. 2015;110:1265–87.
36. Morrison TC, Wells M, Fidler JL, Soto JA. Imaging workup of acute and occult lower gastrointestinal bleeding. Radiol Clin N Am. 2018;56:791–804.
37. Nolan D, Traill Z. The current role of the barium examination of the small intestine. Clin Radiol. 1997 Nov;52(11):809–20.
38. Chung SY, Park SH, Lee SS, Lee JH, Kim AY, Park SK, Han DJ, Ha HK. Comparison between CT colonography and double-contrast barium enema for colonic evaluation in patients with renal insufficiency. Korean J Radiol. 2012 May–Jun;13(3):290–9.
39. Bunker SR, Brown JM, McAuley RJ, et al. Detection of gastrointestinal bleeding sites: use of in vitro technetium Tc99m-labeled RBCs. JAMA. 1982;247:789–92.
40. Howarth DM. The role of nuclear medicine in the detection of acute gastrointestinal bleeding. Semin Nucl Med. 2006;36(2):133–46.
41. Thorne DA, Datz FL, Remley K, Christian PE. Bleeding rates necessary for detecting active gastrointestinal bleeding with Tc-99m labeled red blood cells in an experimental model. Clin Nucl Med. 1987;28(4):514–20.
42. Ziessman H, O'Malley J, Thrall J. Nuclear medicine: the requisites. 4th ed. Philadelphia: Elsevier Saunders; 2013. p. 307–21.
43. Bunker SR, Lull RJ, Tanasescu DE, et al. Scintigraphy of gastrointestinal hemorrhage: superiority of Tc-99m red blood cells over Tc-99m sulfur colloid. AJR. 1984;143:543–8.
44. Siddiqui AR, Schauwecker DS, Wellman HN, et al. Comparison of technetium-99m sulfur colloid and in vitro labeled technetium-99m RBCs in the detection of gastro-intestinal bleeding. Clin Nucl Med. 1985;10:546–9.
45. Dam HQ, Brandon DC, Graham VV, et al. The SNMMI procedure standard/ EANM practice guideline for gastrointestinal bleeding scintigraphy 2.0. J Nucl Med Technol. 2014;42:308–17.
46. Otomi Y, Otsuka H, Terazawa K, Yamanaka M, Obama Y, Arase M, et al. The diagnostic ability of SPECT/CT fusion imaging for gastrointestinal bleeding: a retrospective study. BMC Gastroenterol. 2018;18(1):183:1–7. https://doi.org/10.1186/s12876-018-0915-7.
47. Zahid A, Young CJ. Making decisions using radiology in lower GI hemorrhage. Int J Surg. 2016;31:100–3.
48. Zuckier LS. Acute gastrointestinal bleeding. Semin Nucl Med. 2003;33(4):297–311.
49. Singh PR, Russell CD, Dubovsky EV, et al. Technique of scanning for Meckel's diverticulum. Clin Nucl Med. 1978;3:188–92.

50. Lin S, Suhocki PV, Ludwig KA, Shetzline MA. Gastrointestinal bleeding in adult patients with Meckel's diverticulum: the role of technetium 99m pertechnetate scan. South Med J. 2002;95(11):1338–41.
51. Heyman S. Meckel's diverticulum: possible detection by combining pentagastrin with histamine H2 receptor blocker. J Nucl Med. 1994;35:1656–8.
52. Treves S, Grand RJ, Eraklis AJ. Pentagastrin stimulation of technetium-99m uptake by ectopic gastric mucosa in a Meckel's diverticulum. J Nucl Med. 1991;32:1422–4.
53. Chen Y, Tang Y, Hu C, Chen S. Bleeding meckel diverticulum. J Comput Assist Tomogr. 2019;43:220–7.
54. Platon A, Gervaz P, Becker CD, Morel P, Poletti PA. Computer tomography of complicated Meckel's diverticulum in adults: a pictorial review. Insights Imaging. 2010 May;1(2):53–61.

Part II
Localization

Chapter 5
Esophagus

Omar Tageldin, Virali Shah, Neeha Kalakota, Hwajeong Lee, Micheal Tadros, and James Litynski

Introduction

Occult gastrointestinal (GI) bleeding is defined as any GI bleeding that presents as positive fecal occult blood and/or iron deficiency anemia without being visible to the patient or the physician [1]. The source of occult GI bleeding can be any part of the GI tract including esophagus, stomach, small intestine and large intestine. Bleeding from the upper GI tract (including the esophagus, stomach and duodenum) accounts for about 37% of occult GI bleeding [1]. It is difficult to determine the prevalence of occult GI bleeding due to esophageal diseases as individuals with esophageal diseases may be asymptomatic. Moreover, in general medical and gastroenterological practices, esophagus-related symptoms are considered among the most common symptoms. Dysphagia, which is one of the most common symptoms in esophageal diseases,

O. Tageldin
Department of Internal Medicine, Albany Medical Center, Albany, NY, USA
e-mail: tageldo@amc.edu

V. Shah
Albany Medical College, Albany, NY, USA
e-mail: shahv1@amc.edu

N. Kalakota · J. Litynski (✉)
Division of Gastroenterology, Albany Medical Center, Albany, NY, USA
e-mail: kalakon@amc.edu; litynsj@amc.edu

H. Lee
Department of Pathology and Laboratory Medicine, Albany Medical Center,
Albany, NY, USA
e-mail: LeeH5@amc.edu

M. Tadros
Department of Gastroenterology and Hepatology, Albany Medical Center, Albany, NY, USA
e-mail: tadrosm1@amc.edu

© The Author(s), under exclusive license to Springer Nature
Switzerland AG 2021
M. Tadros, G. Y. Wu (eds.), *Management of Occult GI Bleeding*, Clinical
Gastroenterology, https://doi.org/10.1007/978-3-030-71468-0_5

is common with aging and can present in up to 15% of those that are age 87 or older [2]. Heartburn is another common symptom and can present in healthy individuals. A survey of healthy individuals (regardless of gender or age) in Olmsted County, Minnesota, showed that 20% of them experienced heartburn at least weekly [3]. Other less common esophageal symptoms include chest pain, hiccups, globus sensation and belching. Persistent dry cough, wheezing, hoarseness and sore throat may also be related to esophageal diseases. One of the challenges when evaluating esophageal symptoms is that the severity of symptoms often does not correlate well with the degree of the esophageal damage [4]. For example, the severity of mucosal injury induced by gastroesophageal reflux disease (GERD) among older patients may increase despite overall decrease in the severity of the symptoms [5].

Management of occult esophageal bleeding starts with focused and thorough history taking and physical exam. A thorough history includes current symptoms, past medical history, social history including smoking and alcohol use, family history, and current medications that may result in pill esophagitis. A history of intravenous substance abuse, heavy alcohol use and cirrhosis may give clues to the source of occult GI bleeding as well. Patients with developmental disability may not have typical GI symptoms.

Esophagogastroduodenoscopy (EGD) is considered as the initial diagnostic method in patients with occult GI bleeding. Treatment of occult esophageal bleeding depends on the cause. Treatment options include medications such as proton pump inhibitors (PPIs) in patients with reflux esophagitis, antiviral or antifungal medications in infectious esophagitis, cessation of offending medication to treat pill esophagitis, resection of esophageal malignancy, if applicable, and esophageal banding in esophageal varices. We will discuss different esophageal causes of occult GI bleeding focusing on epidemiology, clinical picture, diagnosis and management.

Esophagitis

Reflux Esophagitis/Erosive Reflux Esophagitis

Patients with erosive reflux esophagitis have common reflux symptoms caused by the esophageal reflux of gastric acid and display esophageal mucosal injury that is evident on endoscopy. On the contrary, patients with non-erosive reflux esophagitis have reflux symptoms only without visible esophageal mucosal injury on endoscopy.

Epidemiology

Erosive reflux esophagitis is a common cause of occult esophageal bleeding. It is difficult to determine accurate prevalence and incidence rates because many affected individuals may be asymptomatic. In 2009, there were 8.9 million outpatient clinic visits for GERD in the United States [6]. For GI disorders, GERD was the 13th most common principal diagnosis at discharge, with an estimated 66,000 total number of discharges per year [6]. The prevalence of endoscopic esophagitis is approximately 7% in the United States. Several recent endoscope-based studies have suggested that the overall prevalence of reflux esophagitis in Western Europe and North America was around 10% to 20% [7]. Another large-scale literature review published in 2000 found that the incidence of esophagitis as a cause of occult GI bleeding is 6% to 18% [8].

Clinical Presentation

Erosive reflux esophagitis may be asymptomatic [9]. When associated with symptoms, the symptoms are similar to those of other esophageal disorders and can be divided into typical and atypical symptoms. Typical symptoms include heartburn, regurgitation, chest pain, dysphasia, odynophagia, eructation, and hiccup. Atypical symptoms include dyspepsia, nausea with or without vomiting, hematemesis, globus sensation, coughing, throat clearing, throat pain, throat burning, hoarseness, wheezing/stridor, dyspnea, apnea, halitosis, sleep disturbance, anorexia. Weight loss, and failure to thrive [3, 10, 11].

Complication

Complications of erosive reflux esophagitis include esophageal ulcer, bleeding, strictures, perforation and Barrett's esophagus. In 2017, a Japanese multicenter, prospective, cross-sectional study analyzed 1749 patients diagnosed with erosive esophagitis. Among these patients, 4.8% experienced esophageal bleeding, 2.6% had esophageal strictures, and 0.8% experienced both. The presence of complications was associated with older age, female sex, and being bedridden [12].

Diagnosis

The diagnosis of erosive reflux esophagitis is made by an endoscopy to find mucosal injury of the esophagus (Figs. 5.1, 5.2, 5.3 and 5.4). Biopsy can be done to confirm the diagnosis (Fig. 5.5).

Classification

Followings are the endoscopic images of the 4 grades of LA classifications (Table 5.1):

Fig. 5.1 EGD showing mucosal break, ≤5 mm long, that does not extend between the tops of two mucosal folds (LA grade A)

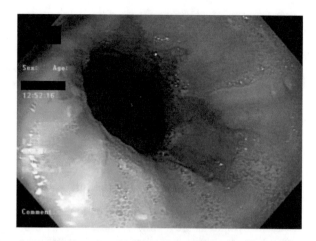

Fig. 5.2 EGD showing mucosal break, >5 mm long, that does not extend between the tops of two mucosal folds (LA grade B)

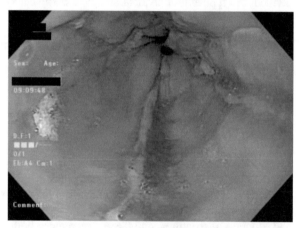

Fig. 5.3 EGD showing mucosal break that is continuous between the tops of two or more mucosal folds, but involves <75% of the circumference (LA grade C)

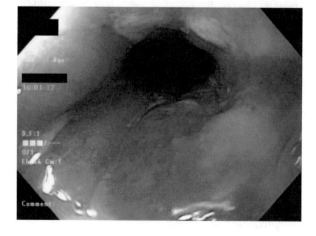

Fig. 5.4 EGD showing mucosal break that involves >75% of the esophageal circumference (LA grade D)

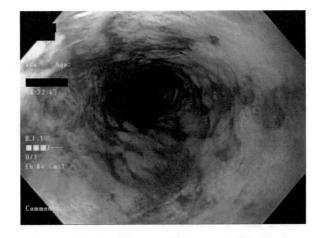

Fig. 5.5 Microscopic image of LA grade D esophagitis. The sample predominantly consists of inflammatory exudate and granulation tissue (Hematoxylin and eosin (H&E), original magnification x100)

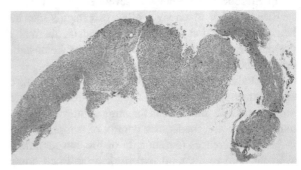

Table 5.1 Los Angeles classification for Erosive Esophagitis [13][a]

Grade	Description
LA grade A	One or more mucosal break, ≤5 mm long, that does not extend between the tops of two mucosal folds
LA grade B	One or more mucosal break, >5 mm long, that does not extend between the tops of two mucosal folds
LA grade C	One or more mucosal break that is continuous between the tops of two or more mucosal folds, but that involves <75% of the circumference
LA grade D	One or more mucosal break that involves at least 75% of the esophageal circumference

[a]Lundell et al. [13]

Management

Management of erosive reflux esophagitis includes lifestyle modifications, PPI, endoscopic therapy, and in rare occasions, surgical interventions. Lifestyle modifications include avoidance of large meals, avoidance of eating shortly before bedtime, avoiding foods that cause symptoms, head-of-the-bed elevation (especially when patient has nighttime symptoms), cessation of smoking, cautious use of non-steroidal drugs, and weight loss in obese patients [14, 15].

PPIs are the mainstay of medical therapy for erosive reflux esophagitis. Sometimes antithrombotic and anticoagulants should be discontinued when treating erosive reflux esophagitis. Typically, a double dose of PPI is prescribed twice daily [16]. In 2012, a meta-analysis that included 4995 eligible references reported thirty-two studies describing the rate of complete relief of heartburn after 4 weeks of PPI therapy in patients with erosive reflux esophagitis. The pooled estimate of complete relief after 4 weeks of PPI therapy was 0.72 (95% CI, 0.69–0.74). Furthermore, six studies in this meta-analysis found complete relief of heartburn after 8 weeks of PPI therapy, and the pooled estimate was 0.73 (95% CI, 0.59–0.8) [17]. H2 blockers are also used for erosive reflux esophagitis but these are not as potent as PPI with limited efficacy for erosive esophagitis. A meta-analysis published in 1997 showed superior effect of PPI compared to H2 blockers in terms of the speed of healing and symptom relief in patients with severe esophagitis (Fig. 5.6) [18].

Bleeding due to erosive reflux esophagitis can be endoscopically treated by hemoclips, injection therapy, fibrin sealant, thermal coagulation and hemostatic powder spray [19]. Among these modalities, hemostatic clips and thermal coagulation are the most commonly used forms [20, 21].

Surgical management of erosive reflux esophagitis consists of open fundoplication or transoral incisionless fundoplication. The latter is a relatively new endoscopic approach. Indications for surgical intervention [22] include failure of medical management (e.g. inadequate control of symptoms or adverse medication effects), patient's preferences (e.g. quality of life considerations, lifelong medication management, and medication expense), established complications (e.g., stricture or Barrett's esophagus), and extra-esophageal symptoms (e.g. asthma, cough, hoarseness, aspiration, and chest pain) [23, 24].

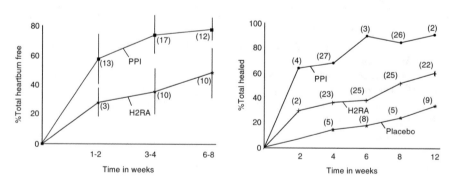

Fig. 5.6 2 graphs showed the difference of speed of healing and symptom relief in severe esophagitis. (Reprinted from "*Speed of healing and symptom relief in grade II to IV gastroesophageal reflux disease: a meta-analysis.*" *By* Chiba, N., et al.. Copyrights 1997, with permission from Elsevier)

Infectious Esophagitis

Epidemiology

While esophageal infections commonly affect immunocompromised patients, some infections affect immunocompetent individuals. Common infectious agents of the esophagus include herpes simplex virus (HSV), cytomegalovirus (CMV) [25–29], and Candida [30]. The reported prevalence of esophageal candida albicans among healthy adults is 20% [31].

Clinical Presentation

These infections typically present with odynophagia. The major complications include stricture with scarring, bleeding, and perforation [25].

Diagnosis

Infectious esophagitis is diagnosed by direct visualization using endoscopy (Fig. 5.7)s with biopsy and/or brushing of the lesion for cytology (Figs. 5.8, 5.9 and 5.10).

Management

Treatment is directed against the causative organism with antiviral or antifungal medicine.

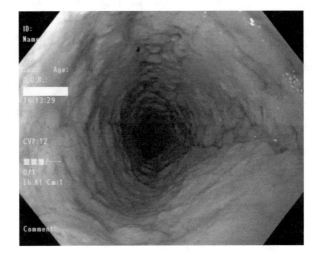

Fig. 5.7 EGD showing lower third of esophagus completely lined with whitish adherent plaques consistent with Candida esophagitis

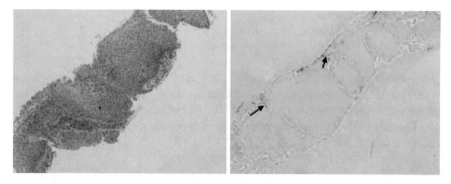

Fig. 5.8 Left, biopsy shows active neutrophilic esophagitis (H&E, original magnification x100). Right, Gomori Methenamine Silver (GMS) special stain shows fungal forms (arrows), consistent with candida (GMS, original magnification x100)

Fig. 5.9 Herpetic esophagitis. Viral inclusions are noted (arrow) (H&E, original magnification x200)

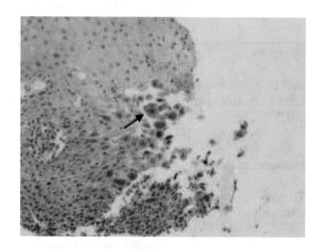

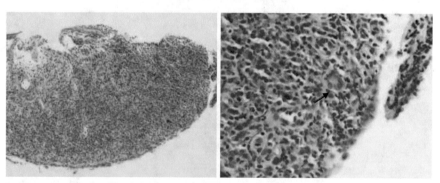

Fig. 5.10 Cytomegaloviral esophagitis. Left, the biopsy shows ulcer and granulation tissue (H&E, original magnification x100). Right, higher magnification view shows stromal cell with viral inclusion (arrow) (H&E, original magnification x400)

Pill Esophagitis

Epidemiology

Medication-induced esophageal ulceration can occur at any age with different types of medications. This condition is usually under-diagnosed because the symptoms may be mistaken for episodes of severe acid reflux. Therefore, it can be challenging to render a correct diagnosis of pill esophagitis for which the main treatment is discontinuation of the offending drug.

Common drugs that cause esophageal ulceration and esophagitis are tetracycline, doxycycline, and bisphosphonate. Other medications include non-steroidal anti-inflammatory drugs (NSAIDs), potassium chloride [32, 33], Quinidine [34], Ferrous sulfate [35], theophylline [36, 37], oral contraceptive pill (OCP) [38], ascorbic acid [39], mycophenolic acid [40], and multivitamins [41].

Clinical Presentation

Patients usually present with acute onset chest pain (with radiating pain to the back), odynophagia, and heartburn. These symptoms associated with history of having incorrectly taken medications that may cause esophagitis, strongly suggest the diagnosis of pill esophagitis [42].

Diagnosis

Diagnosis of pill esophagitis is made by endoscopy or radiography. Endoscopy is more sensitive in rendering the diagnosis of pill esophagitis than radiography. Endoscopic findings range from discrete small ulcers to severe esophagitis that may be associated with pseudomembranes as can be seen in bisphosphonate [43] or Kayexalate [44] use. A diffuse sloughing esophagitis may also be seen on endoscopy [45]. Sometime, stenosis or tumor-like appearance may be seen [34, 46]. Similar findings can be seen on radiography (barium esophagogram) especially when double contrast is used [47, 48].

Treatment

There is no specific treatment that has shown to alter the course of pill esophagitis [42]. Treatment involves symptomatic management with discontinuation of the offending drug. Major complications include stricture, bleeding, and perforation. In the absence of these complications or catastrophic presentation, most patients experience resolution of symptoms within 2–3 weeks and resolution of radiographic findings in 7–10 days [47].

Esophageal Neoplasm

Esophageal Carcinoma [49]

Epidemiology

Esophageal cancer is the sixth leading cause of cancer death worldwide [50]. There are two main subtypes of esophageal cancer: squamous cell carcinoma and adenocarcinoma. Squamous cell cancer arises from the esophageal squamous epithelium usually in the proximal 2/3 of the esophagus, whereas adenocarcinoma arises from metaplastic Barrett's esophagus in the distal end of the esophagus.

Esophageal squamous cell cancer (ESCC) is the most common form of esophageal cancer internationally. About 90% of the 456,000 new cases of esophageal cancer worldwide each year are squamous cell carcinoma. The regions with the highest incidence are Eastern and Central Asia as well as East and South Africa. There are several risk factors associated with the development of ESCC, that vary by region in endemic areas. For example, residents in certain endemic areas consume foods containing high levels of nitrosamines and fungi, which are known risk factors for ESCC. Human papilloma virus may be a risk factor for ESCC as well. In the West, alcohol and tobacco consumption are common risk factors. Certain underlying esophageal diseases may increase the risk of ESCC, such as radiation esophagitis, achalasia, Plummer Vinson syndrome, Fanconi's anemia, and tylosis [51].

Esophageal adenocarcinoma (EAC) is the second most common form of esophageal carcinoma worldwide. In 2012 there were 52,000 new cases of EAC worldwide and 398,000 cases of ESCC. Currently, EAC is the predominant type of esophageal cancer in industrialized countries; about a half of all cases are in Northwestern Europe and North America. Risk factors for developing EAC include age over 65, male gender, GERD, Barrett's metaplasia, scleroderma, tobacco use, and obesity. On the contrary, there appears to be a protective effect with H. pylori gastritis [50].

Clinical Presentation

EAC and ESCC have similar clinical presentations. Most patients are asymptomatic in the early stages; however, as the disease progresses, patients commonly present with weight loss and progressive dysphagisa. Esophageal cancer can present with occult blood loss with either heme positive stool or iron deficient anemia. Less common presentations include odynophagia, cervical lymphadenopathy, chest pain, and voice changes [50].

Complication

Esophageal cancer may be complicated by esophageal-respiratory fistulae and esophageal-aortic fistulae, caused by direct tumor invasion through the esophageal wall and into the mainstem bronchus or aorta. Such patients often present with intractable coughing, frequent pneumonias, or unstable GI bleeding. Life expectancy is less than four weeks following the development of these complications. Metastases are often detected on computed tomography (CT) scans of the chest, abdomen and pelvis. Common sites of distant metastases are liver, lungs, bone, and adrenal glands. Adenocarcinomas frequently metastasize to intraabdominal sites, while metastases from ESCCs are usually intrathoracic [52].

Diagnosis

The diagnosis of esophageal cancer is made by direct visualization with endoscopic biopsies (Figs. 5.11, 5.12, 5.13 and 5.14). Imaging studies, such as chest radiography, barium esophagram, and CT scans, can detect strictures or fistulas but are not sensitive enough to detect early cancers. Other endoscopic techniques such as

Fig. 5.11 EGD showing a mass in the lower third esophagus (EAC)

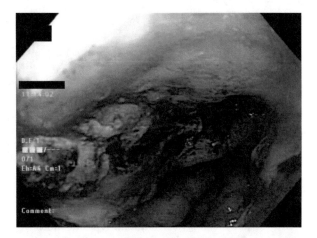

Fig. 5.12 EGD showing a friable ulcer in the mid esophagus (ESCC)

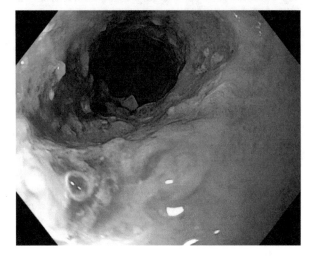

Fig. 5.13 Biopsy showing esophageal adenocarcinoma arising in background Barrett's esophagus. Arrows show goblet cells (intestinal metaplasia) (H&E, original magnification x100)

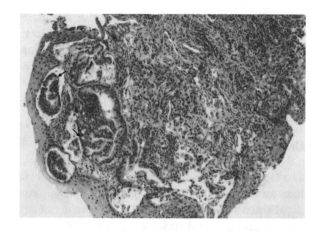

Fig. 5.14 Biopsy showing esophageal squamous cell carcinoma that is moderately differentiated with focal keratin (arrow) formation (H&E, original magnification x100)

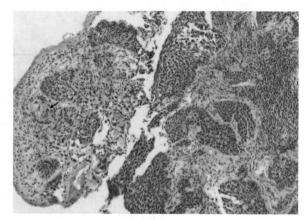

narrow band imaging, conventional chromoendoscopy, electronic chromoendoscopy, autofluorescence imaging, and confocal laser endomicroscopy can also help identify areas of dysplasia and malignancy.

Several other technologies such as optical coherence tomography, endocytoscopy, and high-resolution microendoscopy are also emerging but are not yet commercially available. Indications to refer a patient for endoscopy include progressive dysphagia, weight loss, iron deficiency anemia, heme positive stool, voice changes, and odynophagia [53].

Management

It is essential to implement a multidisciplinary approach to treat esophageal cancer. The treatment planning requires input from experts in gastroenterology, surgical, radiation, and medical oncology team, and often palliative care team. For local disease, initial staging is done with endoscopic ultrasound (EUS) to determine the depth of invasion and lymph node involvement. EUS combined with fine needle aspiration (FNA) has greater than 85% of sensitivity for detecting regional metastases [53].

For Stage 1 and 2 ESCC or EAC, radical surgery is the treatment of choice. Surgeon's preference and location of the tumor are the most important factors in deciding to have a surgery. Endoscopic mucosal resection may be attempted in poor surgical candidates [53]. To improve survival over surgery alone, neoadjuvant chemoradiation may be administered in Stage 2 or 3 cancers. There are preliminary case studies investigating the use of Hemospray (TC 325 hemostatic powder) in cancer related GI bleeding; however more studies are needed prior to standardizing this approach [54]. For patients with metastatic disease (stage 4), palliative care may be considered. Palliative chemoradiation with cisplatin and 5-FU is the standard of care for unresectable disease.

Other Esophageal Malignancies

It is our opinion that other esophageal malignancies such as esophageal lymphoma, GISTs and NETs can cause occult GI bleeding. There are relatively few cases of these diseases in the literature, so the evidence of occult bleeding is scant. We include them for the clinicians to keep them in the differential diagnosis [55].

Esophageal Lymphomas

Epidemiology

Encompassing less than 1% of GI lymphomas, esophageal lymphomas are extremely rare. Primary esophageal non-Hodgkin's lymphomas including diffuse large B-cell lymphoma (DLBCL) and anaplastic large cell lymphoma may occur. Indeed, esophageal lymphomas typically originate from the stomach or mediastinum. Certain tumor suppressor genes such as p53 and MYC, and oncogenes such as BCL-6, have been found to be correlated with DLBCL development. Risk factors for esophageal lymphomas include immunocompromised status and an exposure to HIV [55].

Clinical Presentation

Esophageal lymphomas commonly present with dysphagia, unintentional weight loss and occult GI bleeding [55, 56]. Presentation with epigastric pain and dyspnea has been reported [57].

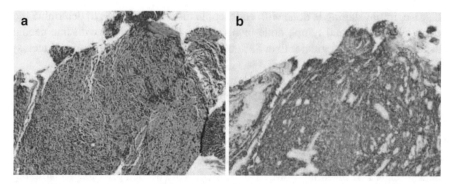

Fig. 5.15 Diffuse large B cell lymphoma of the esophagus. (**a**) biopsy shows a proliferation of dyscohesive, large lymphoid cells (H&E, original magnification x100). (**b**) CD20 immunostain shows that the cells are B cells (CD20 immunostain, x100)

Diagnosis

EGD with biopsy (Fig. 5.15a) is the initial diagnostic modality for detecting esophageal lymphomas [58]. Immunohistochemistry on tissue sample (Fig. 5.15b) can discern lymphomas from other malignant tumors [58]. Transthoracic echocardiography followed by CT with iodinated contrast is an alternative method to visualize and detect a mass-forming esophageal lymphoma [57]. Esophageal lymphomas typically present with esophageal luminal narrowing and soft tissue thickening of the esophageal wall [58].

Management

While management guidelines for esophageal lymphomas are limited, specialized chemotherapy and radiotherapy may be implemented. Surgery may be considered for an early disease [55].

Esophageal Gastrointestinal Stromal Tumors (GIST)

Epidemiology

GISTs are the most common non-epithelial tumors involving GI tract. Esophageal GISTs make up less than 1% of all GIST cases, with an incidence rate of only about 0.1 to 0.3 per million patients [59]. A subset of GISTs is associated with a genetic variation in the PDGFRA proto-oncogene. GISTs are slightly more common in men than women [59].

Clinical Presentation

Symptoms of esophageal GIST include acid reflux, dysphagia, and bleeding [60]. Internal bleeding is common in esophageal GIST as the tumor can metastasize into the peritoneal cavity and cause abdominal pain and bleeding [59].

Diagnosis

EGD is the common diagnostic modality for detecting esophageal GISTs. EUS with FNA can also aid in the diagnosis, while FNA can cause scarring and make subsequent treatment difficult [61].

Management

Esophageal GISTs may be surgically resected or treated by therapeutic endoscopy with luminal closure devices. For malignant esophageal GISTs, thoracoscopic enucleation may be an effective procedure that provides low mortality and favorable oncological outcomes [60]. Tumor enucleation is useful for smaller esophageal GISTs, but larger and malignant esophageal GISTs might require esophagectomy [62]. Research acknowledges the need for further investigation given the limited information available for their surgical management [59].

Neuroendocrine Tumors

Epidemiology

NET is another rare tumor of the esophagus. In the last 20 years about 42 cases of primary esophageal NETs have been published [63]. Thus, our knowledge regarding this tumor is sparse [64]. Current WHO classifies well-differentiated NET of GI tract into 3 grades (G1, G2 and G3) depending on either the mitotic count or ki-67 proliferation index. Small cell and large cell neuroendocrine carcinomas are considered poorly differentiated and are not graded [65]. Mixed neuroendocrine –non neuroendocrine neoplasms (MiNENs) such as adenoneurocrine carcinomas are also recognized [63]. It is critical to detect esophageal NETs before the tumor ruptures into the lymphovascular system [64].

Clinical Presentation

Esophageal NETs are a result of dysfunction involving the neuroendocrine cells (APUD cells). The symptoms include dysphagia, abdominal pain, chest pain, melena and weight loss [63]. Also, NETs may present with esophageal obstruction and occult bleeding [66]. NETs may lead to variceal hemorrhage, hematemesis, and melena [67].

Diagnosis

Esophageal NETs are detected by imaging, such as CT and EUS. Moreover, functional imaging such as somatostatin receptor imaging (OctreoScan) can be performed. Esophageal NETs are prone to misdiagnosis [68]. One study found that endoscopic biopsies of localized esophageal NETS are commonly misdiagnosed; hence, biopsies are not an effective measure of diagnosis [68].

Management

Management of esophageal NETs depends on the size of tumor and the level of metastasis. Smaller NETs are typically resected endoscopically, but larger NETs might require esophagectomy and chemotherapy [64]. The average survival after endoscopic resection of esophageal NETs is about 37 months [68]. Combining surgical treatment with chemotherapy and radiotherapy may improve survival [63].

Vascular Lesions

Esophageal Varices

Epidemiology

In the United States, the reported prevalence of liver cirrhosis is 0.27%. It is estimated that more than 600,000 adults have liver cirrhosis [69]. The incidence of esophageal varices is around 40% in patients with cirrhosis and about 60% in patients with combined cirrhosis and ascites. The annual rate of esophageal variceal bleeding among patients with cirrhosis is 5–15% [70]. Common causes of cirrhosis in developed countries include alcoholism, chronic viral hepatitis, hemochromatosis, and nonalcoholic fatty liver disease [71].

Clinical Presentation

Esophageal varices typically present with hematemesis and/or melena (overt GI bleeding). In rare occasions, esophageal varices may present with occult GI bleeding in the form of positive fecal occult blood test (FOBT) and/or iron deficiency anemia [8]. Furthermore, recurrent variceal bleeding may go unnoticed and patients may present later with iron deficiency anemia or positive FOBT [72].

Diagnosis

The definitive diagnosis of esophageal varices is made by endoscopy (Fig. 5.16), but the diagnosis may be missed in under-resuscitated patients with deflated varices.

Fig. 5.16 EGD showing large varices throughout the entire esophagus

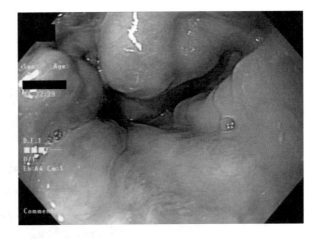

Management

Endoscopic intervention is the definitive therapy for bleeding esophageal varices [73]. The two common endoscopic treatments are: endoscopic variceal ligation (EVL) [74] and endoscopic sclerotherapy (ES) [75]. Previous studies showed that EVL was effective in primary prophylaxis of esophageal variceal bleeding but did not improve overall mortality [76]. Transjugular intrahepatic portosystemic shunt (TIPS) can be offered when endoscopic therapy fails [77].

Potential Missed Lesions

While most of the esophageal causes of occult GI bleeding can be diagnosed with upper endoscopy performed by experienced gastroenterologists, physicians should be aware of esophageal lesions that may be potentially missed.

Lesions right distal to the upper esophageal sphincter (UES) can be easily missed, especially with quick advancement of the scope in the beginning of the endoscopy procedure. Lesions can also be missed when the scope is withdrawn too quickly at the end of the procedure without paying enough attention to the upper part of the esophagus. These two figures (Figs. 5.17 and 5.18) show a granular, laterally spreading lesion that is 2 cm below UES that was missed on initial scope insertion. This lesion turned out to be ESCC. Figure 5.17 shows a subtle granular, laterally spreading lesion on standard high definition endoscopy. The same lesion was better defined/visualized with a narrow band imaging (Fig. 5.18).

Clinicians should be aware about atypical presentations of GERD as it may present with extraesophageal symptoms (e.g. excessive throat clearing, persistent cough, hoarseness, trouble breathing, and sore throat). Patients with cognitive disorders represent a subgroup with diagnostic challenge as they may not

Fig. 5.17 EGD showing a
granular laterally spreading
lesion 2 cm below UES
which was initially missed
on scope insertion

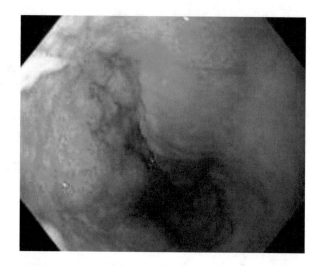

Fig. 5.18 EGD using
narrow band imaging
better visualizing a
granular laterally spreading
lesion 2 cm below UES

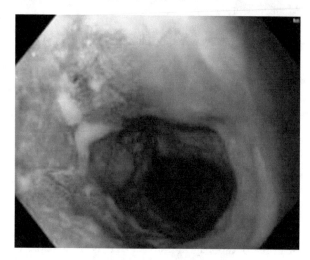

complain of the typical symptoms associated with esophageal disorders [78]. It
is also important to spend adequate amount of time looking for Barrett's esophagus and its complications during EGD. An inadequate or brief examination can
often miss subtle nodular lesions which may represent early cancer [79, 80]. The
diagnosis of esophageal varices can be challenging. If a patient has intravascular
volume depletion (e.g. dehydration or shock), esophageal varices may be deflated
and missed on EGD.

References

1. Mitchell SH, Schaefer DC, Dubagunta S. A new view of occult and obscure gastrointestinal bleeding. Am Fam Physician. 2004;69(4):875–81.
2. Bloem BR, et al. Prevalence of subjective dysphagia in community residents aged over 87. BMJ. 1990;300(6726):721–2.
3. Locke GR 3rd, et al. Prevalence and clinical spectrum of gastroesophageal reflux: a population-based study in Olmsted County, Minnesota. Gastroenterology. 1997;112(5):1448–56.
4. Bredenoord AJ. Mechanisms of reflux perception in gastroesophageal reflux disease: a review. Am J Gastroenterol. 2012;107(1):8–15.
5. Johnson DA, Fennerty MB. Heartburn severity underestimates erosive esophagitis severity in elderly patients with gastroesophageal reflux disease. Gastroenterology. 2004;126(3):660–4.
6. Peery AF, et al. Burden of gastrointestinal disease in the United States: 2012 update. Gastroenterology. 2012;143(5):1179–87. e3
7. Song HJ, et al. The prevalence and clinical characteristics of reflux esophagitis in Koreans and its possible relation to metabolic syndrome. J Korean Med Sci. 2009;24(2):197–202.
8. Zuckerman GR, et al. AGA technical review on the evaluation and management of occult and obscure gastrointestinal bleeding. Gastroenterology. 2000;118(1):201–21.
9. Wang FW, et al. Erosive esophagitis in asymptomatic subjects: risk factors. Dig Dis Sci. 2010;55(5):1320–4.
10. Richter JE, Bradley LA, Castell DO. Esophageal chest pain: current controversies in pathogenesis, diagnosis, and therapy. Ann Intern Med. 1989;110(1):66–78.
11. Smith JA, Abdulqawi R, Houghton LA. GERD-related cough: pathophysiology and diagnostic approach. Curr Gastroenterol Rep. 2011;13(3):247–56.
12. Sakaguchi M, et al. Factors associated with complicated erosive esophagitis: a Japanese multicenter, prospective, cross-sectional study. World J Gastroenterol. 2017;23(2):318–27.
13. Lundell LR, et al. Endoscopic assessment of oesophagitis: clinical and functional correlates and further validation of the Los Angeles classification. Gut. 1999;45(2):172–80.
14. Ness-Jensen E, et al. Tobacco smoking cessation and improved gastroesophageal reflux: a prospective population-based cohort study: the HUNT study. Am J Gastroenterol. 2014;109(2):171–7.
15. Ness-Jensen E, et al. Lifestyle Intervention in Gastroesophageal Reflux Disease. Clin Gastroenterol Hepatol. 2016;14(2):175–82. e1–3
16. Kinoshita Y, Hongo M, Japan TSG. Efficacy of twice-daily rabeprazole for reflux esophagitis patients refractory to standard once-daily administration of PPI: the Japan-based TWICE study. Am J Gastroenterol. 2012;107(4):522–30.
17. Weijenborg PW, et al. PPI therapy is equally effective in well-defined non-erosive reflux disease and in reflux esophagitis: a meta-analysis. Neurogastroenterol Motil. 2012;24(8):747–57, e350
18. Chiba N, et al. Speed of healing and symptom relief in grade II to IV gastroesophageal reflux disease: a meta-analysis. Gastroenterology. 1997;112(6):1798–810.
19. Samuel R, et al. Evaluation and management of non-variceal upper gastrointestinal bleeding. Dis Mon. 2018;64(7):333–43.
20. Marmo R, et al. Dual therapy versus monotherapy in the endoscopic treatment of high-risk bleeding ulcers: a meta-analysis of controlled trials. Am J Gastroenterol. 2007;102(2):279–89; quiz 469

21. Laine L, McQuaid KR. Endoscopic therapy for bleeding ulcers: an evidence-based approach based on meta-analyses of randomized controlled trials. Clin Gastroenterol Hepatol. 2009;7(1):33–47; quiz 1–2

22. Stefanidis D, et al. Guidelines for surgical treatment of gastroesophageal reflux disease. Surg Endosc. 2010;24(11):2647–69.

23. Rakita S, et al. Laparoscopic Nissen fundoplication offers high patient satisfaction with relief of extraesophageal symptoms of gastroesophageal reflux disease. Am Surg. 2006;72(3):207–12.

24. Oelschlager BK, et al. Symptomatic and physiologic outcomes after operative treatment for extraesophageal reflux. Surg Endosc. 2002;16(7):1032–6.

25. Ramanathan J, et al. Herpes simplex virus esophagitis in the immunocompetent host: an overview. Am J Gastroenterol. 2000;95(9):2171–6.

26. Kato S, et al. Herpes simplex esophagitis in the immunocompetent host. Dis Esophagus. 2005;18(5):340–4.

27. Lee B, Caddy G. A rare cause of dysphagia: herpes simplex esophagitis. World J Gastroenterol. 2007;13(19):2756–7.

28. de-la-Riva, S., et al. Herpetic esophagitis: a case report on an immunocompetent adolescent. Rev Esp Enferm Dig. 2012;104(4):214–7.

29. Bando T, et al. Herpes simplex esophagitis in the elderly. Dig Endosc. 2009;21(3):205–7.

30. Badarinarayanan G, Gowrisankar R, Muthulakshmi K. Esophageal candidiasis in non-immune suppressed patients in a semi-urban town, southern India. Mycopathologia. 2000;149(1):1–4.

31. Andersen LI, Frederiksen HJ, Appleyard M. Prevalence of esophageal Candida colonization in a Danish population: special reference to esophageal symptoms, benign esophageal disorders, and pulmonary disease. J Infect Dis. 1992;165(2):389–92.

32. Learmonth I, Weaver PC. Letter: potassium stricture of the upper alimentary tract. Lancet. 1976;1(7953):251–2.

33. Peters JL. Benign oesophageal stricture following oral potassium chloride therapy. Br J Surg. 1976;63(9):698–9.

34. Wong RK, Kikendall JW, Dachman AH. Quinaglute-induced esophagitis mimicking an esophageal mass. Ann Intern Med. 1986;105(1):62–3.

35. Abbarah TR, Fredell JE, Ellenz GB. Ulceration by oral ferrous sulfate. JAMA. 1976;236(20):2320.

36. Stoller JL. Oesophageal ulceration and theophylline. Lancet. 1985;2(8450):328–9.

37. Enzenauer RW, Bass JW, McDonnell JT. Esophageal ulceration associated with oral theophylline. N Engl J Med. 1984;310(4):261.

38. Oren R, Fich A. Oral contraceptive-induced esophageal ulcer. Two cases and literature review. Dig Dis Sci. 1991;36(10):1489–90.

39. Bova JG, et al. Medication-induced esophagitis: diagnosis by double-contrast esophagography. AJR Am J Roentgenol. 1987;148(4):731–2.

40. Nguyen T, et al. Mycophenolic acid (cellcept and myfortic) induced injury of the upper GI tract. Am J Surg Pathol. 2009;33(9):1355–63.

41. Perry PA, Dean BS, Krenzelok EP. Drug induced esophageal injury. J Toxicol Clin Toxicol. 1989;27(4–5):281–6.

42. Katzka DA. Esophageal disorders caused by medications, trauma, and infection. In: Friedman LFM, Brandt LJ, editors. Sleisenger and Fordtran's gastrointestinal and liver disease: Saunders Elsevier; 2010. p. 763–72.

43. Ribeiro A, et al. Alendronate-associated esophagitis: endoscopic and pathologic features. Gastrointest Endosc. 1998;47(6):525–8.

44. Abraham SC, et al. Upper gastrointestinal tract injury in patients receiving kayexalate (sodium polystyrene sulfonate) in sorbitol: clinical, endoscopic, and histopathologic findings. Am J Surg Pathol. 2001;25(5):637–44.

45. Purdy JK, Appelman HD, McKenna BJ. Sloughing esophagitis is associated with chronic debilitation and medications that injure the esophageal mucosa. Mod Pathol. 2012;25(5):767–75.

46. Ravich WJ, Kashima H, Donner MW. Drug-induced esophagitis simulating esophageal carcinoma. Dysphagia. 1986;1(1):13–8.

47. Creteur V, et al. Drug-induced esophagitis detected by double-contrast radiography. Radiology. 1983;147(2):365–8.
48. Agha FP, Wilson JA, Nostrand TT. Medication-induced esophagitis. Gastrointest Radiol. 1986;11(1):7–11.
49. Jung BH. Gastrointestinal cancers. In: Sweetser S, editor. Digestive disease self-education program: American Gastroenterological Association: American Gastroenterological Association; 2016. p. 433–6.
50. Rubenstein JH, Shaheen NJ. Epidemiology, diagnosis, and management of esophageal adenocarcinoma. Gastroenterology. 2015;149(2):302–17. e1
51. Abnet CC, Arnold M, Wei WQ. Epidemiology of esophageal squamous cell carcinoma. Gastroenterology. 2018;154(2):360–73.
52. Sohda M, Kuwano H. Current status and future prospects for esophageal cancer treatment. Ann Thorac Cardiovasc Surg. 2017;23(1):1–11.
53. Wang KK, Wongkeesong M, Buttar NS. American Gastroenterological Association technical review on the role of the gastroenterologist in the management of esophageal carcinoma. Gastroenterology. 2005;128(5):1471–505.
54. Aziz M, et al. Efficacy of Hemospray in non-variceal upper gastrointestinal bleeding: a systematic review with meta-analysis. Ann Gastroenterol. 2020;33(2):145–54.
55. Inayat F, et al. Primary esophageal diffuse large B-Cell lymphoma: a comparative review of 15 cases. J Investig Med High Impact Case Rep. 2018;6:2324709618820887.
56. Schatz RA, Rockey DC. Gastrointestinal bleeding due to gastrointestinal tract malignancy: natural history, management, and outcomes. Dig Dis Sci. 2017;62(2):491–501.
57. Pellecchia R, et al. An esophageal lymphoma discovered by echocardiography. Rev Port Cardiol. 2016;35(6):381–2.
58. Mrad RA, et al. The elusive diagnosis of primary esophageal lymphoma. Turk J Haematol. 2018;35(3):199.
59. Theiss L, Contreras CM. Gastrointestinal stromal tumors of the stomach and esophagus. Surg Clin North Am. 2019;99(3):543–53.
60. Cohen C, et al. Is there a place for thoracoscopic enucleation of esophageal gastrointestinal stromal tumors? Thorac Cardiovasc Surg. 2019;67(7):585–8.
61. Baysal B, et al. The role of EUS and EUS-guided FNA in the management of subepithelial lesions of the esophagus: a large, single-center experience. Endosc Ultrasound. 2017;6(5):308–16.
62. Hihara J, Mukaida H, Hirabayashi N. Gastrointestinal stromal tumor of the esophagus: current issues of diagnosis, surgery and drug therapy. Transl Gastro Hepatol. 2018;3:6.
63. Ma Z, Cai H, Cui Y. Progress in the treatment of esophageal neuroendocrine carcinoma. Tumour Biol. 2017;39(6):1010428317711313.
64. Schizas D, et al. Neuroendocrine tumors of the esophagus: state of the art in diagnostic and therapeutic management. J Gastrointest Cancer. 2017;48(4):299–304.
65. Nagtegaal ID, et al. The 2019 WHO classification of tumours of the digestive system. Histopathology. 2020;76(2):182–8.
66. Giannetta E, et al. A rare rarity: neuroendocrine tumor of the esophagus. Crit Rev Oncol Hematol. 2019;137:92–107.
67. Farley HA, Pommier RF. Surgical treatment of small bowel neuroendocrine tumors. Hematol Oncol Clin North Am. 2016;30(1):49–61.
68. van der Veen A, et al. Management of resectable esophageal and gastric (mixed adeno)neuroendocrine carcinoma: a nationwide cohort study. Eur J Surg Oncol. 2018;44(12):1955–62.
69. Scaglione S, et al. The epidemiology of cirrhosis in the United States: a population-based study. J Clin Gastroenterol. 2015;49(8):690–6.
70. Garcia-Tsao G, et al. Prevention and management of gastroesophageal varices and variceal hemorrhage in cirrhosis. Hepatology. 2007;46(3):922–38.
71. Naveau S, Perlemuter G, Balian A. Epidemiology and natural history of cirrhosis. Rev Prat. 2005;55(14):1527–32.

72. Gkamprela E, Deutsch M, Pectasides D. Iron deficiency anemia in chronic liver disease: etio-pathogenesis, diagnosis and treatment. Ann Gastroenterol. 2017;30(4):405–13.
73. Grace ND. Diagnosis and treatment of gastrointestinal bleeding secondary to portal hyper-tension. American College of Gastroenterology Practice Parameters Committee. Am J Gastroenterol. 1997;92(7):1081–91.
74. de Franchis R, Baveno VIF. Expanding consensus in portal hypertension: report of the Baveno VI Consensus Workshop: stratifying risk and individualizing care for portal hypertension. J Hepatol. 2015;63(3):743–52.
75. Saeed ZA, et al. Endoscopic variceal ligation in patients who have failed endoscopic sclero-therapy. Gastrointest Endosc. 1990;36(6):572–4.
76. Je D, et al. The comparison of esophageal variceal ligation plus propranolol versus propran-olol alone for the primary prophylaxis of esophageal variceal bleeding. Clin Mol Hepatol. 2014;20(3):283–90.
77. Zhu Y, et al. Emergency transjugular intrahepatic portosystemic shunt: an effective and safe treatment for uncontrolled variceal bleeding. J Gastrointest Surg. 2019;23(11):2193–200.
78. Orchard JL, et al. Upper gastrointestinal tract bleeding in institutionalized mentally retarded adults. Primary role of esophagitis. Arch Fam Med. 1995;4(1):30–3.
79. Gupta N, et al. Longer inspection time is associated with increased detection of high-grade dysplasia and esophageal adenocarcinoma in Barrett's esophagus. Gastrointest Endosc. 2012;76(3):531–8.
80. Everson MA, et al. How to perform a high-quality examination in patients with Barrett's esophagus. Gastroenterology. 2018;154(5):1222–6.

Chapter 6
Gastroduodenum

Abbey Barnard, Hwajeong Lee, and Ethan Bortniker

Introduction

Proximal lesions within the reach of a standard upper endoscope may account for occult gastrointestinal bleeding. Prospective studies of patients who underwent both upper endoscopy and colonoscopy for evaluation of occult gastrointestinal blood loss report that 36–71% of culprit lesions were readily identifiable on upper endoscopy [1]. As such, both an upper and lower endoscopy are recommended as part of the initial investigation for occult gastrointestinal bleeding in an adult with iron deficiency anemia. Causative lesions vary depending on patient's age, comorbidities and risk factors. This chapter aims to highlight both common and uncommon etiologies of upper gastrointestinal bleeding with special attention to relevant patient factors and the potential for missed lesions on initial evaluation.

Peptic Ulcer Disease

Peptic ulcer disease is defined as a defect in the mucosal lining with a diameter of equal to or greater than 5 mm extending into the submucosa. Broadly speaking, these lesions occur in the setting of an imbalance in acid secretion and muscosal

A. Barnard · E. Bortniker (✉)
Veterans Affairs San Diego Healthcare System, San Diego, CA, USA

University of California-San Diego, Division of Gastroenterology, La Jolla, CA, USA
e-mail: ebortniker@health.ucsd.edu

H. Lee
Department of Pathology and Laboratory Medicine, Albany Medical Center,
Albany, NY, USA
e-mail: LeeH5@amc.edu

© The Author(s), under exclusive license to Springer Nature
Switzerland AG 2021
M. Tadros, G. Y. Wu (eds.), *Management of Occult GI Bleeding*, Clinical
Gastroenterology, https://doi.org/10.1007/978-3-030-71468-0_6

barrier function. The lifetime risk of an individual developing peptic ulcer disease ranges from 5% to 10%. Two most common etiologies for peptic ulcer disease include *Helicobacter pylori* infection and non-steroidal anti-inflammatory drug (NSAID)s [2] (Figs. 6.1, 6.2, 6.3 and 6.4). While the incidence of peptic ulcer disease has decreased with improved hygiene and increased use of proton pump inhibitors, it remains the most common cause of hospitalization for upper gastrointestinal bleeding. Presentation is variable; some patients present with abdominal pain and acute gastrointestinal hemorrhage manifested by hematemesis and melena, while others present with iron deficiency anemia only. The diagnostic test of choice is esophagogastroduodenoscopy (EGD) which readily identifies the majority of culprit lesions and allows for concurrent therapeutic intervention. Prospective studies report that following investigation with EGD and colonoscopy, the incidence of gastric ulcers as the etiology of occult bleeding ranges from 3% to 13% [1]. However, despite the relatively high sensitivity of endoscopy, these lesions can be missed. A review of enteroscopies performed for obscure gastrointestinal bleeding found that of the 25 culprit proximal lesions, one was a duodenal ulcer that was not visualized on initial upper endoscopy [3]. A number of factors may contribute to missed ulcers on upper endoscopy or capsule endoscopy, including retained clot and blood, insufficient insufflation, ulcer location (especially pyloric channel) and duodenal sweep. We recommend a careful endoscopic evaluation with special attention to the duodenal bulb. While endoscopic treatment may be offered following identification of the culprit lesion, endoscopic therapy is associated with high risk of complication. Therefore, proton pump inhibitor (PPI) therapy remains the mainstay of medical therapy. Patients should receive high dose PPI therapy and undergo follow up endoscopy as indicated, specifically in the setting of gastric ulceration to assess for healing and rule out malignancy [2]. In addition, when indicated, testing for *H. pylori* and antibiotic treatment should be pursued. Eradication of *H. pylori* should be confirmed following therapy [2, 4, 5].

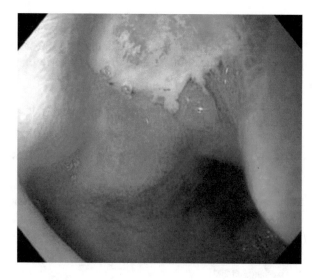

Fig. 6.1 Duodenal bulb ulcer identified on upper endoscopy as etiology of symptomatic anemia in young male patient on NSAIDs

Fig. 6.2 Peptic duodenal
ulcer due to concurrent
Helicobacter gastritis
[Hematoxylin and eosin
(H&E), x100]

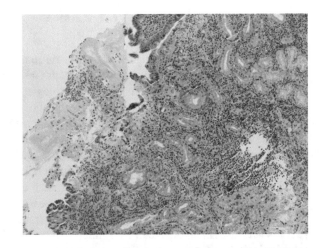

Fig. 6.3 Biopsy of gastric
antrum demonstrates
chronic active Helicobacter
gastritis [H&E, x100]

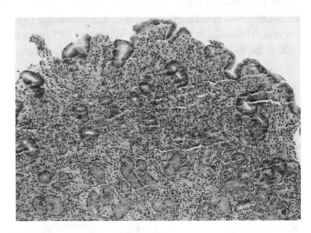

Fig. 6.4 Helicobacter
gastritis. Immunohisto-
chemical stain for
Helicobacter organisms
shows microorganisms
(brown staining) in the
foveolar glands [Helico-
bacter immunostain, x200]

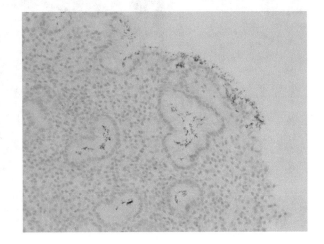

Gastritis

Gastritis is defined as inflammation of the gastric mucosa [6]. Current epidemiological data suggest that chronic gastritis is perhaps one of the most common chronic conditions worldwide [7]. While a number of etiologies have been implicated in the development of gastritis including excessive alcohol consumption, tobacco use, NSAIDs, bile reflux and critical illness, two of the most important clinical entities in regards to both prevalence and clinical sequelae are autoimmune gastritis leading to pernicious anemia and *H. pylori* gastritis. Both have been recognized as important drivers of intestinal metaplasia that is a known risk factor for gastric adenocarcinoma [8]. In reviews of upper endoscopy and colonoscopy performed for investigation of occult gastrointestinal bleeding, gastritis was identified as the culprit pathology in 3–16% of patients. As previously stated, the presence of *H. pylori* gastritis is a significant risk factor for future malignancy. Therefore, random gastric biopsies including the antrum, corpus and angularis are recommended when gastritis is identified and *H. pylori* infection is suspected [9]. When *H. pylori* infection is present, it should be eradicated. When no infection is present, potential inciting factors for gastritis, such as NSAIDs, alcohol, etc., should be identified and removed.

Cameron's Lesions

Cameron's lesions, also referred to as Cameron's erosions, are defined as linear lesions or oval ulcerations visualized on the crests of gastric mucosal folds at the level of the diaphragm in patients with hiatal hernias [10–12] (Fig. 6.5). These lesions are uncommon in small hiatal hernias, but the prevalence ranges from 10%

Fig. 6.5 Cameron's Lesion (arrow) associated with hiatal hernia

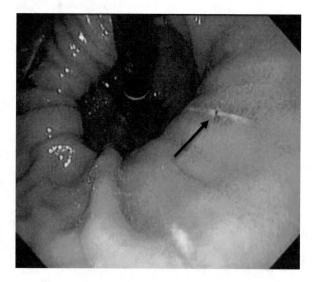

to 20% in patients with large (>5 cm) hiatal hernias. Its prevalence has also been found to be higher in patients taking NSAIDs compared to those who are not taking them [13]. Clinically, it is important to recognize these lesions as they can lead to both overt and occult gastrointestinal bleeding. A number of mechanisms that lead to the development of Cameron's lesions have been proposed, to include trauma at the level of diaphragm resulting in contact between adjacent or opposite gastric folds, mucosal ischemia, and mucosal injury secondary to gastric acid.

While Cameron's lesions are typically associated with iron deficiency anemia, studies have reported overall bleeding rates to be as high as 58% [14]. During an endoscopic evaluation, careful antegrade and retrograde evaluation is required with sufficient insufflation to avoid missing these often subtle lesions. It has been reported that up to 69% of patients with Cameron's lesions undergo one or more upper endoscopies prior to identification of the lesions as the etiology of their gastrointestinal blood loss.

Debate exists as to whether surgical correction of the hiatal hernia is absolutely indicated in these cases or whether simply a trial of medical therapy composed of proton pump inhibitors, iron supplementation and NSAID avoidance is sufficient to prevent future bleeding. Prior studies suggest that in patients with known Cameron's lesions and refractory iron deficiency anemia, surgical hernia correction can be effective in achieving resolution of anemia and thus, surgical intervention should be considered in this population [15].

Portal Hypertensive Gastropathy

Portal hypertensive gastropathy is an often subtle, but clinically important etiology of occult gastrointestinal blood loss occurring in both cirrhotic and non-cirrhotic patients. Previously it was thought to represent an inflammatory process. However, further study demonstrated that the underlying pathology is vascular ectasia. Thus, this entity may fall within a spectrum of congestive gastropathy [16]. This is different from gastric antral vascular ectasia (GAVE) discussed later in this chapter in that the vascular dilation is mild to moderate and no abnormality is appreciated within the vascular lumina or wall on pathology [17]. Overall, the reported prevalence of portal hypertensive gastropathy in the cirrhotic population varies widely throughout the literature with studies reporting ranges from 20% to 98% [17]. This likely is due to the often subtle nature of the lesions and the variability of diagnostic criteria. Portal hypertensive gastropathy can occur in the absence of esophageal varices and its presence is strongly correlated with severity of portal hypertension [18]. Portal hypertensive gastropathy diagnosis is made endoscopically. It is characterized by a mosaic or snakeskin pattern of the gastric mucosa [16–23] on endoscopy (Figs. 6.6 and 6.7). In severe cases cherry spots or active hemorrhage can be noted.

Portal hypertensive gastropathy is an uncommon cause of acute hemorrhage in the cirrhotic population accounting for only 8% of non-variceal hemorrhage. However, it has been recognized as an important etiology of subacute to chronic

Fig. 6.6 Portal
hypertensive gastropathy
as etiology of subacute
anemia

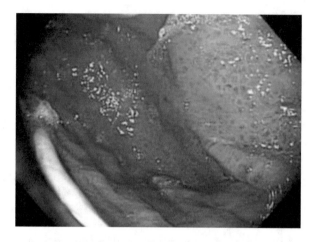

Fig. 6.7 Portal
hypertensive gastropathy
with dilated capillaries
(arrow) in the gastric body
[H&E, x100]

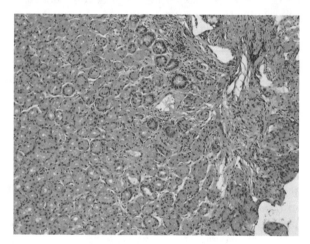

occult gastrointestinal hemorrhage [21]. It is difficult to estimate the exact incidence of occult bleeding secondary to portal hypertensive gastropathy in the cirrhotic population as patients with chronic liver disease have multiple risk factors for anemia. In the literature, its incidence ranges from 3% to 26% [17].

Unfortunately, there are limited treatment options for portal hypertensive gastropathy. Given the diffuse nature of this lesion, endoscopic therapy is not considered to be effective in mitigating blood loss. Octreotide can be effective in the setting of acute bleeding secondary to portal hypertension; however its administration and cost can be limiting factors. Certainly, liver transplantation can reverse the portal hypertension and can resolve portal hypertensive gastropathy. However, this option is not available to all patients given the shortage of the organs. Transjugular intrahepatic portosystemic shunt (TIPS) can be offered to ameliorate portal hypertensive gastropathy, but again, not all patients are eligible for this intervention [23]. Beta blockade has also been utilized with mixed results in regard to efficacy [22]. Typically, supportive care in the form of blood transfusions and aggressive iron repletion are the mainstay of therapy.

Angioectasia

Angioectasia is defined as a collection of dilated blood vessels in the mucosa or submucosa of the bowel wall [24] (Figs. 6.8 and 6.9). Angioectasia is also referred to as arteriovenous malformation (AVM), venous ectasia, angioma, or angiodysplasia [25]. These lesions are very common on upper endoscopy and colonoscopy. It is estimated that less than 10% of patients with angioectasia will experience gastrointestinal bleeding. However, studies report AVMs as the culprit lesions of obscure

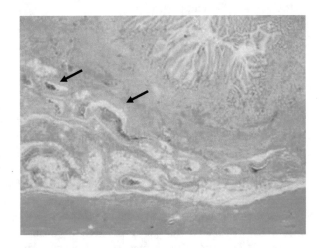

Fig. 6.8 Arteriovenous malformation in the stomach. Scanning view of gastric arteriovenous malformation. Dilated arteries and veins (arrows) are noted in the submucosa [H&E, x20]

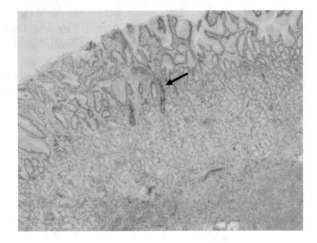

Fig. 6.9 Higher magnification of arteriovenous malformation in the stomach. Overlying mucosa shows dilated capillaries with congestion (arrow) [H&E, x40]

gastrointestinal bleeding in 30–60% of cases [25]. A number of medical conditions increase the risk of bleeding from angioectasia including aortic stenosis, cirrhosis, chronic renal failure, left ventricular assist device (LVAD) placement and von Willebrand disease, in some of which the mechanisms of bleeding remain ill defined. The association between aortic stenosis and hemorrhagic angioectasia is well demonstrated in Heyde's syndrome [26, 27]. While multiple mechanisms have been proposed to account for this association, it is postulated that the high shear stress caused by the aortic stenosis leads an increase in the von Willebrand factor clearing metalloprotease activity, which result in degradation or clearance of von Willebrand factor. Heyde's syndrome and its associations are of particular interest as studies have suggested that valvular repair may ameliorate the angioectasia bleeding [26].

Gastric and duodenal AVMs may be missed on upper endoscopy or capsule endoscopy when the lesions are small. Ongoing occult gastrointestinal bleeding should prompt repeat endoscopic evaluation and consideration for enteroscopy to better define the extent of disease.

Varices

Variceal bleeding is a well-known etiology of potentially life threatening gastrointestinal hemorrhage [28]. Esophageal variceal hemorrhage is readily detected by an upper endoscopy, while its management can be challenging. However, duodenal and gastric varices can pose diagnostic and management dilemmas. Gastric varices are responsible for 20–30% of variceal hemorrhage. Isolated gastric varices may not be detected as the lesion may be obscured by a pool of blood in the fundus due to hemorrhage. In subacute presentation, this portion of the stomach may not be thoroughly examined during endoscopy. In addition, gastric varices can occur in the absence of cirrhosis in association with pancreatic pathology, such as pancreatic malignancy or pancreatitis. Pancreatic disease may lead to isolated splenic vein thrombosis and portal hypertension [29]. Duodenal varices are less common than esophageal or gastric counterparts and account for only 1% of variceal bleeding. They usually occur in the duodenal bulb, but have also been reported in the distal duodenum (Fig. 6.10). In this case, the lesion may not be detected during upper endoscopy [30]. Management of gastric and duodenal varices varies depending on patient presentation, etiology of varices and liver function. The management options include transhepatic intrahepatic portosystemic shunt and endoscopic interventions including glue injection and coiling [31, 32].

Dieulafoy's Lesions

Dieulafoy's lesions are rare, but an important etiology of occult and obscure gastrointestinal hemorrhage. It is caused by an erosion of mucosa by a dilated submucosal artery in the absence of other pathologic processes such as an ulcer or aneurysm

Fig. 6.10 Duodenal
varices identified as a
cause of subacute
gastrointestinal
hemorrhage

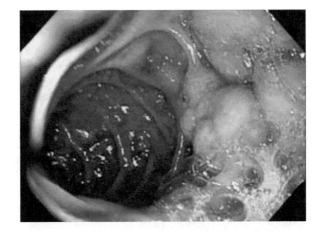

Fig. 6.11 Dieulafoy lesion
in the duodenum which
was ultimately clipped for
hemostasis

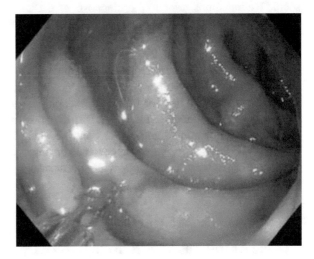

[33]. The arteries in these lesions are up to ten times larger than their normal submucosal counterparts. Approximately 75% of Dieulafoy lesions are identified in the
stomach, but have been described in the esophagus, small intestine and colon. In the
stomach, these lesions are most frequently encountered within 6 cm of the gastroesophageal junction along the lesser curvature. On endoscopy, these appear as a
small visible vessel or an area of pigmentation without surrounding erosion or
ulceration (Fig. 6.11). Given their location and size, it appears that these lesions are
very sensitive to even mild mechanical trauma, such as the passage of a food bolus.
Several mechanisms leading to mucosal rupture have been proposed, but studies
have failed to demonstrate an association with aneurysm, arteriosclerosis, elastic
tissue dysfunction or vasculitis [34]. Dieulafoy lesions have been associated with
advanced age; however, it remains unclear whether these lesions are truly an
acquired phenomena or a congenital defect as they have been reported even in
infants [35]. While many patients who bleed from Dieulafoy lesions are taking

NSAIDs or on therapeutic anti-coagulation, there is no data to support direct association between the development of these lesions and the medications. Studies suggest that patients receiving these medications are simply more likely to bleed from any given lesion [36]. A 2:1 male to female ratio has been observed, but the driving force of this gender predilection is unknown.

The classical presentation of a Dieulafoy lesion is brisk upper gastrointestinal bleeding typically requiring packed red blood cell transfusion. Oftentimes patients present with hemodynamic instability in the absence of abdominal pain. These lesions can also account for occult gastrointestinal bleeding. Retrospective analyses estimate that only 1% of all gastrointestinal hemorrhage may be attributed to Dieulafoy lesions [37]. Upper endoscopy is the test of choice to localize and treat Dieulafoy lesions, but studies have demonstrated only a 70% diagnostic yield on first endoscopic evaluation, likely owing to the subtle nature of these lesions [38]. Other studies have reported that up to 6% of patients may require 3 or more endoscopic examinations prior to the diagnosis of a Dieulafoy lesion as the cause of obscure gastrointestinal hemorrhage [39]. As the lesions are likely to be located near the gastroesophageal junction, a careful retroflexed examination with sufficient insufflation is essential. Insufflation also allows for a better visualization of any lesions in between the gastric rugae, which may escape initial detection given their location. Given the difficulty of endoscopic localization, some experts advocate tattooing the lesion to allow for future endoscopic intervention and help localize if surgery is ultimately required [33, 39]. If the lesion is not localized despite repeat endoscopic examinations, angiography may be helpful to localize and treat the lesion. While there is no specific appearance on angiography that is diagnostic of a Dieulafoy lesion, a tortuous artery with non-tapering, persistent caliber is suggestive of the diagnosis [40].

Gastric Antral Vascular Ectasia (GAVE)

GAVE is an uncommon, but important etiology of upper gastrointestinal blood loss [41]. It is characterized by marked dilation of the mucosal capillaries and venules associated with focal fibrin thrombi and vascular wall alteration such as spindle cell proliferation and fibrohyalinosis (Figs. 6.12, 6.13 and 6.14). GAVE is a rare etiology of upper gastrointestinal bleeding accounting for approximately 4% of all non-variceal upper gastrointestinal bleeding. Studies have demonstrated a female predominance; approximately 71% of cases occur in women. Typically GAVE occurs in the setting of chronic illness, specifically liver disease and connective tissue disorders such as systemic sclerosis [42]. The precise pathogenesis of GAVE remains unclear though a number of mechanisms have been proposed including mechanical stress, hemodynamic alterations, hormonal and autoimmune factors [43]. Most frequently GAVE presents as occult bleeding which manifests as recurrent or refractory iron deficiency anemia. However, there are reports of GAVE manifesting as acute gastrointestinal hemorrhage [44]. Acute bleeding has been associated with male gender and cirrhosis. In cirrhotic patients, it is likely owing to

Fig. 6.12 GAVE identified as etiology of occult gastrointestinal bleeding in patient with nonalcoholic steatohepatitis (NASH) cirrhosis and end stage renal disease

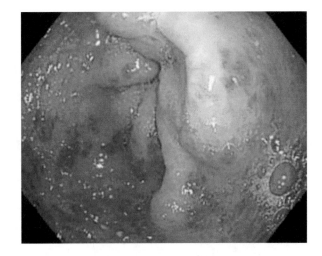

Fig. 6.13 GAVE with fibrin thrombi within mucosal capillaries (arrow) [H&E, x200]. Images courtesy of Dr. Jingmei Lin, Indiana University

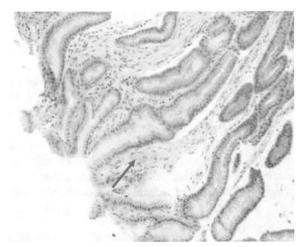

Fig. 6.14 Higher magnification of GAVE with fibrin thrombi within the mucosal capillaries (arrow) [H&E, x400]. Images courtesy of Dr. Jingmei Lin, Indiana University

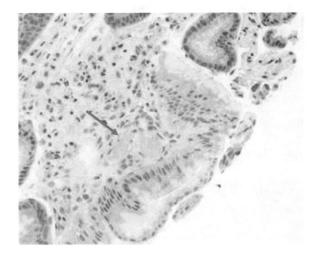

the underlying coagulopathy [45]. There are two distinct endoscopic appearances of GAVE that are well described. GAVE can present as diffuse punctuate lesions throughout the antrum or as the "watermelon stomach" appearance which is created by erythematous lesions emanating radially from the pylorus. The former appearance may be confused with, or obscured by gastritis or portal hypertensive gastropathy delaying the appropriate diagnosis and treatment. Pathologic examination can assist in rendering the diagnosis of GAVE and differentiating if from the aforementioned etiologies.

Endoscopy is the best tool for the diagnosis of GAVE. However, this diagnosis is not always apparent on the initial endoscopic evaluation. One series reported that 4.7% of patients referred for capsule endoscopy (CE) for obscure gastrointestinal bleeding were ultimately found to have GAVE on CE [46]. It is not entirely clear why GAVE was missed on upper endoscopy and later was visualized on CE. Possibly, resuscitation and increased hemoglobin level may allow better visualization of these vascular lesions [43].

Malignancy

Gastric cancer is the fourth most common type of cancer worldwide and second most common cause of cancer death worldwide [47, 48]. Changes in cooking practices and eradication of *Helicobacter pylori* have been associated with reductions in incidence in developed countries. However, it remains an important clinical entity and cause of occult gastrointestinal bleeding. Usual gastric cancer is an adenocarcinoma of intestinal or diffuse type (Figs. 6.15 and 6.16), but it is important to note that other non-epithelial tumors such as mucosa-associated lymphoid tissue (MALT) lymphomas and leiomyosarcomas can also be observed [49]. In addition, metastasis from other sites can also result in occult gastric bleeding. Breast and renal cell

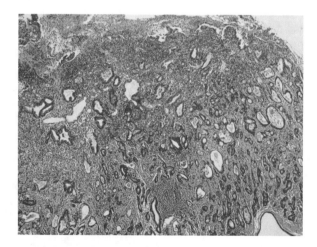

Fig. 6.15 Intestinal type gastric adenocarcinoma [H&E, x40]

Fig. 6.16 Diffuse type gastric adenocarcinoma with signet ring cells [H&E, x100]

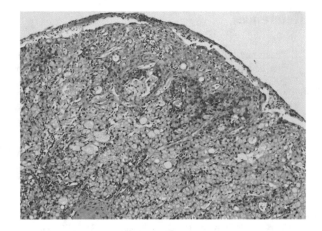

carcinoma are known to have a propensity to metastasize to the stomach and progression of the diseases can present in this manner [50].

Endoscopy remains the test of choice for diagnosis of gastric malignancies. Japan employs nationwide screening upper endoscopy to identify early gastric cancers. However, in the majority of clinical settings, upper endoscopy is pursued when "alarm features" such as new- onset dyspepsia, weight loss, and anemia, are present [51]. In some cases, the culprit gastric lesion is readily apparent. However, a recent meta-analysis found that approximately 1 in 10 gastric cancers are potentially missed on initial upper endoscopy [52]. A number of factors were implicated in missed diagnoses including insufficient number of biopsies from the abnormal tissue, location within the cardia or lesser curvature, and retained food during initial endoscopy.

Management of gastric cancer-related blood loss primarily depends on the extent of the disease. In cases of unresectable disease, options are limited. Supportive care with transfusions and iron therapy can help stabilize the patients while they pursue definitive treatment for their malignancy in the form of surgery, radiation, chemotherapy or immunotherapy. Hemospray, which became widely available in the United States recently, has also been employed for short term hemostasis as a bridge to the aforementioned more definitive therapies. Further clinical experience and research is necessary to better define the role of this intervention.

Conclusions

A number of important etiologies of occult gastrointestinal blood loss exist within the reach of the standard diagnostic upper endoscope. A high index of suspicion and careful endoscopic evaluation is essential to ensure that relevant pathology is identified on initial endoscopy and the patient is treated appropriately, subsequently. We encourage a careful forward and retroflexed examination with sufficient time spent investigating sites of frequently missed lesions, including the duodenal bulb.

References

1. Zuckerman GR, Prakash C, Askin MP, Lewis BS. AGA technical review on the evaluation and management of occult and obscure gastrointestinal bleeding. Gastroenterology. 2000;118:201–21.
2. Malfertheiner P, Chan FK, McColl KE. Peptic ulcer disease. Lancet. 2009;374:1449–61.
3. Zaman A, Katon RM. Push enteroscopy for obscure gastrointestinal bleeding yields a high incidence of proximal lesions within reach of a standard endoscope. Gastrointest Endosc. 1998;47:372–6.
4. Laine L, Jensen DM. Management of patients with ulcer bleeding. Am J Gastroenterol. 2012;107:345–60.
5. Soll AH. Consensus conference. Medical treatment of peptic ulcer disease. Practice guidelines. Practice parameters committee of the American College of Gastroenterology. JAMA. 1996; 275:622–9.
6. Taylor KB. Gastritis. N Engl J Med. 1969;280:818–20.
7. Sipponen P, Maaroos HI. Chronic gastritis. Scand J Gastroenterol. 2015;50:657–67.
8. Toh BH, Van Driel IR, Gleeson PA. Pernicious anemia. N Engl J Med. 1997;337:1441–8.
9. Standards ASGE. Of practice committee. Endoscopic mucosal tissue sampling. Gastrointest Endosc. 2013;78:216–24.
10. Cameron AJ, Higgins JA. Linear gastric erosion. A lesion associated with large diaphragmatic hernia and chronic blood loss anemia. Gastroenterology. 1986;91:338–42.
11. Nguyen N, Tam W, Kimber R, Roberts-Thomson IC. Gastrointestinal: Cameron's erosions. J Gastroenterol Hepatol. 2002;17:343.
12. Zullo A, Manta R, De Francesco V, Fiorini G, Lahner E, Vaira D, Annibale B. Cameron lesions: a still overlooked diagnosis. Case report and systematic review of literature. Clin Res Hepatol Gastroenterol. 2018;42:604–9.
13. Gray DM, Kushnir V, Kalra G, et al. Cameron lesions in patients with hiatal hernias: prevalence, presentation and treatment outcome. Dis Esophagus. 2015;28:448–52.
14. Hocking BV, Alp MH, Grant AK. Gastric ulceration within hiatus hernia. Med J Aust. 1976;2:207–8.
15. Lebenthal A, Waterford SD, Fisichella PM. Treatment and controversies in paraesophageal hernia repair. Front Surg. 2015;2:13.
16. McCormack T, Sims J, Eyre-Brook I, et al. Gastric lesions in portal hypertension: inflammatory gastritis or congestive gastropathy? Gut. 1985;26:1226–32.
17. Cubillas R, Rockey DC. Portal hypertensive gastropathy: a review. Liver Int. 2010;30:1094–102.
18. Taranto D, Suozzo R, Romano M, et al. Gastric endoscopic features in patients with liver cirrhosis: correlation with esophageal varices, intravariceal pressure, and liver dysfunction. Digestion. 1994;55:115–20.
19. Cales P, Zabotto B, Meskens C, et al. Gastroesophageal endoscopic features in cirrhosis. Gastroenterology. 1990;98:156–62.
20. Vigeneri S, Termini R, Piraino A, et al. The stomach in liver cirrhosis. Gastroenterology. 1991;101:472–8.
21. Gjeorgjievski M, Cappell MS. Portal hypertensive gastropathy: a systematic review of the pathophysiology, clinical presentation, natural history and therapy. World J Hepatol. 2016;8:231–62.
22. Pérez-Ayuso RM, Piqué JM, Bosch J, et al. Propranolol in prevention of recurrent bleeding from severe portal hypertensive gastropathy in cirrhosis. Lancet. 1991;337:1431–4.
23. Mezawa S, Homma H, Ohta H, et al. Effect of transjugular intrahepatic portosystemic shunt formation on portal hypertensive gastropathy and gastric circulation. Am J Gastroenterol. 2001;96:1155–9.
24. Igawa A, Oka S, Tanaka S, et al. Major predictors and management of small-bowel angioectasia. BMC Gastroenterol. 2015;15:108.

25. Romagnulo J, Brock AS, Ranney N. Is endscopic therapy effective for angioectasia in obscure gastrointestinal bleeding?: a systematic review of the literature. J Clin Gastroenterol. 2015;49:823–30.
26. Shibamoto A, Kawaratani H, Kubo T, et al. Aortic valve replacement for the management of Heyde syndrome: a case report. J Nippon Med Schol. 2017;84:193–7.
27. Hudzik B, Wilczek K, Gasior M. Heyde syndrome: gastrointestinal bleeding and aortic stenosis. CMAJ. 2016;188:135–8.
28. Kovacs TO, Jensen DM. Recent advances in the endoscopic diagnosis and therapy of upper gastrointestinal, small intestinal and colonic bleeding. Med Clin North Am. 2002;86:1319–56.
29. Mullan FJ, McKelvey ST. Pancreatic carcinoma presenting as bleeding from segmental gastric varices: pitfalls in diagnosis. Postgrad Med J. 1990;66:401–3.
30. Bhagani S, Winters C, Moreea S. Duodenal variceal bleed: unusual case of upper gastrointestinal bleed and a difficulty diagnosis to make. BMJ Case Rep. 2017;27:2017.
31. Levy MJ, Wong Kee Song LM, Kendrick ML, Misra S, Gostout CJ. EUS-guided coil embolization for refractory ectopic variceal bleeding (with videos). Gastrointest Endosc. 2008;67:572–4.
32. Norton ID, Andrews JC, Kamath PS. Management of ectopic varices. Hepatology. 1998;28:1154–8.
33. Lee YT, Walmsley RS, Leong RW, Sung JJ. Dieulafoy's lesion. Gastrointest Endosc. 2003;58:236–43.
34. Juler GL, Labitzke HG, Lamb R, Allen R. The pathogenesis of Dieulafoy's gastric erosion. Am J Gastroenterol. 1984;79:195–200.
35. Mikó TL, Thomázy VA. The caliber persistent artery of the stomach: a unifying approach to gastric aneurysm, Dieulafoy's lesion, and submucosal arterial malformation. Hum Pathol. 1988;19:914–21.
36. Luis LF, Sreenarasimhaiah J, Jiang TS. Localization, efficacy of therapy, and outcomes of Dieulafoy lesions of the GI tract – The UT Southwestern GI Bleed Team experience. Gastrointest Endosc. 2008;67:AB 87.
37. Khan R, Mahmad A, Gobrial M, Onwochei F, Shah K. The diagnostic dilemma of Dieulafoy's lesion. Gastroenterology Res. 2015;8:201–6.
38. Reilly HF 3rd. al-Kawas FH. Dieulafoy's lesion. Diagnosis and management. Dig Dis Sci. 1991;36:1702–7.
39. Baxter M, Aly EH. Dieulafoy's lesion: current trends in diagnosis and management. Ann R Coll Surg Engl. 2010;92:548–54.
40. Nojkov B, Cappell MS. Gastrointestinal bleeding from Dieulafoy's lesion:clinical presentation, endoscopic findings and endoscopic therapy. World J Gastrointest Endosc. 2015;16(7):295–307.
41. Gilliam JH, Geisinger KR, Wu WC, Weidner N, Richter JE. Endoscopic biopsy is diagnostic in gastric antral vascular ectasia. The "watermelon stomach". Dig Dis Sci. 1989;34:885–8.
42. Watson M, Hally RJ, McCue PA, Varga J, Jiménez SA. Gastric antral vascular ectasia (watermelon stomach) in patients with systemic sclerosis. Arthritis Rheum. 1996;39:341–6.
43. Alkhormi AM, Memon MY, Alqarawi A. Gastric antral vascular ectasia: A case report and literature review. J Transl Int Med. 2018;28(6):47–51.
44. Gostout CJ, Viggiano TR, Ahlquist DA, Wang KK, Larson MV, Balm R. The clinical and endoscopic spectrum of the watermelon stomach. J Clin Gastroenterol. 1992;15:256–63.
45. Ito M, Uchida Y, Kamano S, Kawabata H, Nishioka M. Clinical comparisons between two subsets of gastric antral vascular ectasia. Gastrointest Endosc. 2001;53:764–70.
46. Sidhu R, Sanders DS, McAlindon ME. Does capsule endoscopy recognise gastric antral vascular ectasia more frequently than conventional endoscopy? J Gastrointestin Liver Dis. 2006;15:375–7.
47. Ferlay J, Shin HR, Bray F, Forman D, Mathers C, Parkin DM. Estimates of worldwide burden of cancer in 2008: GLOBOCAN 2008. Int J Cancer. 2010;127:2893–917.

48. Jemal A, Center MM, DeSantis C, Ward EM. Global patterns of cancer incidence and mortality rates and trends. Cancer Epidemiol Biomark Prev. 2010;19:1893–907.
49. Karimi P, Islami F, Anandasabapathy S, Freedman ND, Kamangar F. Gastric Cancer: descriptive epidemiology, risk factors, screening, and prevention. Cancer Epidemiol Biomark Prev. 2014;23:700–13.
50. Weigt J, Malfertheiner P. Metastatic disease in the stomach. Gastrointest Tumors. 2015;2:61–4.
51. Maconi G, Manes G, Porro GB. Role of symptoms in diagnosis and outcome of gastric cancer. World J Gastroenterol. 2008;14:1149055.
52. Pimenta-Melo AR, Monteiro-Soares M, Libânio D, et al. Missing rate for gastric cancer during upper gastrointestinal endoscopy: a systematic review and meta-analysis. Eur J Gastroenterol Hepatol. 2016;28:1041–9.

Chapter 7
Small Bowel

Perry K. Pratt and Haleh Vaziri

Epidemiology and Natural History

The reported prevalence of a SB lesion in patients presenting with either occult or overt GIB is about 5–10% [2]. Regarding occult GIB specifically, combined data from four different studies of patients with IDA (total 381 patients) by *Rockey et al*, found a pooled prevalence of SB bleeding in 3% [3].

As one might expect, occult SB bleeding has been shown to have a lower recurrence rate compared to that of overt bleeding. One study demonstrated a 12-month re-bleeding rate of 19.5% in untreated occult bleeding compared to 38.9% in overt bleeding, as well as lower rates of subsequent hospitalization and blood transfusion in occult bleeding [4]. Use of medications such as anticoagulant and/or anti-platelet agents are a risk factor for recurrent SB bleeding, though interestingly, there is no prospective data to support clinical benefit in discontinuation of such medications. [5]

Etiology

Regarding the etiology of SB bleeding, patient age has been demonstrated to be associated with the type of underlying lesion. Younger patients are more likely to be diagnosed with occult SB bleeding related to inflammatory bowel disease, Meckel's diverticulum, and various polyposis syndromes (e.g., familial adenomatous polyposis (FAP), Peutz-Jeghers), while older patients are more likely to be diagnosed with

P. K. Pratt · H. Vaziri (✉)
University of Connecticut Health, Division of Gastroenterology & Hepatology, Farmington, CT, USA
e-mail: pepratt@uchc.edu; hvaziri@uchc.edu

© The Author(s), under exclusive license to Springer Nature Switzerland AG 2021
M. Tadros, G. Y. Wu (eds.), *Management of Occult GI Bleeding*, Clinical Gastroenterology, https://doi.org/10.1007/978-3-030-71468-0_7

Table 7.1 Etiologies of occult small bowel bleeding

Common etiologies in patients younger than 40 years	Common etiologies in patients older than 40 years	Rare etiologies in all ages
Crohn's disease	Angiodysplasia	Telangiectasias (sporadic or congenital)
Small bowel neoplasia	Small bowel neoplasia	Small bowel varices and/or portal hypertensive enteropathy
Dieulafoy's lesion	Dieulafoy's lesion	Blue rubber bleb nevus syndrome
Polyposis syndromes	NSAID-induced ulcers	Amyloidosis
Meckel's diverticulum		Henoch-Schonlein purpura
		Hematobilia
		Hemosuccus entericus
		Kaposi's sarcoma

NSAID; nonsteroidal anti-inflammatory drug

angiodysplasia and NSAID-induced enteropathy. Patients of any age can develop bleeding related to SB neoplasia (GI stromal tumor (GIST), carcinoid, lymphoma, and adenocarcinoma) and Dieulafoy's lesions [2, 6, 7]. Rarer causes of SB bleeding include Henoch-Schoenlein purpura, blue rubber bleb nevus syndrome, Kaposi's sarcoma, amyloidosis, hereditary hemorrhagic telangiectasias, and hematobilia, among others (see Table 7.1). There is no data available to suggest patient ethnicity is associated with specific SB pathology [2].

Vascular Lesions

Small intestinal vascular lesions, including angiodysplasia, telangiectasia, and Dieulafoy's lesions, are a group of heterogeneous diseases, which are the most common causes of occult SB bleeding [8, 9]. The true prevalence of vascular lesions in occult bleeding has not been well studied, but in patients with possible small bowel bleeding (PSBB), SB vascular lesions are reported in about 40–50% of cases [10, 11].

Angiodysplasia (AD; otherwise known as angioectasia) is the formation of aberrant and abnormally dilated, thin-walled (little or no smooth muscle), and tortuous blood vessels, which form within the mucosa or submucosa of the GI tract and have a propensity to bleed [9]. Studies have suggested that these lesions form due to either mechanical dilation related to vessel congestion, sphincter failure from chronically increased intestinal wall pressure, or increased angiogenesis from overexpression of vascular endothelial growth factor (VEGF) due to hypoxia from chronic low-grade vessel obstruction [8].

Clinical risk factors for development of AD include older age and presence of medical comorbidities, such as chronic kidney disease, valvular or ischemic heart disease, congestive heart failure, and hypertension [12–15]. Bleeding from AD in patients with aortic valve stenosis is well-described and known as Heyde's syndrome. This association is theorized to be due to an acquired von Willibrand's factor (vWF) deficiency related to loss of high molecular-weight vWF multimers from high shear stress in the aorta [10, 16–18]. Although not limited to the SB, patients with left ventricular assist devices have also been shown to have increased GI bleeding from AD, thought to be related to a similar mechanism of acquired vWF-deficiency [19].

Telangiectasias (otherwise known as arteriovenous malformations, AVMs) are typically larger than AD, thick-walled with excessive smooth muscle, and without capillaries, involving direct connections between arteries and veins. Telangiectasias can be sporadic or congenital [16]. The autosomal dominant vascular disorder, hereditary hemorrhagic telangiectasias (HHT; otherwise known as Osler-Weber-Rendu syndrome), is most commonly associated with presence of telangiectasias, and presents most typically as epistaxis in childhood, with development of chronic GI bleeding (overt or occult) and IDA later in life. Systemic sclerosis (scleroderma) and Turner's syndrome are also associated with telangiectasias (Fig. 7.1) [16].

Dieulafoy's lesion (DL) is another vascular cause of GIB, which can present as occult bleeding or as a life-threatening overt hemorrhage. The etiology of this lesion is poorly understood, but may be similar to that of AD described above. DLs are much more commonly identified in the stomach, rather than the duodenum or jejunum [7, 8, 16, 20, 21].

Fig. 7.1 A small bowel telangiectasia (also known as arteriovenous malformation, AVM) identified during video capsule endoscopy in a patient with systemic sclerosis. (Image courtesy of Micheal Tadros, M.D)

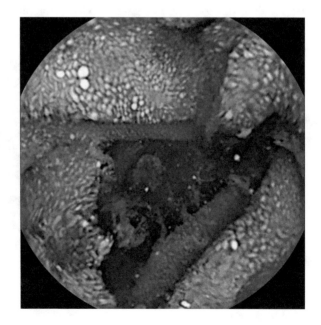

Small Bowel Ulcers

One of the most common etiologies for ulcer formation in the small intestines is Crohn's disease (CD), a chronic progressive inflammatory disease which can involve any segment of the gastrointestinal tract [22]. Although its exact etiology remains unclear, it seems to result from the complex interplay between genetic factors, environmental influences, and the gut microbiota. The prevalence of CD is highest in Europe (322 cases per 100,000), Canada (319 per 100,000) and the USA (214 per 100,000) It is equally distributed among men and women and most commonly presents between the second and fourth decades of life [22].

Around 30% of patients with CD have isolated SB disease (Fig. 7.2) [22]. Ulcer formation is one manifestation of the transmural inflammation that characterizes CD, and is not specific to the small intestines. A significant percentage of patients will go on to develop complications from this chronic inflammation, including fistulas, abscess, and strictures [22, 23]. symptoms including abdominal pain, diarrhea, fatigue, weight loss, growth failure, or extra-intestinal manifestations such rash, arthropathy, ocular inflammation, or hepatobiliary disease [22, 23]. IDA which may result from chronic GI blood loss and/or intestinal malabsorption, is not uncommon in these patients (Fig. 7.3).

Non-steroidal anti-inflammatory drug (NSAID) enteropathy is another common but under-diagnosed cause of small bowel ulceration. Patients commonly self-prescribe NSAIDs owing to their well-demonstrated anti-inflammatory and analgesic effects, though frequently underreport their use [24]. While commonly prescribed acid suppressive regimens (e.g., proton pump inhibitors, H2-receptors antagonists) have reduced NSAID-related gastroduodenal complications, more distal small intestinal complications out of reach of a standard upper endoscope are more

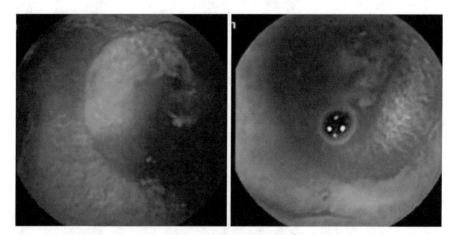

Fig. 7.2 Small bowel ulcerations identified during video capsule endoscopy in a patient with IDA who was ultimately diagnosed with isolated small bowel Crohn's disease. (Images courtesy of Haleh Vaziri, M.D)

Fig. 7.3 Crohn's disease with fissuring ulcer involving the ileum [Hematoxylin and eosin, x20]. (Image courtesy of Dr. Hwa Jeong Lee)

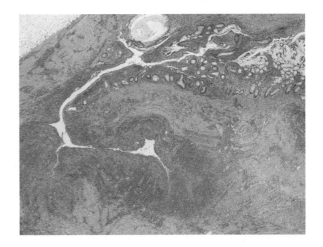

difficult to diagnose. Studies have demonstrated a high incidence of NSAID enteropathy, occurring in 53–80% of healthy short-term users, and 50–71% of long-term users [24]. Iron deficiency anemia can result from occult or overt blood loss, as well as impaired mucosal iron absorption. Protein-losing enteropathy, NSAID-induced small bowel strictures, and small bowel diaphragm disease (pathognomonic, with predilection for the distal small bowel) can all occur secondary to more chronic NSAID use [24].

Meckel's Diverticulum

Meckel's diverticulum (MD) is a congenital malformation that affects between 2–4% of the general population, and occurs due to incomplete closure of the vitelline duct. Bleeding originating from the MD is generally uncommon, but relatively more common in children than adults, and most often results from ulceration of ileal mucosa due to acid production from ectopic gastric mucosa located within the diverticulum [34] (Fig. 7.4).

Small Bowel Tumors

Small bowel tumors, both benign and malignant, are relatively rare, accounting for only 2–5% of all GI tumors [36]. A large retrospective chart review in 2013 examined the incidence of SB tumor types in patients referred for double balloon enteroscopy (DBE) due to occult GIB. In patients with malignant tumors, SB neuroendocrine tumor (NET, formerly known as carcinoid) was the most prevalent (11.1% of patients), followed by GIST, lymphoma, and adenocarcinoma (8.3% each). In the patients who had benign tumors, adenoma (8.3%) and hamartoma (5.6%) were most common [6].

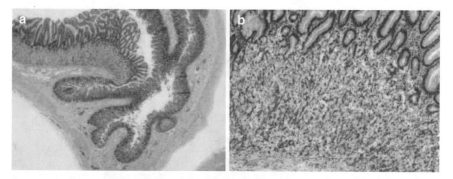

Fig. 7.4 (A on the left & B on the right): (**a**) Meckel's diverticulum of the ileum [Hematoxylin and eosin, x20]. (**b**) Higher magnification of the Meckel's diverticulum showing gastric type oxyntic mucosa within the diverticulum [Hematoxylin and eosin, x100]. (Images courtesy of Dr. Hwa Jeong Lee)

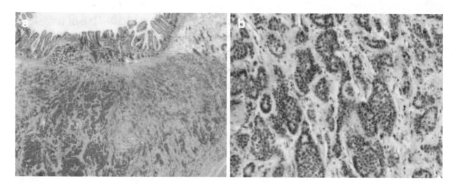

Fig. 7.5 (A on the left & B on the right): (**a**) Well-differentiated neuroendocrine neoplasm of the small bowel [Hematoxylin and eosin, x20]. (**b**) Same tumor under higher magnification showing "salt and pepper" pattern chromatin of the nuclei [Hematoxylin and eosin, x200]. (Images courtesy of Dr. Hwa Jeong Lee)

Neuroendocrine Tumors (NETs)

Neuroendocrine tumors of the small bowel are rare. The SEER (Surveillance, Epidemiology, and End Results) database reported an incidence of jejunal/ileal NETs of 0.67 per 100,000 per year [25]. The median age of diagnosis is 64 years, with most patients presenting with non-specific symptoms. Given their indolent course, 60–80% of patients with SB NETs have metastatic disease to the liver at the time of diagnosis [25]. The overall prognosis for locally advanced and metastatic small bowel NETs is favorable, with 10-year survival rates between 40–70% [26]. Treatment typically involves surgical resection for localized disease and/or soma-tostatin analogue therapy for metastatic disease [26, 27] (Fig. 7.5).

Sporadic Adenocarcinoma

Sporadic adenocarcinoma of the small bowel is also rare, with the majority of tumors occurring within the duodenum and with incidence decreasing distally throughout the jejunum and ileum. One exception is a significantly higher rate of ileal adenocarcinoma in Crohn's ileitis, though it should be noted that patients with CD in general have a 20–30 times higher rate of developing any SB adenocarcinoma [27]. The molecular phenotype of SB adenocarcinoma has been shown to be similar to that of colorectal adenocarcinoma with several similar molecular mutations involved in their malignant transformation [28]. Similar to NETs, the median age at diagnosis of SB adenocarcinoma is the sixth decade of life. Also, patients typically present with non-specific symptoms and are at an advanced disease stage at the time of diagnosis. Unfortunately, in contrast to NETs, the prognosis is generally poor, with a median 5-year survival of 10–40% for stage-III disease and 3–5% for stage-IV disease [27, 28]. Management typically involves surgical resection, with limited data available to guide adjuvant or neoadjuvant chemotherapy [27, 28].

Other Neoplastic Conditions

Several inherited conditions including Lynch syndrome, familial adenomatous polyposis, Peutz-Jeghers syndrome, MUTYH-associated polyposis, serrated polyposis syndrome, juvenile polyposis syndrome, and Cowden syndrome are associated with an increased risk of SB malignancies, highlighting the importance of prompt disease recognition and initiation of relevant screening protocols [29].

Primary gastrointestinal lymphoma is the most common extra-nodal presentation of lymphoma, with the majority of tumors located within the stomach and, less commonly, the small intestines. Management is typically similar to that of lymphomas arising from outside the GI tract [27].

Gastrointestinal stromal tumors (GISTs) are the most common type of mesenchymal tumor, up to a third of which occur within the small bowel (most commonly in the jejunum). They are characterized by a positive CD117 antigen with expression of c-kit receptor tyrosine kinase [27]. These tumors are most commonly benign, though tumor size, high mitotic rate, and presence of necrosis increase risk of malignancy. Treatment options include close observation, surgical resection, adjuvant/neoadjuvant imatinib, and/or locoregional therapy for liver metastasis [30] (Fig. 7.6).

Portal Hypertensive Bleeding

Portal hypertension (PH) is very common and develops secondary to a number of disorders, with cirrhosis being the most common etiology in western countries, and schistosomiasis and portal vein thrombosis the most common in non-western

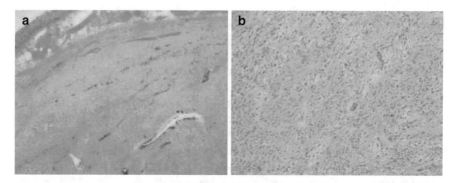

Fig. 7.6 (A on the left, B on the right) (**a**) GIST of the small bowel with involvement of the bowel wall [Hematoxylin and eosin, x40]. (**b**) Higher magnification of the same tumor showing the proliferation of spindle cells [Hematoxylin and eosin, x100]. (Images courtesy of Dr. Hwa Jeong Lee)

countries [31]. PH occurs due to increased resistance to portal blood flow secondary to structural and dynamic changes (vasoconstriction) within the liver and leads to an increase in the portal pressure gradient [31]. Increases in splanchnic blood flow result in systemic hypotension and angiogenesis, and often lead to formation of portosystemic collaterals (varices) and microcirculatory changes within the gastro-intestinal mucosa [31–33]. When varices form within the SB, they are referred to as ectopic or SB varices, and though they are rare (only 5% of all variceal bleeding), they may result in life-threatening overt bleeding [32, 33].

Alternatively, microcirculatory changes within the SB can occur secondary to portal hypertension and are referred to as portal hypertensive enteropathy (PHE). PHE commonly leads to occult bleeding [33]. The reported prevalence of PHE is variable (15–82% of cirrhotic patients), and should be suspected in advanced cirrhosis (Child-Pugh class C) in the presence of portal hypertensive gastropathy [33]. Endoscopically, PHE has a variable appearance, including mucosal edema, loss of vascularity, friability, mosaic-like pattern, inflammatory polyps, and angiodysplasia-like lesions. Unfortunately, histopathologic findings are non-specific and the diagnosis must be made in conjunction with other clinical data [33]. There is insufficient evidence to guide management at this time, though vasoactive medications (beta-blockers, octreotide), argon plasma coagulation, transvenous intrahepatic portosystemic shunting (TIPS), surgical resection of affected SB segment, and liver transplantation have all been described [33].

Celiac Disease

Though celiac disease has previously been thought to be a potential cause for occult SB bleeding with IDA, more recent data has suggested otherwise. A 2006 study using radiolabeled red blood cells, found no evidence of significant gastrointestinal blood loss in patients with untreated celiac disease, and at this time, IDA seen in patients with celiac disease is thought to be a result of intestinal iron malabsorption, rather than occult SB blood loss [37].

Diagnostic Work Up

Second-Look Endoscopy

A long list of factors can potentially influence the quality of any given endoscopic exam, including the endoscopist's experience, skill level or fatigue; the patient's clinical stability and movement; type of anesthetic used and complications related to anesthesia; the quality of bowel preparation and presence of food/blood within the lumen; as well as procedure environment, presence and quality of support staff, and the available equipment. Given these potential limitations, it is not surprising that a significant number of upper and lower GIB sources may be missed during initial endoscopic workup for occult GIB.

The incidence of a missed lesion within reach of a standard endoscope is between 10–40%, while that within reach of a standard colonoscope is between 2–14% [38–42]. The most commonly reported missed lesions are vascular lesions, but others include Cameron ulcers, portal hypertensive gastropathy, peptic ulcer disease, erosive mucosal disease (esophagitis, gastritis, duodenitis), and malignancy [38, 41, 42].

The decision regarding whether to perform a repeat upper and/or lower endoscopy before proceeding with a SB evaluation is complicated. As stated above, repeat upper endoscopy has been shown to have a higher diagnostic yield than repeat lower endoscopy. Factors which may affect this decision include the timing and quality of the prior procedure, the presence of blood or food in the upper GI tract, the quality of the prior colon preparation and the type and severity of bleeding. Repeat colonoscopy should always include an examination of the terminal ileum, to evaluate for a more proximal source of SB bleeding [42].

If the decision is made to repeat an evaluation of the proximal GI tract, consideration should be given to performing a push enteroscopy, where either a specialized commercially-available endoscope or pediatric colonoscope is used to perform a more extensive proximal SB evaluation (including the distal duodenum and proximal jejunum). Studies have demonstrated repeat evaluation with push enteroscopy to have a 38–70% higher diagnostic yield when compared with EGD alone [38, 39]. While a pediatric colonoscope can typically advance 45–60 cm beyond the ligament of Treitz, a push enteroscope may be advanced 70–90 cm beyond the ligament of Treitz if variable stiffness design is utilized [43, 44].

Video Capsule Endoscopy

Up until 2001, the SB was studied non-invasively using relatively ineffective radiographic and nuclear medicine modalities such as SB follow-through (SBFT), SB enteroclysis, CT, MRI, and radionuclide imaging. While CT and MRI without enterography can visualize abdominal masses, vasculature, and solid organs with high sensitivity and specificity, they are unable to provide adequate information regarding the small intestinal wall and the etiology for occult PSBB in most instances [45]. SBFT and SB enteroclysis specifically have been found to have low sensitivity and specificity in diagnosing SB sources of occult bleeding [46]. The introduction of video capsule endoscopy (VCE) in the United States in 2001 drastically changed the field of gastroenterology by allowing for near-complete non-invasive visualization of the entire SB mucosa in the majority of patients [45].

VCE is a procedure that involves swallowing or having endoscopically deployed a small capsule which contains a wireless camera programmed to take thousands of pictures as it traverses the GI tract. The size of a VCE varies by model but typically measures between 10–13 mm in diameter by 24–31 mm in length [47]. Most models incorporate a single camera lens associated with a 140–170-degree field of view, though one model has four different laterally-placed cameras with a reported 360-degree field of view. The capsule emits light and images are taken either at a predetermined frequency or, more recently, at an adaptive rate with fewer images taken during slower transit to avoid redundant imaging. Images are transmitted by radiofrequency to a wireless recorder carried by the patient and later interpreted by a physician [47].

Though most VCE manufacturers recommend a 12-hour clear liquid diet leading up to the study, a 2008 meta-analysis demonstrated superior SB visualization and diagnostic yield in patients who had undergone a bowel purge prior to VCE [48]. Low volume bowel purges provide a similar preparation quality when compared with higher volume preparations [49]. Medications that can cause gastroparesis, such as narcotics, anticholinergics, and antihistamines, should be discontinued 2–3 days prior to VCE administration. If this is not possible, pro-kinetic agents can be prescribed to reduce the risk of delayed gastric passage and an incomplete study [47].

A complete study is defined as the capsule reaching the cecum within the available recording time. Battery life ranges from 8–15 hours, with studies demonstrating an overall completion rate of 79–90% [45, 47]. The most important VCE complication to consider is capsule retention, defined as non-passage within 2 weeks, and which occurs in only 1–2% of those being evaluated for SB bleeding [47]. Though known SB luminal obstruction or ileus are the only absolute contraindications to VCE, caution should be exercised in patients with a history of abdominal radiation, heavy NSAID use, or a history of IBD, specifically Crohn's enteritis and bowel strictures, with a reported capsule retention rate of up to 13% in these cases. In patients at increased risk for capsule retention, luminal patency should first be demonstrated with either SB imaging or a patency capsule [47, 50]. Finally, intestinal perforation due to capsule impaction is very rare, with only a few cases reported [51–53].

PSBB remains the most common indication for performing VCE with a higher diagnostic yield observed in overt compared to occult SB bleeding [2, 54]. Other factors found to be predictive of a positive capsule study include test performance within 2 weeks of bleeding episode, male sex, age >60 years, cardiac and renal comorbidities, and inpatient status [2, 55, 56]. It should be noted that recent guidelines have supported a trial of oral iron supplementation prior to routine use of VCE in asymptomatic patients with IDA, though this recommendation is based upon very low quality evidence [35].

The widespread use of VCE as the initial diagnostic modality in PSBB is largely related to its high positive (94–97%) and negative predictive value (83–100%), though this data pertains to both occult and overt bleeding with data specific to occult bleeding not available [2, 54, 57]. The overall reported diagnostic yield of VCE in occult bleeding specifically following initial negative bidirectional endoscopy is variable and has been reported to range between 32–76% [58–61].

One possible explanation for this reported variability is that studies performed soon after introduction of VCE in 2001 included many patients with longstanding history of obscure GIB, associated with significant anemia and repeated negative testing due to limited diagnostic options. This likely resulted in a higher pre-test probability for SB lesions in this cohort of patients undergoing VCE. Recent larger studies showing a diagnostic yield of 50% is likely a more accurate reflection of current everyday clinical practice [45, 59].

Patient selection, including clinical factors such as type of bleeding (overt versus occult), presence of IDA, minimum hemoglobin value, previous transfusion requirements, and duration of suspected bleeding, have also been shown to significantly impact the diagnostic yield of VCE [62].

Several studies, including a large 2017 systematic review and meta-analysis, have demonstrated a low overall re-bleeding rate in GI bleeding following a negative VCE [63]. The indications or clinical benefit of a repeat VCE in the setting of occult bleeding following an initial non-diagnostic VCE remain controversial. Patients who may benefit from a repeat VCE include those with a further drop in hemoglobin >4 gm/dL, and/or a transition from occult to overt bleeding [64, 65]. In the absence of these criteria, there also has been no demonstrated improvement in the diagnostic yield of VCE when repeated immediately following an initial negative study [66].

Limitations of VCE include a moderate false positive rate, with findings reported in ~15% of healthy individuals [67] and a false negative rate between 10–36% [56, 68]. Of note, VCE has been reported to miss up to 56% of clinically important lesions within the duodenum and proximal jejunum, probably due to the greater transit speed of the capsule within the sharply angulated duodenal sweep and active peristalsis [69]. This known limitation lends additional support to performing push enteroscopy during second-look endoscopy to obtain a more thorough evaluation of the proximal SB.

Radiography of the SB

Despite the medical advances related to VCE described above, there is still no clear consensus on how best to proceed following non-diagnostic or ambiguous VCE results. While several older radiographic techniques (SBFT, SB enteroclysis, radionuclide imaging) offer limited diagnostic utility, more recent developments in cross-sectional imaging have helped CT enterography (CTE) and MR enterography (MRE) to emerge as useful diagnostic tools in certain clinical situations [59].

CTE has been shown to possess diagnostic utility in patients with SB bleeding. A large meta-analysis has shown an overall pooled diagnostic yield of about 40%, with a range between 13–83% for this modality in combined occult and overt PSBB, which is lower than that reported for VCE (see above) [59]. Given the significantly lower diagnostic yield, in the absence of contraindications to VCE, CTE has been utilized mostly as second-line diagnostic test for this indication.

In occult PSBB following a non-diagnostic VCE, the diagnostic utility of CTE is somewhat uncertain, but probably low. Following non-diagnostic VCE, several small studies have demonstrated a diagnostic yield between 0–15% in patients with occult bleeding specifically, whereas patients with overt bleeding were found to have a significantly higher yield between 50–67% [70, 71].

While VCE has been demonstrated to be superior to CTE in diagnosing SB vascular lesions [72–75], studies have shown CTE to be more accurate in diagnosing SB masses [73, 75, 76]. Specifically, studies of patients simultaneously undergoing both CTE and VCE have identified CTE to have a higher sensitivity and VCE to have a higher false positive rate in the evaluation of SB tumors [75, 76].

In general, while data have shown CTE and VCE to be complimentary diagnostic modalities in occult PSBB (i.e., CTE superior in diagnosing masses; VCE superior in diagnosing vascular abnormalities), the overall diagnostic yield of CTE is greater in overt compared to occult bleeding, and several studies have challenged the clinical necessity of reflexively following-up a non-diagnostic VCE study with CTE. Ultimately, clinical judgement must be used to guide study selection, with consideration given to patient age, persistent/progressive anemia, likelihood of SB malignancy, and patient preference.

Very few studies have investigated the use of MRE in evaluating SB sources of bleeding, but this modality may have a role in patients who have a contraindication to CT or when trying to limit radiation exposure. [72, 73]

Deep Enteroscopy

Deep enteroscopy is a combined diagnostic and therapeutic procedure involving an endoscopic evaluation of the proximal and distal SB, accomplished either by an oral or rectal approach. Deep enteroscopy is accomplished with either of two techniques: (i) balloon-assisted enteroscopy, including double-balloon enteroscopy (DBE) and single-balloon enteroscopy (SBE); and (ii) spiral enteroscopy (SE). This section will review the technique, diagnostic utility, and potential complications of these two approaches.

Balloon-Assisted Enteroscopy

DBE was first reported in 2001 by *Yamamoto et al*, and introduced in the United States for clinical practice in 2004 [77]. Shortly thereafter, SBE was introduced in the U.S. in 2007 [78]. A single- and double-balloon enteroscope can be inserted to a depth of 240–360 cm distal to the pylorus using the antegrade (oral) approach, and alternatively, up to 140 cm proximal to the ileocecal valve using the retrograde (rectal) approach. The standard accessory channel within each scope allows for passage of nearly all standard diagnostic and therapeutic endoscopic equipment [2]. DBE includes two latex balloons, one positioned on the distal end of an overtube and the second, on the distal end of the enteroscope. The SBE includes a silicone balloon at the distal end of an overtube but utilizes the tip of the enteroscope to anchor in place of a second balloon in DBE. Patients with a latex allergy should not undergo DBE [2].

Both DBE and SBE utilize the technique of push and pull enteroscopy, effectively shortening the SB to prevent looping, accomplished by drawing/pleating the SB back onto the enteroscope using the balloons, overtubes, and, in SBE specifically, enteroscope tip deflection [77].

Unfortunately, the overwhelming majority of studies investigating the diagnostic yield of balloon-assisted enteroscopy do not distinguish between occult and overt bleeding. However, based upon the select few studies which do specify outcomes, the diagnostic yield of DBE in occult bleeding following negative bidirectional endoscopy and VCE appears to range between 60–80% (Fig. 7.7) [79–82]. While there is conflicting data regarding the difference in diagnostic yield between occult and overt bleeding, several studies have demonstrated an overall lower diagnostic yield of DBE in patients with occult bleeding [2, 83–92].

Several meta-analyses have demonstrated similar diagnostic yields between VCE and DBE. One meta-analysis demonstrated pooled diagnostic yields in VCE and DBE of 61.4% and 56.3%, respectively [93]. Other data has shown that VCE and DBE diagnose vascular, inflammatory, and mass lesions in similar percentages of patients (24%/24%, 18%/16%, and 11%/11%, respectively) [1]. Given VCE commonly precedes DBE, with its result being available to the endoscopists performing DBE, one might expect a detection bias to affect the reported diagnostic yields of DBE. However, in two small studies comparing the diagnostic yields of VCE and DBE in which the endoscopists were blinded to the results of VCE, the

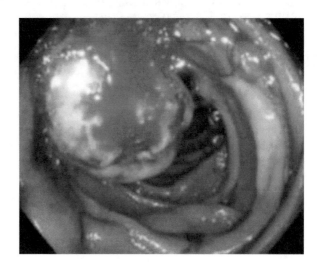

Fig. 7.7 A friable, ulcerated, and bleeding proximal small bowel tumor identified during double-balloon enteroscopy in a patient with iron-deficiency anemia and prior negative EGD, colonoscopy, and video capsule endoscopy. Biopsies confirmed the diagnosis of GIST. (Image courtesy of Micheal Tadros, M.D)

pooled data demonstrated no significant difference in diagnostic yield between the two methods [94–96].

The diagnostic yield of DBE in combined overt and occult bleeding has been shown to increase significantly when preceded by a positive VCE, a diagnostic sequence referred to as 'VCE-guided DBE' or 'targeted DBE' [88, 96]. On the other hand, data has demonstrated significantly lower diagnostic yields in DBE following a non-diagnostic VCE, ranging between 27.5–39.6% [88, 97].

Given the similar diagnostic yields of VCE and DBE, the high positive and negative predictive value of VCE in preceding DBE, along with the more invasive nature of DBE, VCE should be performed first in the vast majority of patients with occult PSBB.

Similar to DBE, there is very little data describing outcomes of SBE in patients with occult PSBB, specifically. Based upon the few studies that do specify outcomes in occult bleeding, the diagnostic yield ranges between 52–67% [98–100]. When evaluating patients with occult or overt PSBB, SBE has been demonstrated to have a similar diagnostic yield compared to DBE [99–106]. Interestingly, the diagnostic yield of enteroscopy has not been shown to correlate with length of SB visualized and complete enteroscopy is often unnecessary [103, 106].

The main limitations of both DBE and SBE are their invasive nature, prolonged procedural time, and need for additional endoscopic personnel [2]. However, these procedures have been demonstrated to have low rates of complication overall [2, 86, 87]. Most of the available data regarding frequency of adverse events is based upon DBE, which may also apply to SBE. According to the ASGE technology committee, the most common adverse events experienced following DBE include pancreatitis, bleeding, ileus, and perforation, occurring in between 1.2–1.6% of cases. Specifically, pancreatitis has been reported in 0.3% and perforation in between 0.3–0.4% of cases, most often occurring following large polypectomies. Complication rates can be higher (up to 4%) when therapeutic interventions are performed or with a history of surgically altered anatomy. Complications following SBE are also rare and include abdominal pain, fever, mucosal tears, bleeding, pancreatitis, and perforation. Perforation, specifically, has been reported in about 0.3% of SBE cases [2, 87]. A 2017 meta-analysis comparing DBE and SBE showed no significant difference in complication profiles [86].

Spiral Enteroscopy

Developed in 2007, SE is a unique method of examining the SB, which utilizes a disposable overtube with soft raised spiral ridges rather than balloons. A single- or double-balloon enteroscope can be used along with this overtube, though the enteroscope balloons are not needed during the procedure. The enteroscope is advanced through the SB with the assistance of a second person, who continuously rotates the spiral overtube in a clockwise fashion, slowly drawing the SB over the overtube, while the endoscopist keeps the enteroscope tip centered within the intestinal lumen.

As with DBE and SBE, this procedure can be performed via both the antegrade (oral) or retrograde (rectal) approach [2, 87].

In studies looking at both occult and overt bleeding, SE has a reported diagnostic yield of between 33–59% [87, 107, 108]. Despite this lower reported yield, a 2017 meta-analysis comparing balloon enteroscopy (DBE and SBE) and SE found no significant difference in diagnostic yield between these techniques [109].

Although pooled data has identified no significant difference between balloon-assisted and SE in depth of maximal insertion, significantly shorter procedural time has been reported with SE [109, 110]. Similar to balloon-assisted enteroscopy, SE has been very well tolerated overall. More common potential adverse events include mucosal tearing and abrasions. Perforation has been reported in about 0.3% of cases. There have been no reported cases of pancreatitis [2, 87].

In patients with occult PSBB, there are several indications for pursuing deep enteroscopy, including a positive VCE requiring endoscopic intervention or tissue sampling, unclear diagnosis with contraindication to VCE, and negative VCE with high clinical suspicion for SB pathology [2]. While the management of patients with occult bleeding following a negative VCE study remains largely unclear at this time, with some data supporting close observation or repeat VCE study, total enteroscopy with DBE/either balloon-assisted or spiral enteroscopy may be pursued if there is a high clinical suspicious for a SB lesion.

Radionuclide Imaging of the SB

Although much less commonly utilized in the workup of obscure PSBB, radionuclide imaging techniques can be considered under proper circumstances. Generally, radionuclide imaging is the generation of images that detect the radioactive emissions (scintigraphy) of an injected radionuclide tracer that is taken up into different tissues at differing rates [111].

Occult SB bleeding occurs infrequently due to a bleeding Meckel's diverticulum (MD), which is typically worked up with the technetium-99 m (^{99m}Tc) pertechnate scan (commonly referred to as the Meckel's scan). This type of scintigraphy is effective because of the tracer's ability to concentrate within ectopic gastric mucosa, often present within a MD. Due to this tracer quality, Meckel's scans will typically be falsely positive in gut duplication cysts [34]. As bleeding is more common in children than adults with MD, the scan has a higher diagnostic yield in children [34, 112, 113].

Scintigraphy using ^{99m}Tc–labeled red blood cells (commonly referred as a 'tagged red blood cell scan') has been commonly utilized to workup suspected overt GI bleeding, though has a limited role in the workup of occult bleeding. Advantages of ^{99m}Tc-labeled RBC scintigraphy include non-invasive nature, identification of both arterial and venous bleeding, recognition of delayed bleeding through use of delayed imaging, and detection of very slow rates of active bleeding (as low as 0.1 mL/minutes in some studies). Studies investigating the clinical utility of this test have reported a wide range of sensitivity (33–93%), specificity (30–95%), and diagnostic yield (26–87%) in the workup of GI bleeding, with increased difficulty localizing bleeding sources within the stomach or SB [2, 111, 114]. Furthermore, all studies investigating diagnostic yield have been performed in patients with acute or overt GI bleeding, rather than chronic occult bleeding, [115–120] and given the slower rate of chronic blood loss in occult GIB, the overall clinical utility of the scan would be very limited.

Missed Lesions of the SB

While recent advances in small bowel diagnostics have revolutionized our ability to identify and treat symptomatic and otherwise worrisome small bowel lesions, physicians need to remain aware of the potential for missed lesions. While VCE does have a high negative predictive value, it also carries a false negative rate of between 10–36% [68]. Missed lesions with VCE can occur in a few ways: the video capsule may not reach the cecum (incomplete study or capsule retention), the capsule may fail to capture necessary images, and/or physicians may misinterpret the images obtained. CT enterography has also been demonstrated to have higher sensitivity for small bowel luminal masses, and should be pursued following negative VCE, if appropriate clinical suspicion exists for such a mass [73, 75, 76]. While the sensitivity and negative predictive value of balloon- and spiral-enteroscopy for occult bleeding have not been reported, these procedures carry a wide (likely operator-dependent) diagnostic yield.

Overall, as there is limited literature available to guide when to repeat a diagnostic study following an initial negative result, providers should use their clinical suspicion to direct subsequent workup. Close attention should be paid to the quality of the index diagnostic test, patients' clinical presentation, laboratory abnormalities, disease course, and response to therapy, patient risk factors for alternate potential underlying etiologies, and development of overt GI bleeding or other new GI symptoms.

Treatment of Occult Bleeding of the SB

Given the broad array of possible diagnoses that can lead to SB bleeding, treatment options are typically tailored to specific pathology, and as a result are equally variable. Potential treatment options for small bowel neoplasia include surgical resection, chemotherapy, radiation, and palliation, with specific management recommendations dependent upon tumor type, metastasis, complications, and patient factors [27]. The management of small intestinal Crohn's disease involves a shifting balance between immunosuppressive therapy and surgical resection, while the treatment of choice for a symptomatic MD is surgical excision [34]. This section will focus on the treatment of vascular lesions within the SB, the most common etiology of occult SB bleeding. While SB vascular lesions thought to be the source of blood loss can be treated with endoscopic therapy, pharmacologic therapy, or close observation, there is very limited data on efficacy of these treatment modalities, with available studies demonstrating overall disappointing reduction in rates of subsequent bleeding [2].

The natural history of occult GIB due to untreated small bowel angiodysplasia (SBAD) has been difficult to define, partly because it is challenging to define an occult bleeding event, and also due to the unethical nature of withholding potentially life-saving therapeutic procedures from patients with bleeding. However, data from the placebo arm of a 2010 trial found rebleeding rates of only 18–21% within 12 months in untreated patients initially presenting with occult bleeding [121]. This is compared with a much higher recurrence rate of 49.2%, reported in a cohort of patients with SBAD presenting with either occult or overt bleeding [122].

Endoscopic Therapy of SB Lesions

While the advent of VCE has significantly improved our diagnostic ability in occult PSBB, the subsequent introduction of balloon-assisted and SE has enabled physicians to intervene upon vascular lesions in the SB. Double-balloon, single-balloon, and spiral enteroscopes are capable of passing nearly all standard diagnostic and therapeutic endoscopic through-the-scope equipment, enabling the endoscopist to perform tissue biopsy, tattoo, hemostasis (using argon plasma coagulation (APC), electrocautery, hemostatic clips), snare polypectomy, balloon dilatation, and foreign body removal (Fig. 7.8) [2].

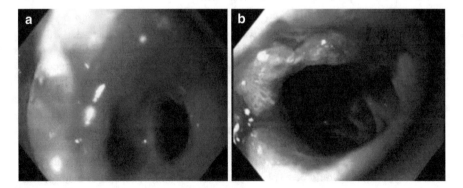

Fig. 7.8 (A on the left, B on the right): (**a**) NSAIDS induced diaphragm-like small bowel stricture identified during double balloon enteroscopy in a patient with occult GI bleeding and a history of heavy chronic NSAID use. (**b**) The same stricture after successful through-the-scope balloon dilation. (Images courtesy of Micheal Tadros, M.D)

The overall therapeutic yield for DBE has been reported to be between 15–55% which is similar to what has been reported for SBE (7–50%) [87]. Pooled data has also shown no significant difference in therapeutic yield between balloon-assisted and spiral enteroscopy [109].

Most studies have used 'recurrence of bleeding' as an indicator to assess the efficacy of the interventions, with disappointing results. A recent systematic review demonstrated a high rate of recurrent bleeding, with no significant difference in recurrence following endoscopically-treated AD (42.7%) versus untreated AD (49.2%) over a mean follow-up of almost 2 years [122, 123]. Risk of recurrent bleeding is greater in the presence of multiple vascular lesions and also appears to increase with time elapsed since endoscopic therapy [124, 125].

Although there is no consensus on the most effective type of endoscopic therapy in treatment of SBAD, argon plasma coagulation (APC) is the most commonly utilized technique [126]. APC is a non-contact thermal coagulation technique utilizing a stream of ionized argon gas directed through an endoscopic probe, resulting in superficial coagulation at a depth of 0.5–3 mm [126]. Rates of recurrent bleeding following APC therapy in SBAD have also been shown to be high (42%) [127]. Electrocautery of AD, where current is delivered through tissue to achieve coagulation, was the standard of care in the 1980s prior to the introduction of APC, but is now mainly used as a second line treatment modality for SBAD, due to the reported increased risk of perforation (~3%) [126, 128]. Hemostatic clip placement for treatment of AD in the stomach or colon has been described in case reports, though not in SBAD specifically. Hemostatic clips can be used alone or in combination with other techniques [129, 130]. To this point, there are no prospective, randomized studies comparing the different techniques described above, though expert opinion favors APC as first line endoscopic therapy [126].

Medical Therapy of SB Occult Bleeding

A significant proportion of patients with occult SB bleeding due to AD will have associated IDA. This can be addressed with iron supplementation, although some patients may need packed red blood cell (pRBC) transfusion and/or correction of underlying coagulopathies, with the ultimate goal being normalization of hemoglobin and iron stores [126]. Oral iron therapy should be considered in patients with normal intestinal absorptive capacity and absent intestinal inflammation, though patients need to be monitored closely for treatment failure. Intravenous iron supplementation should be considered in patients with suspected intestinal inflammation and/or malabsorption, side effects to oral iron, or when rapid repletion of iron stores is needed [126]. As would be expected, data from the placebo arm of a single randomized controlled trial showed little to no improvement in frequency of recurrent bleeding from vascular lesions in patients who received oral iron administered four times daily [131]. Transfusions of pRBC can be essential and should be considered in acutely ill or symptomatic patients (especially those with cardiovascular comorbidities), patients who have failed other medical or endoscopic therapy, and patients who require medical optimization prior to scheduled endoscopic procedures.

Several studies in the 1990s demonstrated conflicting evidence regarding the clinical benefit of hormonal therapy for the treatment of bleeding gastrointestinal AD, generating some interest in their use at that time [132–134]. However, a well-designed study performed in 2001 demonstrated hormonal therapy to be ineffective, with no significant reduction in rates of recurrent bleeding, total number of bleeding episodes, or transfusion requirements between patients on ethinylestradiol or norethisterone versus placebo [135]. Hormonal therapy is not currently recommended for the treatment of SB bleeding from AD [2].

Somatostatin analogs were first investigated as treatment for bleeding AD in 1999 and are thought to work by decreasing splanchnic blood flow, decreasing angiogenesis, and increasing platelet aggregation [136, 137]. Several other studies have demonstrated promising findings since. A 2012 study showed significantly lowered rates of recurrent bleeding from gastrointestinal AD in a small cohort of patients with refractory bleeding treated with long-acting somatostatin analog therapy (73% pre-treatment vs. 20% during treatment) [138]. In a more recent 2016 study, 70% of patients with refractory bleeding from SBAD demonstrated a complete response (no re-bleeding or transfusion requirements) and 20% a partial response (>50% reduction in re-bleeding/transfusion) while on long-acting somatostatin analog therapy, with a significant rise in median hemoglobin levels [139]. Systematic reviews performed in 2010 and 2014 support these findings and restate the importance of somatostatin analog therapy in refractory disease, while at least one multicenter, randomized superiority study (the OCEAN trial) is underway at this time, [123, 140, 141].

Thalidomide has recently generated interest as a treatment for refractory SBAD, despite concerns related to its side effect profile. The mechanism of action in the treatment of bleeding AD is thought to be due to antiangiogenic properties related to suppression of VEGF [131, 142]. In a 2011 randomized controlled trial of patients with refractory bleeding due to gastrointestinal AD, more than 70% of patients treated with thalidomide achieved the primary end point of >50% reduction in bleeding episodes, compared with only 4% of patients treated with iron supplementation. Serum levels of VEGF were significantly reduced during treatment with thalidomide, supporting the proposed mechanism of drug action [131]. The same study group went on to report the long-term outcomes of thalidomide therapy from the above patient cohort. Over a median follow-up period of 46.2 months, a greater than 50% reduction in bleeding episodes was reported in 79.5% of patients [143].

Surgical Therapy of SB Occult Bleeding

Surgical management of occult SB bleeding is now rarely indicated. However, prior to the introduction of VCE and deep enteroscopy, intraoperative enteroscopy (IOE) was considered a gold-standard first-line investigation in patients with PSBB, achieving complete SB evaluation in the majority of patients [144]. Several studies recommend IOE as a crucial step in localizing bleeding site, sometimes in combination with VCE, prior to performing a targeted endoscopic intervention or surgical resection [2, 145, 146]. Published patient series have demonstrated higher diagnostic yields in ongoing overt bleeding (100%), when compared with previous overt bleeding (70%) and occult bleeding (50%), with IOE leading to an endoscopic or surgical therapeutic intervention in between 40–100% of cases [144]. Reported mortality rates have varied between 2–17%, though considerable morbidity related to surgical and non-surgical complications can also occur [144, 147, 148].

There are limited data on long-term outcomes for patients undergoing IOE. One study described a 30% re-bleeding rate in patients with both occult and overt bleeding [149]. Similar re-bleeding rates may be expected even when endoscopic techniques such as APC are employed during IOE to achieve hemostasis [2]. Given the similar rate of re-bleeding and higher procedure-related morbidity and mortality, IOE is reserved for those patients with recurrent severe SB bleeding who have failed less invasive methods. In patients with Heyde's syndrome – the presence of aortic valve stenosis and gastrointestinal AD – there may be a role for performing aortic valve replacement [123].

Conclusions

Occult small bowel bleeding remains a relatively uncommon condition. While vascular lesions are the most common etiology, the differential diagnosis is long. Few studies have focused specifically on the diagnosis and treatment of occult bleeding in particular, and though the workup is similar to that of overt bleeding, including second-look endoscopy, push enteroscopy, VCE, and deep enteroscopy as appropriate, the diagnostic and therapeutic yields are typically lower than what has been reported with overt bleeding. As the risk for recurrent bleeding following appropriate endoscopic therapy remains significant, concomitant medical therapy, such as iron supplementation, pRBC transfusion, somatostatin analogs, and thalidomide, need to be considered in some cases, although additional prospective data will be helpful in the future to better define its role. Surgical management should be reserved for those patients with disease refractory to endoscopic and medical therapy.

References

1. Pasha SF, Leighton JA, Das A, et al. Double-balloon enteroscopy and capsule endoscopy have comparable diagnostic yield in small-bowel disease: a meta-analysis. Clin Gastroenterol Hepatol. 2008;6:671–6.
2. Gerson L, et al. ACG clinical guideline: diagnosis and Management of Small Bowel Bleeding. Am J Gastroenterol. 2015;110:1265–87.

3. Rockey DC. Occult gastrointestinal bleeding. Gastroenterol Clin N Am. 2005;34(4):699–718.
4. Lane L, et al. Does capsule endoscopy improve outcomes in obscure gastrointestinal bleeding? Randomized trial versus dedicated small bowel radiography. Gastroenterology. 2010 May;138(5):1673–80.
5. Koh SJ, Im JP, Kim JW, et al. Long-term outcome in patients with obscure gastrointestinal bleeding after negative capsule endoscopy. World J Gastroenterol. 2013;19:1632–8.
6. Cangemi DJ, Patel MK, Gomez V, et al. Small bowel tumors discovered during double-balloon enteroscopy: analysis of a large prospectively collected single-center database. J Clin Gastroenterol. 2013;47:769–72.
7. Schmulewitz N, Baillie J. Dieulafoy lesions: a review of 6 years of experience at a tertiary referral center. Am J Gastroenterol. 2001;96:688–94.
8. Sakai E, Ohata K, Nakajima A, et al. Diagnosis and therapeutic strategies for small bowel vascular lesions. World J Gastroenterol. 2019 Jun 14;25(22):2720–33.
9. Zammit SC, Koulaouzidis A, Sanders DS, et al. Overview of small bowel angioectasias: clinical presentation and treatment options. Expert Rev Gastroenterol Hepatol. 2018;12(2):125–39.
10. Raju GS, Gerson L, Das A, et al. American Gastroenterological Association (AGA) institute medical position statement on obscure gastrointestinal bleeding. Gastroenterology. 2007;133:1694–6.
11. Liao Z, Gao R, Xu C, et al. Indications and detection, completion, and retention rates of small bowel capsule endoscopy: a systematic review. Gastrointest Endosc. 2010;71:280–6.
12. Igawa A, Oka S, Tanaka S, et al. Major predictors and management of small-bowel angioectasia. BMC Gastroenterol. 2015;15:108.
13. Karagiannis S, Goulas S, Kosmadakis G, et al. Wireless capsule endoscopy in the investigation of patients with chronic renal failure and obscure gastrointestinal bleeding (preliminary data). World J Gastroenterol. 2006;12:5182–5.
14. Holleran G, Hall B, Hussey M, et al. Small bowel angiodysplasia and novel disease associations: a cohort study. Scand J Gastroenterol. 2013;48:433–8.
15. Ohmori T, Konishi H, Nakamura S, et al. Abnormalities of the small intestine detected by capsule endoscopy in haemodialysis patients. Intern Med. 2012;51:1455–60.
16. Gunjan D, Sharma V, Rana SS, et al. Small bowel bleeding: a comprehensive review. Gastroenterol Rep (Oxf). 2014 Nov;2(4):262–75.
17. King RM, Pluth JR, Giuliani ER, et al. The association of unexplained gastrointestinal bleeding with calcific aortic stenosis. Ann Thorac Surg. 1987;44:514–6.
18. Thompson JL, Schaff HV, Dearani JA, et al. Risk of recurrent gastrointestinal bleeding after aortic valve replacement in patients with Heyde syndrome. J Thorac Cardiovasc Surg. 2012;144:112–6.
19. Shrode CW, Draper KV, Huang RJ, et al. Significantly higher rates of gastrointestinal bleeding and thromboembolic events with left ventricular assist devices. Clin Gastroenterol Hepatol. 2014;12:1461–7.
20. Norton ID, Petersen BT, Sorbi D, et al. Management and long-term prognosis of Dieulafoy lesion. Gastrointest Endosc. 1999;50:762–7.
21. Lee YT, Walmsley RS, Leong RW, et al. Dieulafoy's lesion. Gastrointest Endosc. 2003;58:236–43.
22. Torres J, Mehandru S, Colombel JF, et al. Crohn's disease. Lancet. 2017;389(10080):1741–55.
23. Lichtenstein GR, Loftus EV, Isaacs KL, et al. ACG clinical guidelines: management of Crohn's disease in adults. Am J Gastroenterol. 2018;113(4):481–517.
24. Srinivasan A, De Cruz P. A practical approach to the clinical management of NSAID enteropathy. Scand J Gastroenterol. 2017;52(9):941–7.
25. Byrne RM, Pommier RF. Small bowel and colorectal carcinoids. Cli Colon Rectal Surg. 2018;31(5):301–8.
26. Kunz PL, Reidy-Lagunes D, Anthony LB, et al. Consensus guidelines for the management and treatment of neuroendocrine tumors. Pancreas. 2013;42(4):557–77.
27. Pourmand K, Itzkowitz SH. Small bowel neoplasms and polyps. Curr Gastroenterol Rep. 2016;18:23.

28. Aparicio T, Zaanan A, Mary F, et al. Small bowel adenocarcinoma. Gastroenterol Clinic North Am. 2016;45(3):447–57.
29. Syngal S, Brand RE, Church JM, et al. ACG clinical guideline: genetic testing and management of hereditary gastrointestinal cancer syndromes. Am J Gastroenterol. 2015;110(2):223–62.
30. Lim KT, Tan KY. Current research and treatment for gastrointestinal stromal tumors. World J Gastroenterol. 2017;23(27):4856–66.
31. Berzigotti A, Seijo S, Reverter E, et al. Assessing portal hypertension in liver diseases. Expert Rev Gastroenterol Hepatol. 2013;7(2):141–55.
32. Sato T. Treatment of ectopic varices with portal hypertension. World J Hepatol. 2015;7(12):1601–5.
33. Mekaroonkamol P, Cohen R, Chawla S. Portal hypertensive enteropathy. World J Hepatol. 2015;7(2):127–38.
34. Sagar J, Kumar V, Shah DK. Meckel's diverticulum: a systematic review. J R Soc Med. 2006;99:501–5.
35. Ko CW, Siddique SM, Patel A, et al. AGA clinical practice guidelines on the gastrointestinal evaluation of iron deficiency anemia. Gastro. 2020;S0016-5085(20)34847-2
36. Schwartz GD, Barkin JS. Small bowel tumors. Gastrointest Endoscopy Clin N Am. 2006;16:267–75.
37. Mant MJ, Bain VG, Maguire CG, et al. Prevalence of occult gastrointestinal bleeding in celiac disease. Clin Gastroenterol Hepatol. 2006;4:451–4.
38. Zaman A, Katon RM. Push enteroscopy for obscure gastrointestinal bleeding yields a high incidence of proximal lesions within reach of a standard endoscope. Gastrointest Endosc. 1998;47:372–6.
39. Lara LF, Bloomfeld RS, Pineau BC. The rate of lesions found within reach of esophagogastroduodenoscopy during push enteroscopy depends on the type of obscure gastrointestinal bleeding. Endoscopy. 2005;37:745–50.
40. Fry LC, Bellutti M, Neumann H, et al. Incidence of bleeding lesions within reach of conventional upper and lower endoscopes in patients undergoing double balloon enteroscopy for obscure gastrointestinal bleeding. Aliment Pharmacol Ther. 2009;29:342–9.
41. van Turenhout ST, Jacobs MA, van Weyenberg SJ, et al. Diagnostic yield of capsule endoscopy in a tertiary hospital in patients with obscure gastrointestinal bleeding. J Gastrointestin Liver Dis. 2010;19:141–5.
42. Gerson L. Small bowel bleeding: updated algorithm and outcomes. Gastrointest Endoscopy Clin N Am. 2017;27:171–80.
43. Foutch PG, Sawyer R, Sanowski RA. Push-enteroscopy for diagnosis of patients with gastrointestinal bleeding of obscure origin. Gastrointest Endosc. 1990;36:337–41.
44. Harewood GC, Gostout CJ, Farrell MA, et al. Prospective controlled assessment of variable stiffness enteroscopy. Gastrointest Endosc. 2003;58:267–71.
45. Rondonotti E, Villa F, Mulder CJ, et al. Small bowel capsule endoscopy in 2007: indications, risks and limitations. World J Gastroenterol. 2007;13:6140–9.
46. Liangpunsakul S, Maglinte DD, Rex DK. Comparison of wireless capsule endoscopy and conventional radiologic methods in the diagnosis of small bowel disease. Gastrointest Endosc Clin N Am. 2004;14:43–50.
47. Barkin JA, Barkin JS. Video capsule endoscopy: technology, reading, and troubleshooting. Gastrointest Endoscopy Clin N Am. 2017;27:15–27.
48. Rokkas T, Papaxoinis K, Triantafyllou K, et al. Does purgative preparation influence the diagnostic yield of small bowel video capsule endoscopy?: a meta-analysis. Am J Gastroenterol. 2009 Jan;104(1):219–27.
49. Park SC, Keum B, Seo YS, et al. Effect of bowel preparation with polyethylene glycol on quality of capsule endoscopy. Dig Dis Sci. 2011;56(6):1769–75.
50. Cheifetz AS, Kornbluth AA, Legnani P, et al. The risk of retention of the capsule endoscope in patients with known or suspected Crohn's disease. Am J Gastroenterol. 2006;101:2218–22.
51. Repici A, Barbon V, De Angelis C, et al. Acute small-bowel perforation secondary to capsule endoscopy. Gastrointest Endosc. 2008;67:180–3.

52. Simon M, Barge S, Jeune F, et al. Small-bowel perforation caused by AdvanCE capsule endoscopy delivery device. Endoscopy. 2016;0(48(S01)):E342.
53. Skovsen AP, Burcharth J, Burgdorf SK. Capsule endoscopy: a cause of late small bowel obstruction and perforation. Case Rep Surg. 2013:458108.
54. Pennazio M, Santucci R, Rondonotti E, et al. Outcome of patients with obscure gastrointestinal bleeding after capsule endoscopy: report of 100 consecutive cases. Gastroenterology. 2004;126:643–53.
55. Bresci G, Parisi G, Bertoni M, et al. The role of video capsule endoscopy for evaluating obscure gastrointestinal bleeding: usefulness of early use. J Gastroenterol. 2005;40:256–9.
56. Lepileur L, Dray X, Antonietti M, et al. Factors associated with diagnosis of obscure gastrointestinal bleeding by video capsule enteroscopy. Clin Gastroenterol Hepatol. 2012;10:1376–80.
57. Delvaux M, et al. Clinical usefulness of the endoscopic video capsule as the initial intestinal investigation in patients with obscure digestive bleeding: validation of a diagnostic strategy based on the patient outcome after 12 months. Endoscopy. 2004;36(12):1067–73.
58. Koulaouzidis A, Rondonotti E, Giannakou A, et al. Diagnostic yield of small-bowel capsule endoscopy in patients with iron-deficiency anemia: a systematic review. Gastrointest Endosc. 2012;76:983–92.
59. Fireman Z, Kopelman Y. The role of video capsule endoscopy in the evaluation of iron deficiency anaemia. Dig and Liver Disease. 2004;36:97–102.
60. Apostolopoulos P, Liatsos C, Gralnek IM, et al. The role of wireless capsule endoscopy in investigating unexplained iron deficiency anemia after negative endoscopic evaluation of the upper and lower gastrointestinal tract. Endoscopy. 2006;38(11):1127–32.
61. Sturniolo GC, DiLeo V, Vettorato MG, et al. Small bowel exploration by wireless capsule endoscopy: results from 314 procedures. Am J Med. 2006;119:341–7.
62. May A, Wardak A, Nachbar L, et al. Influence of patient selection on the outcome of capsule endoscopy in patients with chronic gastrointestinal bleeding. J Clin Gastroenterol. 2005;39:684–8.
63. Yung DE, Koulaouxidis A, Avni T, et al. Clinical outcomes of negative small-bowel capsule endoscopy for small-bowel bleeding: a systematic review and meta-analysis. Gastrointest Endosc. 2017 Feb;85(2):305–17.
64. Viazis N, Papaxoinis K, Vlachogiannakos J, et al. Is there a role for second-look capsule endoscopy in patients with obscure GI bleeding after a nondiagnostic first test? Gastrointest Endosc. 2009;69:850–6.
65. Robertson AR, Yung DE, Douglas S, et al. Repeat capsule endoscopy in suspected gastrointestinal bleeding. Scand J Gastroenterol. 2019 May;54(5):656–61.
66. Min BH, Chang DK, Kim BJ, et al. Does back-to-back capsule endoscopy increase the diagnostic yield over a single examination in patients with obscure gastrointestinal bleeding? Gut Liver. 2010;4:54–9.
67. Goldstein JL, Eisen GM, Lewis B, et al. Video capsule endoscopy to prospectively assess small bowel injury with celecoxib, naproxen plus omeprazole, and placebo. Clin Gastroenterol Hepatol. 2005;3:133–41.
68. Appleyard M, Fireman Z, Glukhovsky A, et al. A randomized trial comparing wireless capsule endoscopy with push enteroscopy for the detection of small-bowel lesions. Gastroenterology. 2000;119:1431–8.
69. Kong H, Kim YS, Hyun JJ, et al. Limited ability of capsule endoscopy to detect normally positioned duodenal papilla. Gastrointest Endosc. 2006 Oct;64(4):538–41.
70. Huprich JE, Fletcher JG, Alexander JA, et al. Obscure gastrointestinal bleeding: evaluation with 64-section multiphase CT enterography—initial experience. Radiology. 2008;246:562–71.
71. Agrawal JR, Travis AC, Mortele KJ, et al. Diagnostic yield of dual-phase computed tomography enterography in patients with obscure gastrointestinal bleeding and a non-diagnostic capsule endoscopy. J Gastroenterol Hepatol. 2012;27:75–9.
72. Bocker U, Dinter D, Litterer C, et al. Comparison of magnetic resonance imaging and video capsule enteroscopy in diagnosing small-bowel pathology: localization-dependent diagnostic yield. Scand J Gastroenterol. 2010;45:490–500.

73. Wiarda BM, Heine DG, Mensink P, et al. Comparison of magnetic resonance enteroclysis and capsule endoscopy with balloon-assisted enteroscopy in patients with obscure gastrointestinal bleeding. Endoscopy. 2012;44:668–73.
74. Leighton JA, Triester SL, Sharma VK. Capsule endoscopy: a meta-analysis for use with obscure gastrointestinal bleeding and Crohn's disease. Gastrointest Endosc Clin N Am. 2006;16:229–50.
75. Huprich JE, Fletcher JG, Fidler JL, et al. Prospective blinded comparison of wireless capsule endoscopy and multiphase CT enterography in obscure gastrointestinal bleeding. Radiology. 2011;260:744–51.
76. Khalife S, Soyer P, Alatawi A, et al. Obscure gastrointestinal bleeding: preliminary comparison of 64-section CT enteroclysis with video capsule endoscopy. Eur Radiol. 2011;21:79–86.
77. Yamamoto H, Sekine Y, Sato Y, et al. Total enteroscopy with a nonsurgical steerable double-balloon method. Gastrointest Endosc. 2001;53:216–20.
78. Gerson L. Outcomes associated with deep enteroscopy. Gastrointest Endoscopy Clin N Am. 2009;19:481–96.
79. Ohmiya N, Yano T, Yamamoto H, et al. Diagnosis and treatment of obscure GI bleeding at double balloon endoscopy. Gastrointest Endosc. 2007;66:S72–7.
80. Shinozaki S, Yamamoto H, Yano T, et al. Long-term outcome of patients with obscure gastrointestinal bleeding investigated by double-balloon endoscopy. Clin Gastroenterol Hepatol. 2010;8:151–8.
81. Sun B, Rajan E, Cheng S, et al. Diagnostic yield and therapeutic impact of double-balloon enteroscopy in a large cohort of patients with obscure gastrointestinal bleeding. Am J Gastroenterol. 2006;101:2011–5.
82. Chen LH, Chen WG, Cao HJ, et al. Double-balloon enteroscopy for obscure gastrointestinal bleeding: a single center experience in China. World J Gastroenterol. 2010 Apr 7;16(13):1655–9.
83. May A, Nachbar L, Ell C, et al. Double-balloon enteroscopy (push-and-pull enteroscopy) of the small bowel: feasibility and diagnostic and therapeutic yield in patients with suspected small bowel disease. Gastrointest Endosc. 2005;62:62–70.
84. Gross SA, Stark ME. Initial experience with double-balloon enteroscopy at a U.S. center. Gastrointest Endosc. 2008;67:890–7.
85. Yamamoto H, Kita H, Sunada K, et al. Clinical outcomes of double-balloon endoscopy for the diagnosis and treatment of small-intestinal diseases. Clin Gastroenterol Hepatol. 2004;2:1010–6.
86. Kim TJ, Kim ER, Chang DK, et al. Comparison of the efficacy and safety of single- versus double-balloon enteroscopy performed by endoscopist experts in single-balloon enteroscopy: a single-center experience and meta-analysis. Gut Liver. 2017 Jul 15;11(4):520–7.
87. ASGE Technology Committee. Chauhan SS, Manfredi MA, et al. Enteroscopy. Gastrointest Endosc. 2015;82:975–90.
88. Brito HP, Ribeiro IB, de Moura DTH, et al. Video capsule endoscopy vs double-balloon enteroscopy in the diagnosis of small bowel bleeding: a systematic review and meta-analysis. World J Gastrointest Endosc. 2018 Dec;10(12):400–21.
89. Shiani A, Nieves J, Lipka S, et al. Degree of concordance between single balloon enteroscopy and capsule endoscopy for obscure gastrointestinal bleeding after an initial positive capsule endoscopy finding. Ther Adv Gastroenterol. 2016;9:13–8.
90. Carey EJ, Fleischer DE. Investigation of the small bowel in gastrointestinal bleeding--enteroscopy and capsule endoscopy. Gastroenterol Clin N Am. 2005;34:719–34.
91. Gerson LB, Van Dam J. Wireless capsule endoscopy and double-balloon enteroscopy for the diagnosis of obscure gastrointestinal bleeding. Tech Vasc Interv Radiol. 2004;7:130–5.
92. Shelnut DJ, Sims OT, Zaibaq JN, et al. Predictors for outcomes and readmission rates following double balloon enteroscopy: a tertiary care experience. Endosc Int Open. 2018 Jun;6(6):E751–7.

93. Chen X, Ran ZH, Tong JL. A meta-analysis of the yield of capsule endoscopy compared to double balloon enteroscopy in patients with small bowel disease. World J Gastroenterol. 2007 Aug 28;13(32):4372–8.
94. Nakamura M, Niwa Y, Ohmiya N, et al. Preliminary comparison of capsule endoscopy and double-balloon enteroscopy in patients with suspected small-bowel bleeding. Endoscopy. 2006;38:59–66.
95. Kameda N, Higuchi K, Shiba M, et al. A prospective, single-blind trial comparing wireless capsule endoscopy and double-balloon enteroscopy in patients with obscure gastrointestinal bleeding. J Gastroenterol. 2008;43:434–40.
96. Teshima CW, Kuipers EJ, van Zanten SV, et al. Double balloon enteroscopy and capsule endoscopy for obscure gastrointestinal bleeding: an updated meta-analysis. J Gastroenterol Hepatol. 2011 May;26(5):796–801.
97. Otani K, Watanabe T, Shimada S, et al. Clinical utility of capsule endoscopy and double-balloon enteroscopy in the management of obscure gastrointestinal bleeding. Digestion. 2018;97:52–8.
98. Ooka S, Kobayashi K, Kawagishi K, et al. Roles of capsule endoscopy and single-balloon enteroscopy in diagnosing unexplained gastrointestinal bleeding. Clin Endosc. 2016 Jan;49(1):56–60.
99. Prachayakul V, Deesomsak M, Aswakul P, et al. The utility of single balloon enteroscopy for the diagnosis and management of small bowel disorders according to their clinical manifestations: a retrospective review. BMC Gastroenterol. 2013;13:103.
100. Kushnir VM, Tang M, Goodwin J, et al. Long-term outcomes after single-balloon enteroscopy in patients with obscure gastrointestinal bleeding. Dig Dis Sci. 2013;58:2572–9.
101. Efthymiou M, Desmond PV, Brown G, et al. SINGLE-01: a randomized, controlled trial comparing the efficacy and depth of insertion of single- and double-balloon enteroscopy by using a novel method to determine insertion depth. Gastrointest Endosc. 2012;76:972–80.
102. Takano N, Yamada A, Watabe H, et al. Single-balloon versus double-balloon endoscopy for achieving total enteroscopy: a randomized, controlled trial. Gastrointest Endosc. 2011;73:734–9.
103. May A, Färber M, Aschmoneit I, et al. Prospective multicenter trial comparing push-and-pull enteroscopy with the single- and double-balloon techniques in patients with small-bowel disorders. Am J Gastroenterol. 2010;105:575–81.
104. Zhu M, Zhang J, Tang J, et al. Diagnostic value of single balloon endoscopy in obscure gastrointestinal bleeding. World Chin J Digestol. 2014:1033–6.
105. Manno M, Riccioni ME, Cannizzaro R, et al. Diagnostic and therapeutic yield of single balloon enteroscopy in patients with suspected small-bowel disease: results of the Italian multicentre study. Dig Liver Dis. 2013;45:211–5.
106. Wadhwa V, Sethi S, Tewani S, et al. A meta-analysis on efficacy and safety: single-balloon vs. double-balloon enteroscopy. Gastroenterol Rep. 2015;3(2):148–55.
107. Akerman PA, Agrawal D, Chen W, et al. Spiral enteroscopy: a novel method of enteroscopy by using the Endo-Ease Discovery SB overtube and a pediatric colonoscope. Gastrointest Endosc. 2009;69:327–32.
108. Judah JR, Draganov PV, Lam Y, et al. Spiral enteroscopy is safe and effective for an elderly United States population of patients with numerous comorbidities. Clin Gastroenterol Hepatol. 2010;8:572–6.
109. Baniya R, Upadhaya S, Subedi SC, et al. Balloon enteroscopy versus spiral enteroscopy for small-bowel disorders: a systematic review and meta-analysis. Gastrointest Endosc. 2017 Dec;86(6):997–1005.
110. Lenz P, Domagk D. Double- vs. single-balloon vs. spiral enteroscopy. Best Pract Res Clin Gastroenterol. 2012;26:303–13.
111. Graca BM, Freire PA, Brito JB, et al. Gastroenterologic and radiologic approach to obscure gastrointestinal bleeding: how, why, and when? Radiographics. 2010 Jan;30(1):235–52.

112. Kong MS, Chen CY, Tzen KY, et al. Technetium-99m pertechnetate scan for ectopic gastric mucosa in children with gastrointestinal bleeding. J Formos Med Assoc. 1993;92:717–20.
113. Lin S, Suhocki PV, Ludwig KA, et al. Gastrointestinal bleeding in adult patients with Meckel's diverticulum: the role of technetium 99m pertechnetate scan. South Med J. 2002;95:1338–41.
114. Howarth DM. The role of nuclear medicine in the detection of acute gastrointestinal bleeding. Semin Nucl Med. 2006;36:133–46.
115. Howarth DM, Tang K, Lees W, et al. The clinical utility of nuclear medicine imaging for the detection of occult gastrointestinal haemorrhage. Nucl Med Commun. 2002;23:591–4.
116. Brunnler T, Klebl F, Mundorff S, et al. Significance of scintigraphy for the localisation of obscure gastrointestinal bleedings. World J Gastroenterol. 2008;14:5015–9.
117. Dolezal J, Vizda J, Bures J, et al. Detection of acute gastrointestinal bleeding by means of technetium-99m in vivo labelled red blood cells. Nat Med Central Eastern Eur. 2002;5:151–4.
118. Dolezal J, Vizda J, Kopacova M, et al. Single-photon emission computed tomography enhanced Tc-99m-pertechnetate disodium-labelled red blood cell scintigraphy in the localization of small intestine bleeding: a single-Centre twelve-year study. Digestion. 2011;84:207–11.
119. Dusold R, Burke K, Carpentier W, et al. The accuracy of technetium-99m labeled red cell scintigraphy in localizing gastrointestinal bleeding. Am J Gastroenterol. 1994;89:345–8.
120. Friebe B, Wieners G. Radiographic techniques for the localization and treatment of gastrointestinal bleeding of obscure origin. Eur J Trauma Emerg Surg. 2011;37:353–63.
121. Laine L, Sahota A, Shah A. Does capsule endoscopy improve outcomes in obscure gastrointestinal bleeding? Randomized trial versus dedicated small bowel radiography. Gastroenterology. 2010;138:1673–80.
122. Romagnuolo J, Andrew S, Brock AS, et al. Is endoscopic therapy effective for angioectasia in obscure gastrointestinal bleeding? A systematic review of the literature. J Clin Gastroenterol. 2015 Nov-Dec;49(10):823–30.
123. Jackson CS, Gerson LB. Management of Gastrointestinal Angiodysplastic Lesions (GIADs): a systematic review and meta-analysis. Am J Gastroenterol. 2014;109:474–83.
124. Pinho R, Ponte A, Rodrigues A, et al. Longterm rebleeding risk following endoscopic therapy of small-bowel vascular lesions with device-assisted enteroscopy. Eur J Gastroenterol Hepatol. 2016 Apr;28(4):479–85.
125. Grooteman KV, Holleran G, Matheeuwsen M, et al. A risk assessment of factors for the presence of angiodysplasias during endoscopy and factors contributing to symptomatic bleeding and rebleeds. Dig Dis Sci. 2019 Oct;64(10):2923–32.
126. Becq A, Rahmi G, Perrod G, et al. Hemorrhagic angiodysplasia of the digestive tract: pathogenesis, diagnosis, and management. Gastrointest Endosc. 2017 Nov;86(5):792–806.
127. May A, Friesing-Sosnik T, Manner H, et al. Long-term outcome after argon plasma coagulation of small-bowel lesions using double-balloon enteroscopy in patients with mid-gastrointestinal bleeding. Endoscopy. 2011 Sep;43(9):759–65.
128. Rogers BH. Endoscopic diagnosis and therapy of mucosal vascular abnormalities of the gastrointestinal tract occurring in elderly patients and associated with cardiac, vascular, and pulmonary disease. Gastrointest Endosc. 1980;26:134–8.
129. Jovanovic I, Knezevic A. Combined endoclipping and argon plasma coagulation (APC)--daisy technique for cecal angiodysplasia. Endoscopy. 2013;45(Suppl 2 UCTN):E384.
130. Moparty B, Raju GS. Role of hemoclips in a patient with cecal angiodysplasia at high risk of recurrent bleeding from antithrombotic therapy to maintain coronary stent patency: a case report. Gastrointest Endosc. 2005 Sep;62(3):468–9.
131. Ge ZZ, Chen HM, Gao YJ, et al. Efficacy of thalidomide for refractory gastrointestinal bleeding from vascular malformation. Gastroenterology. 2011;141:1629–37.
132. Lewis BS, Salomon P, Rivera-MacMurray S, et al. Does hormonal therapy have any benefit for bleeding angiodysplasia? J Clin Gastroenterol. 1992 Sep;15(2):99–103.
133. Barkin JS, Ross BS. Medical therapy for chronic gastrointestinal bleeding of obscure origin. Am J Gastroenterol. 1998 Aug;93(8):1250–4.

134. van Cutsem E, Rutgeerts P, Vantrappen G. Treatment of bleeding gastrointestinal vascular malformations with oestrogen-progesterone. Lancet. 1990 Apr 21;335(8695):953–5.
135. Junquera F, Feu F, Papo M, et al. A multicenter, randomized, clinical trial of hormonal therapy in the prevention of rebleeding from gastrointestinal angiodysplasia. Gastroenterology. 2001 Nov;121(5):1073–9.
136. Nardone G, Rocco A, Balzano T, et al. The efficacy of octreotide therapy in chronic bleeding due to vascular abnormalities of the gastrointestinal tract. Aliment Pharmacol Ther. 1999;13:1429–36.
137. Szilagyi A, Ghali MP. Pharmacological therapy of vascular malformations of the gastrointestinal tract. Can J Gastroenterol. 2006;20:171–8.
138. Bon C, Aparicio T, Vincent M, et al. Long-acting somatostatin analogues decrease blood transfusion requirements in patients with refractory gastrointestinal bleeding associated with angiodysplasia. Aliment Pharmacol Ther. 2012;36:587–93.
139. Holleran G, Hall B, Breslin N, et al. Long-acting somatostatin analogues provide significant beneficial effect in patients with refractory small bowel angiodysplasia: results from a proof of concept open label mono-centre trial. United European Gastroenterol J. 2016;4(1):70–6.
140. Brown C, Subramanian V, Wilcox CM, et al. Somatostatin analogues in the treatment of recurrent bleeding from gastrointestinal vascular malformations: an overview and systematic review of prospective observational studies. Dig Dis Sci. 2010;55:2129–34.
141. Grooteman KV, van Geenen EJM, Drenth JPH. Multicentre, open-label, randomised, parallel-group, superiority study to compare the efficacy of octreotide therapy 40 mg monthly versus standard of care in patients with refractory anaemia due to gastrointestinal bleeding from small bowel angiodysplasias: a protocol of the OCEAN trial. BMJ Open. 2016;6(9):e011442.
142. Stephens TD, Bunde CJ, Fillmore BJ. Mechanism of action in thalidomide teratogenesis. Biochem Pharmacol. 2000;59:1489–99.
143. Chen H, Fu S, Feng N, et al. Bleeding recurrence in patients with gastrointestinal vascular malformation after thalidomide. Medicine (Baltimore). 2016 Aug;95(33):e4606.
144. Monsanto P, Almeida N, Lérias C, et al. Is there still a role for intraoperative enteroscopy in patients with obscure gastrointestinal bleeding? Rev Esp Enferm Dig. 2012;104:190–6.
145. Cave DR, Cooley JS. Intraoperative enteroscopy. Indications and techniques. Gastrointest Endosc Clin N Am. 1996;6:793–802.
146. Hartmann D, Schmidt H, Bolz G, et al. A prospective two-center study comparing wireless capsule endoscopy with intraoperative enteroscopy in patients with obscure GI bleeding. Gastrointest Endosc. 2005;61:826–32.
147. Lewis BS, Wenger JS, Waye JD. Small bowel enteroscopy and intraoperative enteroscopy for obscure gastrointestinal bleeding. Am J Gastroenterol. 1991;86:171–4.
148. Desa LA, Ohri SK, Hutton KA, et al. Role of intraoperative enteroscopy in obscure gastrointestinal bleeding of small bowel origin. Br J Surg. 1991;78:192–5.
149. Douard R, Wind P, Panis Y, et al. Intraoperative enteroscopy for diagnosis and management of unexplained gastrointestinal bleeding. Am J Surg. 2000;180:181–4.

Chapter 8
Lower GI

Robert Smolic, Kristina Bojanic, Martina Smolić, Micheal Tadros, and George Y. Wu

R. Smolic
Department of Pathophysiology, Physiology and Immunology, Faculty of Dental Medicine and Health Osijek, J. J. Strossmayer University of Osijek, Osijek, Croatia

Department of Pathophysiology, Faculty of Medicine Osijek, J. J. Strossmayer University of Osijek, Osijek, Croatia

Department of Medicine, Division of Gastroenterology/Hepatology, University Hospital Osijek, Osijek, Croatia

K. Bojanic
Department of Biophysics and Radiology, Faculty of Dental Medicine and Health Osijek, J. J. Strossmayer University of Osijek, Osijek, Croatia

Department of Biophysics and Radiology, Faculty of Medicine Osijek, J. J. Strossmayer University of Osijek, Osijek, Croatia

Department of Radiology, Health Center Osijek, Osijek, Croatia
e-mail: kbojanic@fdmz.hr

M. Smolić
Department of Pharmacology and Biochemistry, Faculty of Dental Medicine and Health Osijek, J. J. Strossmayer University of Osijek, Osijek, Croatia

Department of Pharmacology, Faculty of Medicine Osijek, J. J. Strossmayer University of Osijek, Osijek, Croatia
e-mail: martina.smolic@fdmz.hr; martina.smolic@mefos.hr

M. Tadros
Department of Gastroenterology and Hepatology, Albany Medical Center, Albany, NY, USA
e-mail: tadrosm1@amc.edu

G. Y. Wu (✉)
Department of Internal Medicine, Division of Gastrenterology/Hepatology, University of Connecticut Health Center, Farmington, CT, USA
e-mail: wu@uchc.edu

© The Author(s), under exclusive license to Springer Nature Switzerland AG 2021
M. Tadros, G. Y. Wu (eds.), *Management of Occult GI Bleeding*, Clinical Gastroenterology, https://doi.org/10.1007/978-3-030-71468-0_8

131

Introduction

Occult lower gastrointestinal bleeding (LGIB) as the initial presentation of a positive FOBT or IDA without evidence of visible bleeding to the patient or clinician [1, 8] can originate from colon, rectum and anus [1], mainly in the setting of a positive fecal occult blood test (FOBT) and/or iron-deficiency anemia (IDA) [2]. Data on the frequency and natural history of the occult lower GI bleeding are scant [10]. In a review of five prospective studies in patients with occult GI bleeding, endoscopy determined a colorectal source in 20 to 30% of patients. Simultaneous causes of occult bleeding in the upper GI tract and the colon or synchronous lesions were found in 1–17% of patients. According to frequency, the most commonly diagnosed colonic lesions were colon cancer (5–11%), colon polyps/adenomas (5–14%), vascular ectasias (1–9%), and colitis (1–2%) [3]. The most common etiologic lesions of occult LGIB are colonic adenomas ≥ 1 cm, colon carcinoma and angiodysplasia [5]. Other etiologies include colonic ulcers, colitis/inflammatory bowel disease (IBD), parasitic infestation, hemorrhoids and recurrent diverticular bleeding.

In patients younger than 40 years, the most common causes of occult LGIB included celiac disease [4] and Crohn disease [5] while in patients older than 40 years, vascular ectasias and non-steroidal anti-inflammatory drug–induced ulcers are common [6]. Long-distance running has been described in the literature as rare cause of occult LGIB probably due to decreased splanchnic perfusion resulting in transient intestinal ischemia during longdistance running induces GI blood loss and anemia [7].

Epidemiology

Epidemiological data on occult LGIBs are unavailable. Recently published studies suggest that 20–30% of all GIBs are LGIBs [2, 8, 9]. However, this is probably an underestimate since research on LGIB incidence are limited, and many patients with milder forms of LGIB do not seek medicalattention or are not admitted to the hospital [10].

The LGIB incidence is higher in men than in women [11]. It may present in patients at any age. Since the bleeding is chronic and slow, patients have microcytic, hypochromic anemia [8]. Increased incidence is seen with advancing age, probably as a consequence of the increasing prevalence of diverticulosis and angiodysplasia in the elderly, both common causes of occult LGIB [9].

The overall mortality rate is estimated to range from 2% to 4% [2, 12], doubtless higher in elderly patients with multiple co-morbid conditions. Some risk factors of increased morbidity and mortality are age >60 years, low hematocrit (<35%), elevated levels of serum creatinine and hemodynamic instability [12].

Specific Etiologies

Diverticular Bleeding

Despite the wide variation among studies, diverticular bleeding is the most common etiology in general [13] accounting for 26–33% of all LGIB [14, 15]. Some studies even report incidence rates between 20–50% [16]. To determine the true incidence of diverticular hemorrhage, it is important to differentiate presumptive from definitive diverticular hemorrhage. The Centre for Ulcer Research and Education (CURE) established three categories; presumptive diverticular bleeding (confirmed diagnosis of diverticulosis, without colonoscopic evidence of bleeding), incidental diverticulosis (confirmed diagnosis of diverticulosis, but with definitive evidence of an other origin of bleeding) and definitive diverticular hemorrhage. Using this classification, definitive diverticular hemorrhage was reported in 20% of patients, while presumptive in 46% [17]. The incidence of diverticular bleeding as a complication of diverticulitis is also different among various studies and ranges from 3–5% [18] to 10–15% [2].

A diverticulum by definition is a protrusion of mucosa through the colon wall at the point of weakness where the blood vessels penetrate trough muscular layer [8]. During the formation of the diverticulum, the perforating vessels become exposed over the fundus and prone to chronic trauma and erosion. Rupture of the branches of the marginal artery occurs eccentrically and toward the lumen of the diverticulum [19]. Diverticular bleeding is mostly unrelated to inflamation, and is not a common feature of diverticulitis [20]. Risk factors include advancing age, NSAID and anticoagulant use, low fiber diet, constipation, hypertension, diabetes mellitus, coronary artery disease [21].

Diverticulosis occurs predominantly (75%) in the sigmoid and descending colon. Studies suggest that diverticular bleeding is more prevalent in the proximal colon because right sided diverticula are characterised with wider necks and domes, thus exposing a longer length of penetrating vessels to injury. The localization of bleeding diverticula also depends on the dignostic modality used. Sixty percent of diverticular bleeding is diagnosed on the left side using colonoscopy while 50–90% on the right side of colon is detected by angiography [23].

The majority of diverticular bleeding episodes are self-limited with spontaneous resolution in 75–90% [18, 23]. The incidence of rebleeding is less than 15% after an initial episode, but much higher after a second episode (50%).

Neoplasia

Colorectal adenocarcinoma (CRC) is the third most common cancer, and second in mortality rates in the USA [24–27]. Historically, CRC has been the leading cause of occult LGIB, typically presenting with IDA and/or positive FOBT [28]. Despite the high prevalence of CRC, there are only a limited number of studies about clinical manifestations in a population-based setting. Studies report overt bleeding (rectal bleeding and/or melena) in a wide range from 37% to 58% of patients with CRC [29, 30]. Other clinical presentations include obstructive symptoms, altered stools (constipation or diarrhea), abdominal pain or discomfort, fatigue, weight loss, nausea or vomiting [29].

Overall symptomatology of CRC largely depends on the location of the mass. Right-sided carcinomas may be asymptomatic with occult bleeding from the erosions on the luminal tumor sufrace, thus resulting in IDA, Fig. 8.1.

Obstructive symptoms are more likely with left-sided carcinomas. For rectal carcinomas hematochezia and decreased stool caliber are common [30, 31].

Histologically, 90% to 95% of CRC are adenocarcinomas, Fig. 8.2 [31].

More than 95% of CRC arise from precursor polyps, Fig. 8.3, [31] which could histologically be separated into neoplastic (adenomatous) and non-neoplastic categories. The latter are further sub-classified into hyperplastic, hamartomatous, and inflammatory [32]. Adenomatous polyps are histologically sub-classified as tubular, villous, or tubulo-villous adenomas.

Clinically, most polyps are asymptomatic and represent incidental findings on screening colonoscopy. It has been shown that adenomatous polyps ≥1–1.5 cm in size are more likely to bleed, Fig. 8.4, as opposed to hyperplasic polyps [33]. Risk factors for adenomatous polyps include increasing age and male gender [34, 35].

Vascular Malformations

The reported percentage of LGIB due to vascular malformations varies in the literature from 3–6% [36], up to 40% [37]. However, their importance lies in the fact that they are among the most commonly missed lesions during colonoscopy, Fig. 8.5 [38].

Fig. 8.1 A small colon cancer detected during colonoscopy

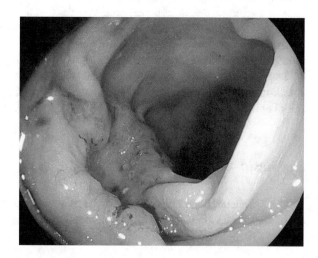

Fig. 8.2 Upper panel: colonic adenocarcinoma undermines benign mucosa [hematoxylin and eosin, ×20], lower panel: higher magnification view shows malignant glands with nuclear stratifications and central dirty necrosis [hematoxylin and eosin, ×100]. Images courtesy of Dr. Hwajeong Lee, Albany Medical Center

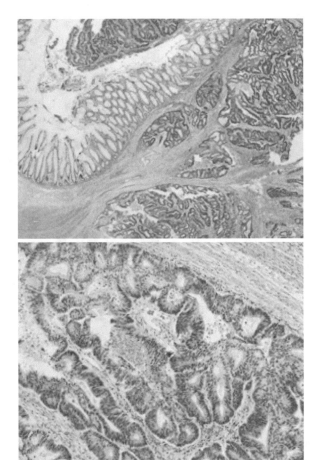

Fig. 8.3 A hepatic flexure polyp (yellow arrow) partially obscured by a fold and seen only on retroflexed view

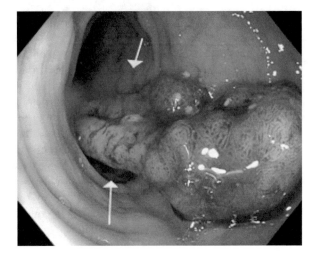

Fig. 8.4 A large friable
pedunculated colonic
polyp in patient with iron
deficiency anemia. Arrows
point to the stalk

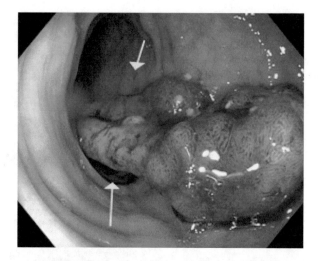

Fig. 8.5 A colonic AVM

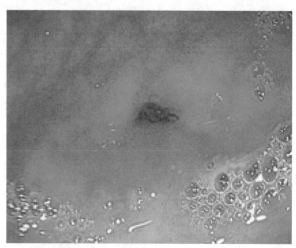

The three main categories are arteriovenous malformations (AVMs), hemangiomas and colonic varices [2]. AVM are ectatic and tortuous thin walled area of existing vessels. According to the Moore et al., they can be classified as: [39]. Type I lesions called angiodysplasias which are the most prevalent, typically solitary lesions, predominantly localized on the right side of the colon [40]. Although their exact etiology is unclear, the assumption is that chronic, intermittent low-grade colonic contractions result in chronic venous congestion, capillary dilation and finally in development of the angiodysplasia. Since these lesions are acquired, their incidence increases with advancing age, particulary beyond sixth decade of life. Bleeding from angiodysplasia is venous and, therefore, is rarely the cause of the massive LGIB [8]. The typical presentation is intermittent bleeding in the setting of IDA. Although in the historical studies angiodysplasia was traditionally associated with the colon, recent studies have shown that it is actually much more common in the small intestine [41]. Type II and III AVMs are congenital in origin, usually in younger patients, multiple and often localised in small intestine [39].

Hemangiomas are subclassified into capillary and cavernous. Cavernous are more common, defined as large endothelium lined, blood filled sinuses, usually localized in the distal colon and rectum. Some rare syndromes include the blue rubber bleb nevus [42].

Colonic varices are a rare entity, defined as continuously dilated submucosal veins, mainly due to portal hypertension or portal vein obstruction. They are uncommon causes of LGIB except in patients with cirrhosis in whom they are a cause of bleeding with frequency of 1 to 8% [43]. The most common sites of colonic varices are the rectum and cecum [44]. When the etiology cannot be ascertained, a colon varix is classified as idiopathic or primary [45].

Hemorrhoids, Anal Fissures and Anal Cancer

Anorectal bleeding is the sixth most common symptom in outpatient clinic visits [2] with a prevalence from 13% to 20% [46]. Anorectal disease encompasses many etiologies, including hemorrhoids, anal fissures and anal cancer.

Hemorrhoids were the fourth leading outpatient digestive system diagnosis in US according to an National Institutes of Health report [47]. As a very common anorectal condition, they are defined as a symptomatic abnormal downward displacement and enlargement of the anal cushions, consequently causing venous dilatation [48].

An epidemiologic study reported a prevalence rate around 4.4% in the United States with a peak age from 45 to 65 years. A significant reduction in incidence was observed after 65 years of life, and they were unusual before 20 years of life. Caucasians were affected more frequently than African Americans, and increased prevalence rates were associated with higher socioeconomic status [49].

Hemorrhoids are categorized on the basis of their location as internal, external and mixed depending on their relationship to the dentate line. Hemorrhoids that originate above the dentate line from the inferior hemorrhoidal venous plexus and covered by mucosa are defined as internal. External hemorrhoids are dilated venules below the dentate line and are covered with squamous epithelium. Mixed (internoexternal) hemorrhoids arise both above and below the dentate line.

A retrospective review of patients from Mayo Clinic from 1976 through 1990 revealed that the incidence of hemmorrhoidal bleeding that caused anemia was 0.5 patients per 100,000 population per year. They concluded that resolution of anemia after definitive treatment with hemorrhoidectomy should be expected take up to six months [50]. Several cases of severe obscure bleeding caused by hemorrhoids have been reported in the literature resulting in anemia and requiring multiple transfusions, Fig. 8.6 [51].

Fig. 8.6 Large
internal hemorrhoids
viewed by retroflexion

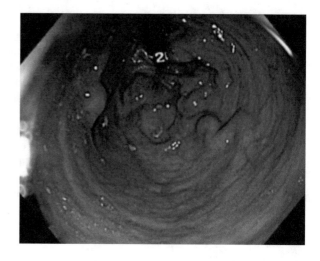

This confirms and highlights the fact that hemorrhoids can cause substantial blood loss during long periods of time, and the assumption that any gastrointestinal bleeding that causes anemia or requires transfusion cannot be a hemorrhoidal bleed is incorrect [51]. Bleeding can also occur as a complication of hemorrhoidectomy. Usually, it is an acute and self-limiting condition presenting with small amounts of bleeding [2].

Anal fissures begin as a tear in the anal mucosa. If a tear spontaneously resolves, it is defined as an acute anal fissure. If a tear persists, the fissure is considered chronic. The most common clinical manifestation is bright red bleeding as a consequence of stool passage and further injury to the mucosa. As a rule, they occur in the midline, and any fissure off the midline requires further diagnostics for underlying etiology [10].

The vast majority (85%) of anal carcinomas are squamous cell cancers linked with human papilloma virus (HPV) infection [55]. It is a rare condition constituting only 0.5% of all cancer diagnoses according to the National Canceer Institute. However, the incidence has increased over the past several decades, particularly in women [52]. Other less common, malignancies of the anal canal that can cause LGIB include anal melanoma and anal adenocarcinoma [53].

Inflammatory Bowel Disease (IBD)

There are no data in the literature on the incidence of occult bleeding due to IBD. A few retrospective studies investigated acute and severe LGIB in Crohn disease and concluded that it is quite uncommon with a prevalence of 4% [54]. The cumulative probability of bleeding increases with duration of Crohn disease, 1.7% after 1 year, 3.6% after 5 years, 6.5% after 10 years, and 10.3% after 20 years [54]. The diagnosis of the bleeding source is limited and only in less than one third of cases, was an origin of bleeding be identified reliably. Fortunately, these bleeding episodes usually resolve spontaneously, or after medical treatment [55].

Ulcerative colitis is characterized by bloody diarrhea in over 95% of cases, Figs. 8.7 and 8.8, but severe or massive hemorrhage is actually quite rare, occurring less commonly than other complications. Most patients with severe LGIB have pancolitis and surgical treatment is indicated [56].

Ischemic Colitis

In the elderly, ischemic colitis is the leading cause of LGIB [2], accounting for 3%–9% of all LGIB [11]. Ischemia commonly affects two watershed areas in colon, the namely the splenic flexure (Griffith point), Fig. 8.9, and the rectosigmoid junction (Sudek point) [22].

Bloody diarrhea and abdominal pain are common symptoms. A study has shown that patients with ischemic colitis usually had left-sided colitis, shorter hospital stay and a lower transfusion requirements compared to patients with other LGIB etiologies. After discharge, patients with ischemic colitis had lower recurrence and rebleeding episodes over the long term than other LGIB patients [57].

In athletes who engage in prolonged exercise, LGIB can occur as a consequence of visceral ischemia. Usually the clinical presentation is chronic with anemia, or positive FOBT with little clinical disease. This clinical condition is usually transient and reversible, but it must be kept in the mind [58].

Fig. 8.7 Fulminant ulcerative colitis viewed during colonoscopy

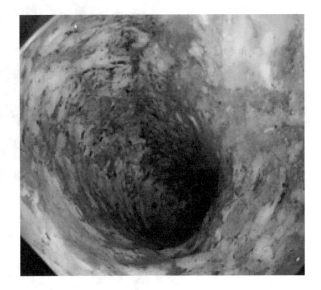

Fig. 8.8 Upper: ulcerative colitis with diffuse mucosal inflammation [hematoxylin and eosin, ×20], lower: higher magnification view shows crypt abscesses and crypt distortion [hematoxylin and eosin, ×40]. Images courtesy of Dr. Hwajeong Lee, Albany Medical Center

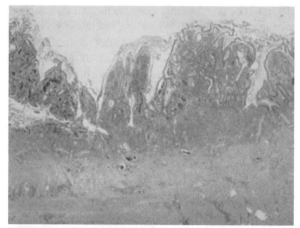

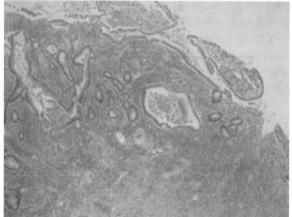

Fig. 8.9 Erythema, submusosal hemmorhage, and edema from ischemia of the splenic flexure as found by colonoscopy

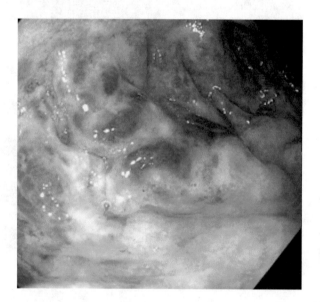

Radiation Colitis

Radiation is one of the major modalities for treatment of malignant disease. Radiation-related colon complications are dose- and time-dependent. The part of the bowel that is most commonly affected by the effects of radiation therapy is the rectum with hematochezia as the most common symptom [2]. Acute symptoms that develop in the first 6 weeks after radiation must be distinguished from chronic ones that develop or persist after 6 to 12 months [2]. Acute radiation colitis is mostly self-limited disease after regional radiotherapy for malignancy. Chronic radiation colitis is a progressive disease with development of fibrosis, edema, fragility and could result in complications like obstruction and perforation. It is even considered as a pre-cancerous lesion with radiation-associated malignancy diagnosed at an advanced stage with poor prognosis. Although radiation colitis may occur at any time during the therapy or after, the median repored time is 6 months to 5 years [58]. Radiation therapy may cause LGIB by several mechanisms including obliterative endarteritis resulting in chronic ischemic changes [59]. It is estimated that 4% to 10% of patients undergoing radiotherapy will develop chronic changes in the subsequent 5 to 10 years, with a rate as high as 15% to 20% after 20 years [60].

Microscopic Colitis

Although microscopic colitis (MC) has become recognized as a common cause of chronic non-bloody diarrhea, it is still under-recognized among physicians with limited knowledge about its pathophysiology, etiology and natural course [61]. It is a worldwide chronic inflammatory bowel disease of unknown cause [62], nearly as common as classic IBD with estimated overall prevalence of 119 per 100,000 [63]. Mainly, MC is a disease of the elderly, with an average age at diagnosis of 65 years, with a striking female predominance [64]. Colonoscopy with biopsy is the gold standard method for making the diagnosis since only histology can differentiate two major subtypes, lymphocytic colitis, Fig. 8.10 and collagenous colitis, Fig. 8.11

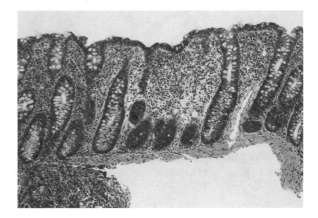

Fig. 8.10 Lymphocytic colitis with numerous intraepithelial lymphocytes associated with surface epithelial damage [hematoxylin and eosin, ×100]

Fig. 8.11 Collagenous colitis with a thick subepithelial collagenous band (arrow) [hematoxylin and eosin, ×100]. Images courtesy of Dr. Hwajeong Lee, Albany Medical Center

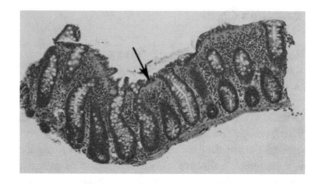

[65] and a third, recently identified subgroup of incomplete MC [61]. It can also to rule out other causes of chronic diarrhea. Biopsies should also be performed in the colon, particularly in patients with diarrhea, as 50% of microscopic colitis have mild anemia [66]. There is a strong association with autoimmune disorders, such as celiac disease, thyroid disorders and polyarthritis [67]. In fact, histological features of MC in the colon are present in 30% of patients with celiac sprue [68]. Thus, new European guidelines recommend that all patients with MC should be screened for celiac disease [61]. Since occult gastrointestinal bleeding can be detected in about half of patients with celiac sprue [4], further basic science and clinical investigations are needed to better understand the underlying mechanisms and to improve general knowledge about the MC.

Diagnosis

Occult GI bleeding by definition is detected as a positive finding of a FOBT or IDA, in the absence of visible blood [1, 69]. According to the latest guidelines of American Gastroenterological Association, it is recommended to use FOBT only in the clinical context of CRC screening, since it has been shown to reduce CRC mortality [1, 28].

Colonoscopy

In general, diagnostic procedure of choice for evaluation of LGIB is colonoscopy due its high diagnostic yield and concurrent ability for therapeutic intervention [8, 70].

Colonoscopy successfully identified the etiology in 80% of cases of severe hematochezia [71], but in only 20% to 30% of cases of occult LGIB [69].

Regarding occult hemorrhage, colonoscopy is indicated after a positive FOBT or a laboratory finding of IDA as part of a routine diagnostic workup. Ideally, it should be done after good bowel preparation with cathartic agents. Colon lesions commonly missed by initial colonoscopy are angiodysplasia and neoplasms [28, 38]. Some of the reasons for false negative findings on colonoscopy are lesions cbaracterized by very slow and intermittent bleeding, cessation of bleeding during the initial colonoscopy and lesions obscured by blood clots. Also, significant anemia and hypovolemia present at the same time can make the lesion difficult to visualize by colonoscopy [1]. Colonoscopy as diagnostic modality is limited to the mucosal surface. Thus, intramural malformations may be overlooked. Also, some technical aspects of colonoscopy could result in missed lesions. This includes failure to intubate the terminal iluem, failure to visualize or mistaken visualization of the cecum, failure to preform retroflexion in the rectum.

According to the review from 2018, computed tomography enterography (CTE) is the most commonly used diagnostic test for occult bleeding, since it can identify lesions missed on colonoscopy [69]. The advantage of CTE as cross-sectional imaging method, is its ability to present intramural lesions, like angiodisplasias [72, 73].

High Quality Colonoscopy and Missed Colonic Lesions

While colonoscopy is an essential tool in the work up of occult GI bleed, the quality of colonoscopy depends on the operator, and the completeness of bowel preparation. The incidence rate of post-colonoscopy colorectal cancers (defined as cancers that are diagnosed less than 10 years after a negative colonoscopy) is closely correlated [74] to the quality of the exam [75]. There are established quality parameters for colonoscopy whic includes proper bowel preparation to consistently allow detection of polyps >5 mm after suctioning residual fluids, Fig. 8.12 [76]. Guidelines suggest a benchmark of 85% adequate bowel rate in clinical practice [75]. Other notable quality parameters include adenoma detection rate, complete polyp removal, and ensuring complete colonoscopy exam with cecal intubations.

There some important technical aspects that the endoscopist can do to increase the diagnostic yield. For example, "retroflexion" where the endoscope is is pointed backwards on itself in a U shape which allows better visualization of areas behind tall haustral folds [77]. This technique can also be performed in the rectum to permit careful inspection of the distal rectum and anus, Fig. 8.13. Also, second look or looking twice in the right side of the colon can improve adenoma detection [78]. Colonoscopy should always start with proper rectal exam as anal pathology can be easily overlooked. The endoscopist should properly examine between the haustral folds as large polyps and cancers can be hidden. Examining the terminal ileum by intubating the ilececal valve can be useful. It is not surprising that studies show that up to 30% of clinically significant non-small bowel lesions are missed on EGD, push enteroscopy, and colonoscopy and are incidentally detected by capsule study [79]. Therefore, second-look or repeat colonoscopy can be warranted to patients with refractory anemia for whom a comprehensive initial exam did not uncover the bleeding source. This should be considered especially if patient is referred for second opinion for unexplained occult GI bleed or IDA after negative prior work up.

Fig. 8.12 A small small right colon cancer that can be easily missed in case of inadequate colon preparation

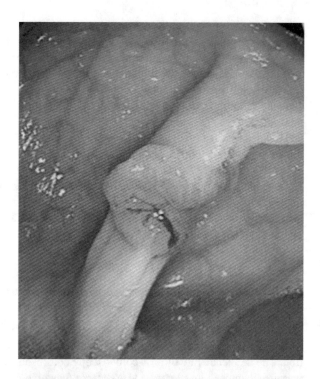

Fig. 8.13 Retroflexed view of the rectum showing a subtle mass (anal cancer) that was missed in at least 2 prior colonoscopies

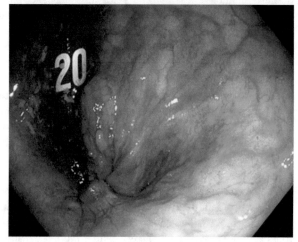

Conclusions

Occult gastrointestinal bleeding from colon is defined as the initial presentation of a positive fecal occult blood test (FOBT) or and/or iron-deficiency anemia (IDA) without evidence of visible bleeding to the patient or clinician. Colonoscopy is the primary diagnostic modality for evaluation of the etiology. The most common etiologic lesions of an occult gastrointestinal bleeding from colon are colonic adenomas ≥ 1 cm, colon carcinoma and angiodysplasia. Other etiologies include colonic ulcers, colitis/inflammatory bowel disease (IBD), parasitic infestation, hemorrhoids and recurrent diverticular bleeding. Since colonoscopy can identify a cause of occult LGIB in 20% to 30% of patients, special attention to all aspects of high quality colonoscopy should be done in order to minimize missed lesions.

References

1. Raju GS, Gerson L, Das A, Lewis B. American Gastroenterological Association (AGA) Institute technical review on obscure gastrointestinal bleeding, (in eng). Gastroenterology. 2007;133(5):1697–717. https://doi.org/10.1053/j.gastro.2007.06.007.
2. Adegboyega T, Rivadeneira D. Lower GI bleeding: an update on incidences and causes, (in eng). Clin Colon Rectal Surg. 2020;33(1):28–34. https://doi.org/10.1055/s-0039-1695035.
3. Zuckerman GR, Prakash C, Askin MP, Lewis BS. AGA technical review on the evaluation and management of occult and obscure gastrointestinal bleeding, (in eng). Gastroenterology. 2000;118(1):201–21. https://doi.org/10.1016/s0016-5085(00)70430-6.
4. Fine KD. The prevalence of occult gastrointestinal bleeding in celiac sprue, (in eng). N Engl J Med. 1996;334(18):1163–7. https://doi.org/10.1056/nejm199605023341804.
5. Rockey DC. Occult and obscure gastrointestinal bleeding: causes and clinical management, (in eng). Nat Rev Gastroenterol Hepatol. 2010;7(5):265–79. https://doi.org/10.1038/nrgastro.2010.42.
6. Bull-Henry K, Al-Kawas FH. Evaluation of occult gastrointestinal bleeding, (in eng). Am Fam Physician. 2013;87(6):430–6.
7. Stewart JG, Ahlquist DA, McGill DB, Ilstrup DM, Schwartz S, Owen RA. Gastrointestinal blood loss and anemia in runners, (in eng). Ann Intern Med. 1984;100(6):843–5. https://doi.org/10.7326/0003-4819-100-6-843.
8. Shah AR, Jala V, Arshad H, Bilal M. Evaluation and management of lower gastrointestinal bleeding, (in eng). Dis Mon. 2018;64(7):321–32. https://doi.org/10.1016/j.disamonth.2018.02.002.
9. Oakland K. Changing epidemiology and etiology of upper and lower gastrointestinal bleeding, (in eng). Best Pract Res Clin Gastroenterol. 2019;42–43:101610. https://doi.org/10.1016/j.bpg.2019.04.003.
10. Feinman M, Haut ER. Lower gastrointestinal bleeding, (in eng). Surg Clin North Am. 2014;94(1):55–63. https://doi.org/10.1016/j.suc.2013.10.005.
11. Longstreth GF. Epidemiology and outcome of patients hospitalized with acute lower gastrointestinal hemorrhage: a population-based study, (in eng). Am J Gastroenterol. 1997;92(3):419–24.
12. Strate LL, Gralnek IM. ACG clinical guideline: management of patients with acute lower gastrointestinal bleeding, (in eng). Am J Gastroenterol. 2016;111(4):459–74. https://doi.org/10.1038/ajg.2016.41.
13. Feldman M, Friedman LS, Brandt LJ. Sleisenger and Fordtran's gastrointestinal and liver disease: pathophysiology/diagnosis/management. 10th ed. Philadelphia: Saunders/Elsevier; 2016. p. xxxi, (various paging)
14. Oakland K, et al. Acute lower GI bleeding in the UK: patient characteristics, interventions and outcomes in the first nationwide audit (in eng). Gut. 2018;67(4):654–62. https://doi.org/10.1136/gutjnl-2016-313428.
15. Strate LL, Ayanian JZ, Kotler G, Syngal S. Risk factors for mortality in lower intestinal bleeding, (in eng). Clin Gastroenterol Hepatol. 2008;6(9):1004–10; quiz 955-. https://doi.org/10.1016/j.cgh.2008.03.021.

16. Marion Y, Lebreton G, Le Pennec V, Hourna E, Viennot S, Alves A. The management of lower gastrointestinal bleeding, (in eng). J Visc Surg. 2014;151(3):191–201. https://doi.org/10.1016/j.jviscsurg.2014.03.008.

17. Jensen DM. The ins and outs of diverticular bleeding. Gastrointest Endosc. 2012;75(2):388–91. United States

18. Zuckerman GR, Prakash C. Acute lower intestinal bleeding: part I: clinical presentation and diagnosis, (in eng). Gastrointest Endosc. 1998;48(6):606–17. https://doi.org/10.1016/s0016-5107(98)70043-4.

19. Lewis M. Bleeding colonic diverticula, (in eng). J Clin Gastroenterol. 2008;42(10):1156–8. https://doi.org/10.1097/MCG.0b013e3181862ad1.

20. Keighley MRB, Williams NS. Surgery of the anus, rectum & colon. 3rd ed. Philadelphia/Edinburgh: Saunders Elsevier; 2008.

21. Nagata N, et al. Risk factors for adverse in-hospital outcomes in acute colonic diverticular hemorrhage, (in eng). World J Gastroenterol. 2015;21(37):10697–703. https://doi.org/10.3748/wjg.v21.i37.10697.

22. Chait MM. Lower gastrointestinal bleeding in the elderly, (in eng). World J Gastrointest Endosc. 2010;2(5):147–54. https://doi.org/10.4253/wjge.v2.i5.147.

23. Bounds BC, Kelsey PB. Lower gastrointestinal bleeding, (in eng). Gastrointest Endosc Clin N Am. 2007;17(2):273–88, vi. https://doi.org/10.1016/j.giec.2007.03.010.

24. Siegel RL, Miller KD, Jemal A. Cancer statistics, 2019, (in eng). CA Cancer J Clin. 2019;69(1):7–34. https://doi.org/10.3322/caac.21551.

25. Siegel RL, Miller KD, Jemal A. Cancer statistics, 2020, (in eng). CA Cancer J Clin. 2020;70(1):7–30. https://doi.org/10.3322/caac.21590.

26. Siegel RL, et al. Colorectal cancer statistics, 2020, (in eng). CA Cancer J Clin. 2020; https://doi.org/10.3322/caac.21601.

27. Bray F, Ferlay J, Soerjomataram I, Siegel RL, Torre LA, Jemal A. Global cancer statistics 2018: GLOBOCAN estimates of incidence and mortality worldwide for 36 cancers in 185 countries, (in eng). CA Cancer J Clin. 2018;68(6):394–424. https://doi.org/10.3322/caac.21492.

28. Rockey DC. Occult gastrointestinal bleeding, (in eng). Gastroenterol Clin N Am. 2005;34(4):699–718. https://doi.org/10.1016/j.gtc.2005.08.010.

29. Hreinsson JP, Jonasson JG, Bjornsson ES. Bleeding-related symptoms in colorectal cancer: a 4-year nationwide population-based study, (in eng). Aliment Pharmacol Ther. 2014;39(1):77–84. https://doi.org/10.1111/apt.12519.

30. Alexiusdottir KK, et al. Association of symptoms of colon cancer patients with tumor location and TNM tumor stage, (in eng). Scand J Gastroenterol. 2012;47(7):795–801. https://doi.org/10.3109/00365521.2012.672589.

31. Sundling KE, Zhang R, Matkowskyj KA. Pathologic features of primary colon, rectal, and anal malignancies (in eng). Cancer Treat Res. 2016;168:309–30. https://doi.org/10.1007/978-3-319-34244-3_15.

32. Shussman N, Wexner SD. Colorectal polyps and polyposis syndromes, (in eng). Gastroenterol Rep. 2014;2(1):1–15. https://doi.org/10.1093/gastro/got041.

33. Macrae FA, John DJS. Relationship between patterns of bleeding and Hemoccult sensitivity in patients with colorectal cancers or adenomas, (in eng). Gastroenterology. 1982;82(5 Pt 1):891–8.

34. Rex DK, et al. Colonic neoplasia in asymptomatic persons with negative fecal occult blood tests: influence of age, gender, and family history, (in eng). Am J Gastroenterol. 1993;88(6):825–31.

35. Johnson DA, et al. A prospective study of the prevalence of colonic neoplasms in asymptomatic patients with an age-related risk, (in eng). Am J Gastroenterol. 1990;85(8):969–74.

36. Ghassemi KA, Jensen DM. Lower GI bleeding: epidemiology and management, (in eng). Curr Gastroenterol Rep. 2013;15(7):333. https://doi.org/10.1007/s11894-013-0333-5.

37. Zuckerman GR, Prakash C. Acute lower intestinal bleeding. Part II: etiology, therapy, and outcomes, (in eng). Gastrointest Endosc. 1999;49(2):228–38. https://doi.org/10.1016/s0016-5107(99)70491-8.

38. Leighton JA, et al. Obscure gastrointestinal bleeding, (in eng). Gastrointest Endosc. 2003;58(5):650–5. https://doi.org/10.1016/s0016-5107(03)01995-3.
39. Moore JD, Thompson NW, Appelman HD, Foley D. Arteriovenous malformations of the gastrointestinal tract, (in eng). Arch Surg. 1976;111(4):381–9. https://doi.org/10.1001/archsurg.1976.01360220077013.
40. Nishimura N, et al. Risk factors for active bleeding from colonic angiodysplasia confirmed by colonoscopic observation, (in eng). Int J Colorectal Dis. 2016;31(12):1869–73. https://doi.org/10.1007/s00384-016-2651-1.
41. Jackson CS, Strong R. Gastrointestinal angiodysplasia: diagnosis and management, (in eng). Gastrointest Endosc Clin N Am. 2017;27(1):51–62. https://doi.org/10.1016/j.giec.2016.08.012.
42. Martinez CA, et al. Blue rubber bleb nevus syndrome as a cause of lower digestive bleeding, (in eng). Case Rep Surg. 2014;2014:683684. https://doi.org/10.1155/2014/683684.
43. Ganguly S, Sarin SK, Bhatia V, Lahoti D. The prevalence and spectrum of colonic lesions in patients with cirrhotic and noncirrhotic portal hypertension, (in eng). Hepatology. 1995;21(5):1226–31.
44. Sato T, Akaike J, Toyota J, Karino Y, Ohmura T. Clinicopathological features and treatment of ectopic varices with portal hypertension, (in eng). Int J Hepatol. 2011;2011:960720. https://doi.org/10.4061/2011/960720.
45. Ko BS, et al. A case of ascending colon variceal bleeding treated with venous coil embolization, (in eng). World J Gastroenterol. 2013;19(2):311–5. https://doi.org/10.3748/wjg.v19.i2.311.
46. Daram SR, Lahr C, Tang SJ. Anorectal bleeding: etiology, evaluation, and management (with videos), (in eng). Gastrointest Endosc. 2012;76(2):406–17. https://doi.org/10.1016/j.gie.2012.03.178.
47. Everhart JE, Ruhl CE. Burden of digestive diseases in the United States part II: lower gastrointestinal diseases, (in eng). Gastroenterology. 2009;136(3):741–54. https://doi.org/10.1053/j.gastro.2009.01.015.
48. Lohsiriwat V. Hemorrhoids: from basic pathophysiology to clinical management, (in eng). World J Gastroenterol. 2012;18(17):2009–17. https://doi.org/10.3748/wjg.v18.i17.2009.
49. Johanson JF, Sonnenberg A. The prevalence of hemorrhoids and chronic constipation. An epidemiologic study, (in eng). Gastroenterology. 1990;98(2):380–6. https://doi.org/10.1016/0016-5085(90)90828-o.
50. Kluiber RM, Wolff BG. Evaluation of anemia caused by hemorrhoidal bleeding, (in eng). Dis Colon Rectum. 1994;37(10):1006–7. https://doi.org/10.1007/bf02049313.
51. Ibrahim AM, Hackford AW, Lee YM, Cave DR. Hemorrhoids can be a source of obscure gastrointestinal bleeding that requires transfusion: report of five patients, (in eng). Dis Colon Rectum. 2008;51(8):1292–4. https://doi.org/10.1007/s10350-008-9376-3.
52. Howlader N, Noone AM, Krapcho M, et al. National Cancer Institute: Cancer Statistics Review. 1975–2014.
53. Symer MM, Yeo HL. Recent advances in the management of anal cancer, (in eng). F1000Res. 2018;7 https://doi.org/10.12688/f1000research.14518.1.
54. Kim KJ, et al. Risk factors and outcome of acute severe lower gastrointestinal bleeding in Crohn's disease, (in eng). Dig Liver Dis. 2012;44(9):723–8. https://doi.org/10.1016/j.dld.2012.03.010.
55. Daperno M, Sostegni R, Rocca R. Lower gastrointestinal bleeding in Crohn's disease: how (un-)common is it and how to tackle it? (in eng). Dig Liver Dis. 2012;44(9):721–2. https://doi.org/10.1016/j.dld.2012.06.006.
56. Robert JH, Sachar DB, Aufses AH Jr, Greenstein AJ. Management of severe hemorrhage in ulcerative colitis, (in eng). Am J Surg. 1990;159(6):550–5. https://doi.org/10.1016/s0002-9610(06)80064-4.
57. Nagata N, et al. Natural history of outpatient-onset ischemic colitis compared with other lower gastrointestinal bleeding: a long-term cohort study, (in eng). Int J Color Dis. 2015;30(2):243–9. https://doi.org/10.1007/s00384-014-2079-4.

58. Moses FM. Gastrointestinal bleeding and the athlete, (in eng). Am J Gastroenterol. 1993;88(8):1157–9.
59. Qayed E, Dagar G, Nanchal RS. Lower gastrointestinal hemorrhage, (in eng). Crit Care Clin. 2016;32(2):241–54. https://doi.org/10.1016/j.ccc.2015.12.004.
60. Bailey HR. Colorectal surgery. Philadelphia: Elsevier/Saunders; 2013. p. xiv, 540 p
61. Bodil O. New European statements and recommendations for the management of microscopic colitis, (in eng). United European Gastroenterol J. 2020:2050640620945811. https://doi.org/10.1177/2050640620945811.
62. Münch A, Langner C. Microscopic colitis: clinical and pathologic perspectives, (in eng). Clin Gastroenterol Hepatol. 2015;13(2):228–36. https://doi.org/10.1016/j.cgh.2013.12.026.
63. Miehlke S, Verhaegh B, Tontini GE, Madisch A, Langner C, Münch A. Microscopic colitis: pathophysiology and clinical management, (in eng). Lancet Gastroenterol Hepatol. 2019;4(4):305–14. https://doi.org/10.1016/s2468-1253(19)30048-2.
64. Münch A, et al. Microscopic colitis: current status, present and future challenges: statements of the European Microscopic Colitis Group, (in eng). J Crohns Colitis. 2012;6(9):932–45. https://doi.org/10.1016/j.crohns.2012.05.014.
65. Pardi DS. Diagnosis and Management of Microscopic Colitis, (in eng). Am J Gastroenterol. 2017;112(1):78–85. https://doi.org/10.1038/ajg.2016.477.
66. Boland K, Nguyen GC. Microscopic colitis: a review of collagenous and lymphocytic colitis, (in eng). Gastroenterol Hepatol (N Y). 2017;13(11):671–7.
67. Vigren L, et al. Celiac disease and other autoimmune diseases in patients with collagenous colitis, (in eng). Scand J Gastroenterol. 2013;48(8):944–50. https://doi.org/10.3109/0036552 1.2013.805809.
68. Pardi DS, et al. Acute major gastrointestinal hemorrhage in inflammatory bowel disease, (in eng). Gastrointest Endosc. 1999;49(2):153–7. https://doi.org/10.1016/s0016-5107(99)70479-7.
69. Morrison TC, Wells M, Fidler JL, Soto JA. Imaging workup of acute and occult lower gastrointestinal bleeding, (in eng). Radiol Clin N Am. 2018;56(5):791–804. https://doi.org/10.1016/j.rcl.2018.04.009.
70. Mekaroonkamol P, et al. Repeat colonoscopy's value in gastrointestinal bleeding, (in eng). World J Gastrointest Endosc. 2013;5(2):56–61. https://doi.org/10.4253/wjge.v5.i2.56.
71. Vernava AM 3rd, Moore BA, Longo WE, Johnson FE. Lower gastrointestinal bleeding, (in eng). Dis Colon Rectum. 1997;40(7):846–58. https://doi.org/10.1007/bf02055445.
72. Huprich JE. Multi-phase CT enterography in obscure GI bleeding, (in eng). Abdom Imaging. 2009;34(3):303–9. https://doi.org/10.1007/s00261-008-9412-8.
73. Huprich JE, Barlow JM, Hansel SL, Alexander JA, Fidler JL. Multiphase CT enterography evaluation of small-bowel vascular lesions, (in eng). AJR Am J Roentgenol. 2013;201(1):65–72. https://doi.org/10.2214/ajr.12.10414.
74. Anderson R, Burr NE, Valori R. Causes of post-colonoscopy colorectal cancers based on world endoscopy organization system of analysis, (in eng). Gastroenterology. 2020;158(5):1287–1299. e2. https://doi.org/10.1053/j.gastro.2019.12.031.
75. Lieberman DA, Rex DK, Winawer SJ, Giardiello FM, Johnson DA, Levin TR. Guidelines for colonoscopy surveillance after screening and polypectomy: a consensus update by the US Multi-Society Task Force on Colorectal Cancer, (in eng). Gastroenterology. 2012;143(3):844–57. https://doi.org/10.1053/j.gastro.2012.06.001.
76. Rex DK, et al. Quality indicators for colonoscopy, (in eng). Gastrointest Endosc. 2015;81(1):31–53. https://doi.org/10.1016/j.gie.2014.07.058.
77. Rex DK, Vemulapalli KC. Retroflexion in colonoscopy: why? Where? When? How? What value? (in eng). Gastroenterology. 2013;144(5):882–3. https://doi.org/10.1053/j.gastro.2013.01.077.
78. Ai X, et al. Results of a second examination of the right side of the colon in screening and surveillance colonoscopy: a systematic review and meta-analysis, (in eng). Eur J Gastroenterol Hepatol. 2018;30(2):181–6. https://doi.org/10.1097/meg.0000000000001009.
79. Koffas A, Laskaratos FM, Epstein O. Non-small bowel lesion detection at small bowel capsule endoscopy: a comprehensive literature review, (in eng). World J Clin Cases. 2018;6(15):901–7. https://doi.org/10.12998/wjcc.v6.i15.901.

Chapter 9
Biliary- Pancreatic System

Cassidy Alexandre, Peter Ells, and Hwajeong Lee

Anatomy and Relevant Vasculature

The right and left hepatic ducts, shortly after leaving the porta hepatis, unite to form the 2- to 3-cm long hepatic duct, which then joins the cystic duct to form the common bile duct (CBD), 10 to 15 cm in length. The CBD is partially or fully covered by pancreatic tissue posteriorly as it descends into the duodenum. In more than 66% of cases, the CBD and the major pancreatic duct share a common channel, 2 to 7 mm in length. The two ducts unite to form the hepatopancreatic ampulla (ampulla of Vater), where the distal end of the ampulla opens into the duodenum through the major duodenal papilla [2]. See Fig. 9.1 for illustration.

Generally, the arterial supply to the pancreas, common bile duct, and adjacent portions of the duodenum comes from branches of the gastroduodenal, superior mesenteric, and splenic arteries. The arteries supplying the bile duct include the posterior superior pancreaticoduodenal artery and gastroduodenal artery, supplying the retroduodenal part of the duct; cystic artery, supplying the proximal part of the duct; and right hepatic artery, supplying the middle part of the duct [3].

C. Alexandre · P. Ells (✉)
Department of Medicine, Division of Gastroenterology, Albany Medical Center, Albany, NY, USA
e-mail: alexanc1@amc.edu; ellsp@amc.edu

H. Lee
Department of Pathology and Laboratory Medicine, Albany Medical Center, Albany, NY, USA
e-mail: LeeH5@amc.edu

© The Author(s), under exclusive license to Springer Nature Switzerland AG 2021
M. Tadros, G. Y. Wu (eds.), *Management of Occult GI Bleeding*, Clinical Gastroenterology, https://doi.org/10.1007/978-3-030-71468-0_9

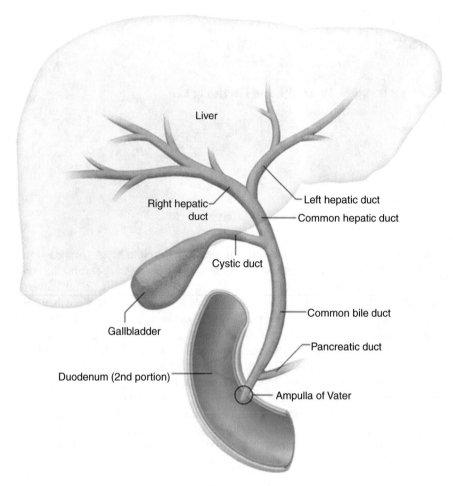

Fig. 9.1 The biliary tree [4]. https://link.springer.com/chapter/10.1007/978-1-4939-1884-3_5

Etiologies

Hemobilia arises where there is a fistula between the surrounding vascular structure and the biliary tree. Bleeding may result from obstruction or injury of any of the organs or structures associated with the hepatobiliary-pancreatic tract. The arterial system is usually the source of the bleeding due to relatively greater intravascular pressure creating unidirectional flow into the biliary tree. However, cases of hemobilia associated with higher venous pressure have been reported in the presence portal hypertension [5]. Most cases of hemobilia result from an iatrogenic injury, through inflammation, trauma, or vascular anomalies and can also occur spontaneously in setting of coagulopathy [6–15]. Malignancy in the hepatobiliary-pancreatic tract can also contribute to obscure nonvariceal upper GI bleeding as it has been demonstrated in cases of ampullary and periampullary tumors [16, 17].

Percutaneous Liver Procedures

Percutaneous liver interventions are of widespread use due to their minimal invasive approach and they can often be performed in the outpatient setting. Some of those procedures include liver biopsy, percutaneous transhepatic cholangiography (PTC), and percutaneous biliary therapies, including radiofrequency ablation. The insertion of a needle through the liver for tissue sampling or intervention can potentially cause inadvertent injury to interior blood vessels which are anatomically near the biliary tree. Formation of fistula and communication between hepatic vasculature and biliary system can ensue. The true incidence of hemobilia due to liver biopsies is unclear. However, a large multicenter retrospective study on 68,267 biopsies only revealed 4 reported cases of hemobilia but no deaths [18]. It has been reported that there is a higher incidence of hemobilia with percutaneous transhepatic biliary drainage (PTBD) in comparison to percutaneous transhepatic cholangiography (PTC) [19]. This is likely due to the increased instrumentation and manipulation prior to drain insertion in PTBD [19].

Hepatobiliary Surgery

Surgery of the hepatobiliary system carries potential risk for hemobilia. Cystic artery and right hepatic artery pseudoaneurysms leading to hemobilia have been reported as complications of laparoscopic and open cholecystectomy [20–22]. Though the exact pathogenesis of the pseudoaneurysm formation has yet to be determined, it is thought to be related to bile leakage causing blood vessels irritation and associated peritoneal infection; hence delaying proper healing of damaged vasculature. Cases of hemobilia have also been reported with liver transplantation and pancreaticoduodenectomy (Whipple procedure) [23, 24].

Endoscopic Hepatobiliary Procedures

Bleeding during endoscopic sphincterotomy or post-sphincterotomy is a common complication, typically from an arterial source associated with the margin of cut sphincter. This is manifested as bright red blood flowing outward from the lesion to the duodenum. Anomalous location of the ampulla creates a set of challenges and difficulties for endoscopic retrograde cholangiopancreatography (ERCP) and is a risk factor for sphincterotomy associated hemobilia [25]. Other clinical settings where ERCP associated hemobilia have been observed include portal biliopathy, metal biliary stenting, and intrahepatic vascular anomalies associated with hereditary hemorrhagic telangiectasia [26–28]. Portal biliopathy refers to abnormalities of the biliary system seen as a late complication of portal hypertension in patients with extrahepatic portal venous obstruction. It gives rise to cavernous transformation of the blood vessels nearing the biliary tree. In essence, this creates choledochal varices that can easily damage or rupture especially in setting intraductal manipulations. Spontaneous hemobilia has also been reported in portal biliopathy without endoscopic intervention. Of note, ERCP-associated hemobilia increases in coagulopathy and biliary stenosis [5].

Accidental Trauma

Liver injury frequently occurs in blunt abdominal trauma victims and the mortality rate related to the liver injury is estimated to range from 4.1% to 11.7% [29]. When the liver sustains a blunt trauma, a shearing injury of the hepatic artery may develop resulting in a hepatic pseudoaneurysm [30]. Intraperitoneal hemorrhage can result if these pseudoaneurysms rupture. They can also drain into the biliary system leading to hemobilia. Cases of hemobilia are seen in less than 3% of liver trauma. Hemobilia related abdominal trauma is more common to the pediatric population [31].

Cholelithiasis

Cholelithiasis can cause minor trauma to the bile duct, hence mild intraductal bleeding. However, significant hemobilia can occur if the stone erodes through the hepatoduodenal ligament or cystic artery, potentially resulting in cystic artery aneurysm [32]. In severe cases, choledocholithiasis can provoke necrotic erosion through the ductal wall and into surrounding blood vessels, leading to significant hemorrhage [33].

Inflammation and Infection

Hemobilia can arise from known complications of chronic pancreatitis; namely pseudoaneurysm of the pancreaticoduodenal, splenic, hepatic, and gastroduodenal arteries. Similarly, chronic cholecystitis may be complicated by cystic artery pseudoaneurysm resulting in hemobilia [34].

Infection of the biliary tree and liver is also a risk factor for hemobilia. Ascaris lumbricoides, Clonorchis sinensis, and Fasciola hepaticum are known parasites that are associated with infection and obstruction in the biliary tree and liver. Some of the clinical manifestations are ascending cholangitis, acute cholecystitis, pancreatitis, hepatic abscess, and hemobilia [34]. The mechanism of hemobilia in that setting is inflammation of perivascular tissue, weakening of vessel walls, and pseudoaneurysm formation [34].

Malignancy

Hepatobiliary tumors (primary or metastatic) are potential causes of hemobilia. Tumor tissue is often friable and hypervascular, which creates the likelihood of spontaneous hemorrhage. Furthermore, the biliary tree can be invaded by those tumors [35]. Minimal invasive procedures, such as radiofrequency ablation, are effective and relatively safe at managing unresectable hepatic tumors, however a range of complication have been reported. Hemobilia is a known potential complication of percutaneous intervention and has been related to radiofrequency ablation. Hepatocellular carcinoma (HCC), cholangiocarcinoma (Fig. 9.2), pancreatic adenocarcinoma, gallbladder cancer, and liver metastases have reportedly caused hemobilia [36–38].

Missed Lesions

Ampullary (Fig. 9.3) and periampullary lesions are rare entities, however they are often missed on routine upper endoscopies. They have also been reported as etiologies of occult GI bleeding, likely related to ulceration and slow blood loss due to the hypervascular and friable nature of those lesions [16, 17]. Radiographic imaging techniques such as CT angiography and radionucleotide tagged red blood cell scan,

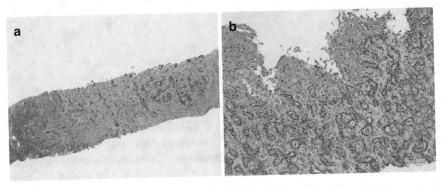

Fig. 9.2 Microscopic images of intrahepatic cholangiocarcinoma. (**a**) the tumor induces marked desmoplastic stromal response [Hematoxylin and eosin (H&E), original magnification ×40]. (**b**) infiltrative neoplastic glands in the hepatic parenchyma [H&E, original magnification ×100]

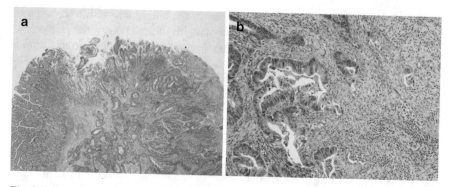

Fig. 9.3 Ampullary adenocarcinoma. (**a**) Scanning view of ampullary adenocarcinoma extending toward duodenal submucosa [H&E, original magnification ×20]. (**b**) Higher magnification view shows neoplastic glands within desmoplastic stroma [H&E, original magnification ×100]

are usually useful only during active bleeding. Side-viewing endoscope should be strongly considered while evaluating the duodenal papilla and the ampullary complex, especially in cases of suspected hemobilia or nonvariceal upper gastrointestinal bleeding.

Hemosuccus Pancreaticus (HP)

Hemosuccus pancreaticus (HP) is a rare entity of gastrointestinal bleeding. It is clinically distinct from hemobilia as bleeding originates from the pancreatic duct instead of the common bile duct. It is often associated with pancreatic diseases. Hemosuccus pancreaticus can be due to chronic pancreatitis, pancreatic pseudocysts, and pancreatic neoplasms where bleeding occurs from an erosion into a blood vessel forming a fistula with the pancreatic duct [39]. Therapeutic endoscopic intervention of the pancreas, such as pancreatic sphincterotomy or stone removal, can contribute to hemosuccus pancreaticus [39].

Clinical Presentation

The classic triad of hemobilia is right upper quadrant pain, jaundice, and bleeding, however all three findings are only present in 22–35% of cases [38]. Most cases of hemobilia are characterized by minor hemorrhage that resolve spontaneously, though profuse bleeding presenting with hematemesis, melena or hematochezia can also occur. Slow oozing in the biliary tract can lead to blood clot, which can then cause obstructive jaundice and is associated with biliary sepsis. The presentation of hemobilia and its timing vary based on the etiology. For instance, hemobilia due to ERCP usually occurs immediately or within the next few days [40, 41]. Presentation can also be delayed in cases pseudoaneurysm formation or following a trauma. In patients with a percutaneous transhepatic biliary drain (PTBD), blood output from the biliary drain is often noted.

Diagnosis

Hemobilia should be suspected in patients presenting with GI bleeding, history of right upper quadrant abdominal pain, jaundice, recent biliary instrumentation and abnormal liver function tests (LFTs). Diagnosis of hemobilia, however, can be delayed or missed due to lack awareness from clinicians. Moreover, given its rare occurrence and sometimes insidious presentation, diagnosis of hemobilia can be challenging. Imaging and endoscopic studies play a crucial role in establishing an initial diagnosis, assessing possible etiology and extent of bleeding, and guiding treatment modalities. Figure 9.4 provides a flow diagram for management of suspected hemobilia.

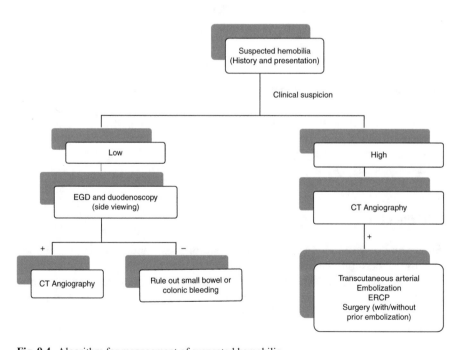

Fig. 9.4 Algorithm for management of suspected hemobilia

Diagnostic Imaging

Computed Tomography Angiography (CTA)

CT angiography of the abdomen has been recognized as the first-line investigative modality in suspected hemobilia due to its noninvasive nature, rapid results, and diagnostic yield and characteristics. CTA can not only help confirm hemobilia but also provide details about potential etiology [42]. Some the pathologies identified on CTA include extravasation into the parenchyma, clots in the gallbladder or biliary system, biliary dilatation, pseudoaneurysms, and other vascular malformations (e.g., aneurysms, angiodysplasia, arteriovenous malformations and hemangiomas).

Angiography

Angiography remains the gold standard for diagnosis and treatment of hemobilia as it can help localize the actual bleeding source and provide detailed visualization of the vasculature and potential anomalies (arteriobiliary fistula, vascular malformations such as aneurysms, pseudoaneurysms, hemangiomas etc.). It does, however, involve higher radiation exposure and endovascular access unlike the CTA. It has been reported that angiography yields the correct etiology of massive hemobilia in more than 90% of cases [43].

Magnetic Resonance Cholangiopancreatography (MRCP)

MRCP is not often used for the diagnosis of hemobilia though it has been reported in cases involving biliary obstruction [8]. It is a noninvasive alternative to endoscopic retrograde cholangiopancreatography (ERCP) that shows imaging of the pancreaticobiliary system [8].

Ultrasound

Abdominal ultrasound is dependent on operator's skill and experience and body habitus can certainly be a detrimental factor in preventing proper visualization of the biliary tree. Moreover, blood clots within the bile ducts lose echogenicity over time and can be missed during ultrasound examination [43]. Therefore, the diagnostic effectiveness of abdominal ultrasound in identifying hemobilia is limited.

Endoscopy

Upper GI endoscopy (esophagogastroduodenoscopy) is commonly used in the evaluation of patients presenting with upper GI bleeding. It is very effective at ruling out common etiologies of upper GI bleeding and can, sometimes incidentally, diagnose cases of hemobilia. When hemobilia is suspected, a duodenoscope (i.e., side-viewing scope) should be used to directly visualize the ampulla for the presence of blood and/or clots or ampullary lesions (Fig. 9.5a).

ERCP helps to visualize the bile ducts, gallbladder and can even play a therapeutic role in cases of hemobilia and/or associated with biliary obstruction. ERCP findings of blood clots to suggest hemobilia are characterized by amorphous, tubular, or cast-like filling defects in the biliary tree or gallbladder (Fig. 9.5b) [43].

Endoscopic ultrasound (EUS) has been used to successfully diagnosed hemobilia from hepatic artery pseudoaneurysm [44]. It can also be helpful at identifying blood within the biliary tree, common bile duct, which would be characterized by mobile, hyperechoic material [45].

Cholangioscopy is an advanced endoscopic technique that has been reported to determine the etiology of hemobilia in rare cases [46]. It provides direct visualization of the biliary tree however endoscopic therapy is limited due to small accessory channel.

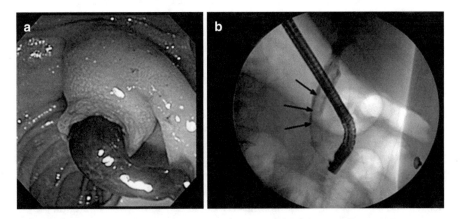

Fig. 9.5 (a) Blood clot at the papilla in a case of hemobilia seen with side-viewing duodenoscopy. (b) ERCP demonstrating radiolucent filling defects in the extrahepatic bile duct in a patient found to have hemobilia [34]. https://link.springer.com/article/10.1007/s11894-010-0092-5

Management

After adequate resuscitation, management of hemobilia comprises of 2 objectives: achieve hemostasis and maintain biliary patency and adequate bile flow. The modalities used in the management of hemobilia depend on the etiology of the bleed, however they mostly encompass conservative therapy, percutaneous radiologic intervention, endoscopic treatment and surgery.

Conservative management is usually reserved for minor hemobilia and interventions usually include correction of coagulopathy if needed, and IV fluid hydration. Minor hemobilia can often be seen in injury related to PTBD catheters where catheter exchange and upsize and position adjustment can help tamponade blood and resolve hemobilia [42].

Angiography

Radiologic interventions for management of hemobilia can serve both diagnostic and therapeutic modalities. Angiography has emerged as the gold standard for management of hemobilia and has a success rate of 80% to 100% [47]. Of note, iatrogenic hemobilia is commonly related to hepatic artery injury. Angiography with transcatheter arterial embolization (TAE) is often considered when hemobilia is secondary to large arterial aneurysms or pseudoaneurysms, arteriobiliary fistulae, and/or intrahepatic or extrahepatic vascular lesions.

After selecting the injured artery, embolization is performed both proximal and distal to the injury to ensure that no back bleeding occurs via intrahepatic arterial collaterals [48]. As the liver receives dual blood supply (portal vein and hepatic artery), TAE is contraindicated when portal vein thrombosis or obstruction is present in order to prevent potential significant hepatic ischemia. TAE should be avoided in patients with liver transplant, cirrhosis with concurrent shock, as more extensive ischemic liver injury can result due to the already compromised collateral blood flow [49]. An alternative to TAE is arterial stenting which works as a tamponade measure. It may be beneficial in cases where preserving blood flow is critical and when TAE is contraindicated. Complications of TAE include hepatic ischemia leading to necrosis, hepatic abscesses, hyperaminotransaminemia, and gallbladder infarction [50].

Percutaneous thrombin injection is a salvage technique used to management pseudoaneurysms when TAE fails [51–53].

ERCP

There is a role for the use of ERCP in management of hemobilia especially in hemodynamically stable patients. Moreover, it can help maintain biliary patency by removing blood clots within the biliary tree; hence preventing obstructive jaundice, acute cholangitis, acute cholecystitis, and acute pancreatitis [43]. Post-sphincterotomy hemobilia arises from injury of the posterior branch of the superior pancreaticoduodenal artery and many endoscopic techniques can be used in the management of this postprocedural bleeding. Balloon tamponade, monopolar or bipolar coagulation, epinephrine injection, hemoclipping, and biliary stenting have been reported to be successful at post-sphincterotomy hemobilia or in cases where the site of bleeding is distal (i.e., at the level of the papilla or ampulla) [54–56].

Biliary stents have been reported to help control bleeding located at the extrahepatic bile duct. They work by providing a tamponade effect on the bile duct wall while maintaining ductal patency to allow bile flow. Metallic and plastic stents have been used successfully in managing hemobilia related to therapeutic maneuvers of sphincterotomy, stent removal, papillary balloon dilation, bile duct biopsy, pancreatic fine-needle aspiration, and malignancy with bile duct invasion [35, 57–62].

Surgery

Surgical intervention is indicated in cases of failed, endoscopic, endovascular, and/or percutaneous therapies. Surgery is also needed when hemobilia is complicated by cholecystitis. When pseudoaneurysms are infected or are compromising surrounding vasculature, surgery is also preferred [43, 44]. When the lesion or injury is located, the damaged vessel is ligated, or the infected pseudoaneurysm is excised. Cholecystectomy can be performed concurrently if indicated. Of note, in setting of uncontrolled intrahepatic bleeding, partial hepatectomy is an option.

References

1. Yoshida J, Donahue PE, Nyhus LM. Hemobilia: review of recent experience with a worldwide problem. Am J Gastroenterol. 1987;82:448–53.
2. Floch MH, et al. Netter's gastroenterology. Philadelphia: Saunders/Elsevier; 2010.
3. Moore KL, Agur AMR, Dalley AF. Essential clinical anatomy. Philadelphia: Lippincott Williams & Wilkins; 2002.
4. Wagner-Bartak NA, Prabhakar AM, Menias CO, Prabhakar HB, Elsayes KM. The biliary tree. In: Elsayes KM, editor. Cross-sectional imaging of the abdomen and pelvis. New York: Springer; 2015. https://doi.org/10.1007/978-1-4939-1884-3_5.
5. Schlansky B, Kaufman JA, Bakis G, et al. Portal biliopathy causing recurrent biliary obstruction and hemobilia. ACG Case Rep J. 2013;1:44–6.
6. Ahn J, Trost DW, Mitty HA, Sos TA. Pseudoaneurysm formation after catheter dissection of the common hepatic artery: report of two cases. Am J Gastroenterol. 1997;92:696–9.
7. Albuquerque W, Arantes V, de Paula FK, Lambertucci JR. Acute pancreatitis and acute cholecystitis caused by hemobilia after percutaneous ultrasound-guided liver biopsy. Endoscopy. 2005;37:1159–60.
8. Asselah T, Condat B, Sibert A, et al. Haemobilia causing acute pancreatitis after percutaneous liver biopsy: diagnosis by magnetic resonance cholangiopancreatography. Eur J Gastroenterol Hepatol. 2001;13:877–9.

9. Attiyeh FF, McSweeney J, Fortner JG. Hemobilia complicating needle liver biopsy: a case report with arteriographic demonstration. Radiology. 1976;118:559–60.

10. Bichile LS, Malkan G, Patel YS, et al. Recurrent haemobilia in a patient with polyarteritis nodosa. J Assoc Physicians India. 1996;44:49–50.

11. de Quinta FR, Moles ML, Docobo DF, et al. Hemobilia secondary to chronic cholecystitis. Rev Esp Enferm Dig. 2004;96:221–5.

12. de Sio I, Castellano L, Calandra M. Hemobilia following percutaneous ethanol injection for hepatocellular carcinoma in a cirrhotic patient. J Clin Ultrasound. 1992;20:621–3.

13. Edden Y, St Hilaire H, Benkov K, Harris MT. Percutaneous liver biopsy complicated by hemobilia-associated acute cholecystitis. World J Gastroenterol. 2006;12:4435–6.

14. Enne M, Pacheco-Moreira LF, Cerqueira A, et al. Fatal hemobilia after radiofrequency thermal ablation for hepatocellular carcinoma. Surgery. 2004;135:460–1.

15. Forlee MV, Krige JE, Welman CJ, Beningfield SJ. Haemobilia after penetrating and blunt liver injury: treatment with selective hepatic artery embolization. Injury. 2004;35:23–8.

16. Janzen RM, Ramj AS, Flint JDA, Scudamore CH, Yoshida EM. Obscure gastrointestinal bleeding from an ampullary tumour in a patient with a remote history of renal cell carcinoma: a diagnostic conundrum. Can J Gastroenterol. 1998;12(1):75–8.

17. Kashani A, Nissen NN, Guindi M, Jamil LH. Metastatic periampullary tumor from hepatocellular carcinoma presenting as gastrointestinal bleeding. Case Rep Gastrointest Med. 2015;2015:732140.

18. Piccinino F, Sagnelli E, Pasquale G, et al. Complications following percutaneous liver biopsy. A multicentre retrospective study on 68,267 biopsies. J Hepatol. 1986;2:165–73.

19. Fidelman N, Bloom AI, Kerlan RK Jr, et al. Hepatic arterial injuries after percutaneous biliary interventions in the era of laparoscopic surgery and liver transplantation: experience with 930 patients. Radiology. 2008;247:880–6.

20. Park JY, Ryu H, Bang S, et al. Hepatic artery pseudoaneurysm associated with plastic biliary stent. Yonsei Med J. 2007;48:546–8.

21. Ribeiro A, Williams H, May G, et al. Hemobilia due to hepatic artery pseudoaneurysm thirteen months after laparoscopic cholecystectomy. J Clin Gastroenterol. 1998;26:50–3.

22. Wen F, Dong Y, Lu ZM, et al. Hemobilia after laparoscopic cholecystectomy: imaging features and management of an unusual complication. Surg Laparosc Endosc Percutan Tech. 2016;26:e18–24.

23. Mori K, Murata S, Yoshioka H, et al. Transcatheter embolization of celiac artery pseudoaneurysm following pancreaticoduodenectomy for pancreatic cancer. A case report. Acta Radiol. 1998;39:690–2.

24. Londono MC, Balderramo D, Cardenas A. Management of biliary complications after orthotopic liver transplantation: the role of endoscopy. World J Gastroenterol. 2008;14:493–7.

25. Tsou YK, Liu NJ, Jan YY. Biliary obstruction caused by hemobilia after endoscopic sphincterotomy in a patient with an anomalous location of papilla of Vater. Gastrointest Endosc. 2008;68:1232–4.

26. Dhiman RK, Behera A, Chawla YK, et al. Portal hypertensive biliopathy. Gut. 2007;56:1001–8.

27. Costa MT, Maldonado R, Valente A, et al. Hemobilia in hereditary hemorrhagic telangiectasia: an unusual complication of endoscopic retrograde cholangiopancreatography. Endoscopy. 2003;35:531–3.

28. Rai R, Rose J, Manas D. Potentially fatal haemobilia due to inappropriate use of an expanding biliary stent. World J Gastroenterol. 2003;9:2377–8.

29. Matthes G, Stengel D, Seifert J, et al. Blunt liver injuries in polytrauma: results from a cohort study with the regular use of whole-body helical computed tomography. World J Surg. 2003;27:1124–30.

30. Croce MA, Fabian TC, Spiers JP, Kudsk KA. Traumatic hepatic artery pseudoaneurysm with hemobilia. Am J Surg. 1994;168:235–8.

31. Jones PM, Subbarao G. Hemobilia caused by hepatic artery pseudoaneurysm following abdominal trauma. J Pediatr Gastroenterol Nutr. 2015;60:e40.

32. Yu YH, Sohn JH, Kim TY, et al. Hepatic artery pseudoaneurysm caused by acute idiopathic pancreatitis. World J Gastroenterol. 2012;18:2291–4.
33. Jee SL, Lim KF, Krishnan R. A rare case of fulminant hemobilia resulting from gallstone erosion of the right hepatic artery. Med J Malaysia. 2014;69:191–2.
34. Chin MW, Enns R. Hemobilia. Curr Gastroenterol Rep. 2010;12:121–9.
35. Kawaguchi Y, Ogawa M, Maruno A, et al. A case of successful placement of a fully covered metallic stent for hemobilia secondary to hepatocellular carcinoma with bile duct invasion. Case Rep Oncol. 2012;5:682–6.
36. Ahmad SS, Basheer FT, Idris SF, et al. Cholangiocarcinoma presenting as hemobilia and recurrent iron-deficiency anemia: a case report. J Med Case Rep. 2010;4:133.
37. Coulier B, Maldague P, Ramboux A, et al. Mass-forming intrahepatic cholangiocarcinoma presenting with painful obstructive hemobilia. JBR-BTR. 2014;97:366–9.
38. Ooishi T, Saeki I, Yamasaki T, et al. Hepatocellular carcinoma-induced hemobilia. Intern Med. 2014;53:1579.
39. Etienne S, Pessaux P, Tuech JJ, et al. Hemosuccus pancreaticus: a rare cause of gastro-intestinal bleeding. Gastroenterol Clin Biol. 2005;29:237–47.
40. Green MHA, Duell RM, Johnson CD, Jamieson NV. Haemobilia. Br J Surg. 2001;88(6):773–86.
41. Goffette PP, Laterre PF. Traumatic injuries: imaging and intervention in post-traumatic complications (delayed intervention). Eur Radiol. 2002;12(5):994–1021.
42. Cathcart S, Birk JW, Tadros M, Schuster M. Hemobilia an uncommon but notable cause of upper gastrointestinal bleeding. J Clin Gastroenterol. 2017;51:796–804.
43. Berry R, Han J, Girotra M, Tabibian JH. Hemobilia: perspective and role of the advanced endoscopist. Gastroenterology research and practice. 2018; vol. 2018, Article ID 3670739, 12 pages.
44. Konerman MA, Zhang Z, Piraka C. Endoscopic ultrasound as a diagnostic tool in a case of obscure hemobilia. ACG Case Rep J. 2016;3:e170.
45. Cattan P, Cuillerier E, Cellier C, et al. Hemobilia caused by a pseudoaneurysm of the hepatic artery diagnosed by EUS. Gastrointest Endosc. 1999;49:252–5.
46. Foong KS, Lee A, Kudakachira S, Ramberan H. Hemobilia from biliary angiodysplasia diagnosed with cholangioscopy. ACG Case Rep J. 2016;3(4):e132.
47. Marynissen T, Maleux G, Heye S, et al. Transcatheter arterial embolization for iatrogenic hemobilia is a safe and effective procedure: case series and review of the literature. Eur J Gastroenterol Hepatol. 2012;24:905–9.
48. Saad WEA, Davies MG, Darcy MD. Management of bleeding after percutaneous transhepatic cholangiography or transhepatic biliary drain placement. Tech Vasc Interv Radiol. 2008;11(1):60–71.
49. Zaydfudim VM, Angle J, Adams R. Current management of hemobilia. Curr Surg Rep. 2014;2:54.
50. Srivastava DN, Sharma S, Pal S, et al. Transcatheter arterial embolization in the management of hemobilia. Abdom Imaging. 2006;31:439–48.
51. Kumar A, Sheikh A, Partyka L, et al. Cystic artery pseudoaneurysm presenting as a complication of laparoscopic cholecystectomy treated with percutaneous thrombin injection. Clin Imaging. 2014;38:522–5.
52. Robert Y, Dubrulle F, Chambon JP, et al. Iatrogenic aneurysm of the hepatic artery. Treatment by percutaneous injection of thrombin and selective arterial embolization. Ann Chir. 1994;48:210–3.
53. Ghassemi A, Javit D, Dillon EH. Thrombin injection of a pancreaticoduodenal artery pseudoaneurysm after failed attempts at transcatheter embolization. J Vasc Surg. 2006;43:618–22.
54. Bagla P, Erim T, Berzin TM, et al. Massive hemobilia during endoscopic retrograde cholangiopancreatography in a patient with cholangiocarcinoma: a case report. Endoscopy. 2012;44(suppl 2 UCTN):E1.
55. Leung JW, Chan FK, Sung JJ, et al. Endoscopic sphincterotomy-induced hemorrhage: a study of risk factorsand the role of epinephrine injection. Gastrointest Endosc. 1995;42:550–4.

56. Katsinelos P, Paroutoglou G, Beltsis A, et al. Endoscopic hemoclip placement for postsphinc-terotomy bleeding refractory to injection therapy: report of two cases. Surg Laparosc Endosc Percutan Tech. 2005;15:238–40.
57. Itoi T, Yasuda I, Doi S, et al. Endoscopic hemostasis using covered metallic stent placement for uncontrolled postendoscopic sphincterotomy bleeding. Endoscopy. 2011;43:369–72.
58. Valats JC, Funakoshi N, Bauret P, et al. Covered selfexpandable biliary stents for the treatment of bleeding after ERCP. Gastrointest Endosc. 2013;78:183–7.
59. Aslinia F, Hawkins L, Darwin P, et al. Temporary placement of a fully covered metal stent to tamponade bleeding from endoscopic papillary balloon dilation. Gastrointest Endosc. 2012;76:911–3.
60. Song JY, Moon JH, Choi HJ, et al. Massive hemobilia following transpapillary bile duct biopsy treated by using a covered self-expandable metal stent. Endoscopy. 2014;46(suppl 1 UCTN):E161–2.
61. Barresi L, Tarantino I, Ligresti D, et al. Fully covered selfexpandable metal stent treatment of spurting bleeding into the biliary tract after endoscopic ultrasound-guided fine-needle aspiration of a solid lesion of the pancreatic head. Endoscopy. 2015;47(suppl 1 UCTN):E87–8.
62. Shinjo K, Matsubayashi H, Matsui T, et al. Biliary hemostasis using an endoscopic plastic stent placement for uncontrolled hemobilia caused by transpapillary forceps biopsy (with video). Clin J Gastroenterol. 2016;9:86–8.

Part III
Treatment Modalities

Chapter 10
Bipolar and Monopolar Cautery, Clips, Bands, Spray, Injections, Embolization, and Minimally Invasive Surgery

Enxhi Rrapi, Sunil Narayan, Gary Siskin, Steven C. Stain, Micheal Tadros, and Marcel Tafen

Introduction

Upon diagnosis of an occult GI bleed through iron deficiency anemia with or without a positive fecal occult blood test, the first step in management of occult GI bleeding is to stabilize the patient. Treatment of underlying anemia should be initiated. A careful review of the patient's medical and surgical history may help localize bleeding to the upper GI tract (esophagus to the ligament of Treitz) or lower GI tract (ligament of Treitz to the rectum) and identify any contributing underlying disease, such as portal hypertension, peptic ulcer disease/gastritis, malignancy, arteriovenous malformation/angiodysplasia, or recent surgery/intervention. In the appropriate clinical context, pharmacotherapy (proton pump inhibitors, somatostatin, etc.) may temporize active bleeding. Once the patient is stable, a variety of treatment options may be considered—including therapeutic endoscopic modalities,

E. Rrapi
Albany Medical College, Albany, NY, USA
e-mail: rrapie@amc.edu

S. Narayan · G. Siskin
Vascular and Interventional Radiology, Albany Medical College, Albany, NY, USA
e-mail: narayas1@amc.edu; sisking@amc.edu

S. C. Stain
Department of Surgery, Albany Medical College, Albany, NY, USA
e-mail: stains@amc.edu

M. Tadros (✉)
Department of Gastroenterology and Hepatology, Albany Medical Center, Albany, NY, USA
e-mail: tadrosm1@amc.edu

M. Tafen
Division of Trauma and Surgical Critical Care, Albany Medical College, Albany, NY, USA
e-mail: tafenwm@amc.edu

© The Author(s), under exclusive license to Springer Nature
Switzerland AG 2021
M. Tadros, G. Y. Wu (eds.), *Management of Occult GI Bleeding*, Clinical
Gastroenterology, https://doi.org/10.1007/978-3-030-71468-0_10

interventional radiology, and surgery. While the book's main focus is on occult GI bleeding, in order to review the principles of endoscopy, interventional radiology, and surgical treatment, there will be some degree of overlap with overt GI bleeding. Sometimes, overt bleeds can be intermittent, recurrent, and go unnoticed, and result in iron deficiency anemia and heme positive stool.

Therapeutic Endoscopic Modalities

Endoscopy is a safe and effective method for treating GI bleeds [1]. Endoscopic hemostatic methods for GI bleeding include thermal, mechanical, topical and injection therapies (Table 10.1). An overview of the treatment modalities follows, along with the effectiveness of each method.

Table 10.1 Summary of therapeutic endoscopic modalities and the lesions they are used to treat

Modality	Type	Use
Thermal	Bipolar and Monopolar Probes (ex, Gold Probe, HeatProbe, and Coagrasper)	Bipolar probes (ex. Gold Probe) are recommended as treatment for hemorrhaging ulcers and nonbleeding visible vessels. HeatProbes are used to treat peptic ulcers in the upper two thirds of the posterior wall of the lesser curvature of the corpus of the stomach and the posterior wall of the duodenal bulb. Monopolar probes (ex. Coagrasper) are effective in treating non-variceal bleeding and managing gastroduodenal ulcer bleeding
	Argon Plasma Coagulation	Recommended for use when treating AVMs, gastric antral vascular ectasias, and CRP
Mechanical	Through the Scope Clips (Endoclips)	Useful in managing non-variceal type bleeding such as Mallory-Weiss tears, Dieulafoy's lesions, diverticular bleeding, bleeding peptic ulcers, postpolyectomy bleeding, and perforations and fistulas
	Over the Scope Clips	Should be used in patients with recurrent bleeding when other therapies have not worked. Typically used to promote hemostasis of perforations and fistulas
	Band Ligation	Primarily recommended as a first treatment variceal bleeding. EBL has been shown to be effective in managing esophageal and duodenal Dieulafoy lesions, and Mallory Weiss tears
Topical	Procoagulant Spray (Hemospray)	Recommended for management of tumoral GI bleeds. Usually used as a second-line intervention when patients experience unsuccessful long-term hemostasis with the standard therapies such as in the case of unresectable cancers. Also, used in combination with thermal therapy for peptic ulcer treatment
Injection	Epinephrine	Should not be used as a monotherapy. Is recommended for use in combination therapy with thermal or mechanical therapy
	Glue (ECGI)	Useful in managing gastric varices
	Sclerosing Agents	Useful in treatment of esophageal varices (obsolete in the United States)

Thermal Therapy

Thermal or thermal coagulation therapy is a technique endoscopists utilize to promote hemostasis through cauterization of the bleeding site, resulting in coagulation of the lesion. Thermal therapy can be further categorized into contact and noncontact techniques.

Contact thermal therapy is performed through direct tissue contact with the cauterizing device. Through direct tissue contact, the device compresses the bleeding site while simultaneously cauterizing the tissue in a process called coaptive coagulation. Cauterizing devices can be further subdivided into bipolar probe (ex. Gold Probe), heater probe (ex. HeatProbe), and monopolar probe (ex. Coagrasper). These devices are especially useful in treating active hemorrhages and nonvisible vessels such as those underlying peptic ulcers.

Bipolar probes generate heat from electrical currents that pass through electrodes; the heat is transferred onto the bleeding tissue through contact (Fig. 10.1). The electrical current must be transferred to the tissue at an angle or perpendicular to the bleeding site to achieve desiccation. The current will automatically stop flowing when it reaches a specified temperature in the tissue. This makes administering thermal therapy easier and more straightforward. An inherent limitation of the probe does not allow for deep tissue penetration; this eliminates the possibility of this device causing perforation of the underlying tissue and increased rates of rebleeding [2]. Thermal therapy works by facilitating tissue damage; therefore, multiple rounds of this therapy to the same bleeding site is not recommended. Additional limitations of the bipolar probe include its dependence on the inherent tissue properties such as tissue water, resistance, or desiccation. Device properties and settings can be altered depending on the lesion that is being treated [3]. Bipolar probes are specifically recommended to manage hemorrhaging ulcers and nonbleeding visible vessels [4].

Heater probes are yet another type of contact diathermy. Although they have similar efficacy to bipolar probes, they are more difficult to use because they require perpendicular application of heat. Furthermore, the design and heating technology of the device make it easier to cause deep tissue coagulation [5]. Therefore, heater probes require experienced endoscopists to minimize the risk of perforation. When used properly, heater probes efficiently achieve hemostasis of peptic ulcers. A study

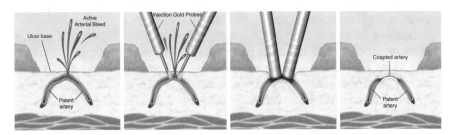

Fig. 10.1 Bipolar thermal hemostasis via Injection Gold Probe™. Copyright Boston Scientific Corporation. Courtesy of Boston Scientific

that compared the efficacy of heater probes and hemoclips (a form of mechanical therapy) found that heater probes are more successful in halting peptic ulcer bleeding in the upper two thirds of the posterior wall of the lesser curvature of the corpus of the stomach and the posterior wall of the duodenal bulb – areas that are hard reach with mechanical therapy [5].

Monopolar probes are another method of performing contact thermal therapy. Like bipolar probes, they promote coagulation through cauterization via an electric current. However, due to their one-electrode device nature, monopolar probes require grounding pads. Furthermore, the technique required to deliver the current to the bleeding site also differs from the bipolar probe technique. For monopolar probes, either the edges of the bleeding site are tautly pulled away from the GI wall and then cauterized or the probe is lightly touched to the center of the stigmata. Monopolar probes have been shown to be effective in treating non-variceal bleeding. Some disadvantages to monopolar probes include that the device has no inherent limitation on the current transferred to the bleeding site. This increases the chances of deep tissue penetration and formation of GI perforations [6]. It is important that endoscopists using this thermal modality have proper training in administering treatment. New monopolar hemostatic forceps, Coagrasper, attempt to address this limitation by maintaining the voltage at a constant level to decrease the chance of deep tissue coagulation and promoting soft coagulation. Although studies are limited, there have been promising outcomes with the use of these new devices in effectively managing gastroduodenal ulcer bleeding [7]. Small comparative studies have preliminarily shown that the Coagrasper is more effective than the heater probe and hemoclips in achieving primary hemostasis with less adverse effects and lower rebleeding rates [7, 8].

Noncontact thermal therapy is performed through indirect tissue contact with the cauterizing device. This technology is used in the Argon Plasma Coagulation (APC) device. APC stimulates hemostasis with an electrical current generated from ionizing argon gas. The ionization energy is then dispersed into the nearby tissue, making this therapy less precise and able to cover large areas. Depending on the clinical situation, this can be an advantage of the APC, when compared to the contact therapy devices, by allowing the device reach to bleeding sites that are in hard-to-reach areas. APC results in more superficial coagulation because coaptive coagulation is not possible with APC treatment due to the nature of noncontact diathermy. Due to its low penetrance of tissue, APC is particularly useful in managing superficial bleeding sites such as Arteriovenous malformations (AVMs), gastric antral vascular ectasias, and chronic radiation proctitis (CRP) [9–11].

Regarding its use in treating CRP, radiofrequency ablation (RFA) is another endoscopic modality that has made headway. As its name suggests, RFA works to ablate tissue with radiofrequency energy delivered through a catheter [10]. This form of intervention has been especially successful in treating CRP in patients who have had recurrent bleeding after APC treatment. The RFA technique offers the advantage of covering broader areas and making even less superficial ablations, further lowering the complications associated with thermal therapy and decreasing the chance of rebleeding [12]. With further research, RFA may emerge as the standard treatment for individuals with complicated cases of CRP.

Mechanical Therapy

Mechanical therapy requires the use of devices that promote hemostasis by physically closing the bleeding source. Clips and Bands are the most common agents used to perform mechanical endoscopic therapy.

Clips can further be categorized as *Through the Scope Endoclips (Endoclips)*, which are widely used, and *Over-The-Scope-Clips (OTSC)* (Fig. 10.2). The endoclips and OTSCs differ in how they are deployed, the amount of area they can compress, and the efficacy of the clips in treating peptic ulcers and recurrent bleeding ulcers [13–15]. The mechanical agent of choice is dependent on recognizing the type of lesion or bleeding site. There are a variety of endoclips which allow for different movements during and after deployment of the clips [4]. Endoclips are deployed through-the-scope and require trained endoscopists for proper placement (Fig. 10.3). In order to properly place the clip, it is important for the hemorrhaging area to be visible and clear to receive the clip. Poor visibility of the stigmata can lead to improper placement of the clip and increased rates of recurrent bleeding. Multimodal therapy that pairs injections with endoclips can help mitigate this problem. In spite of the advancements that have made endoclips more user-friendly, anatomical locations of lesions and difficult deployment of endoclips persist as

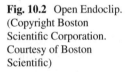
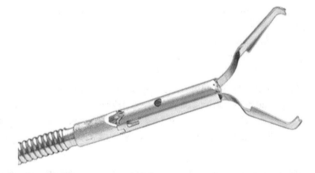

Fig. 10.2 Open Endoclip. (Copyright Boston Scientific Corporation. Courtesy of Boston Scientific)

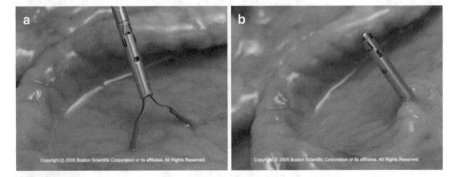

Fig. 10.3 (**a**) Open clip. (**b**) Deployed, closed clip. (Copyright 2005 Boston Scientific Corporation. Courtesy of Boston Scientific)

limiting factors in their efficacy [16]. Endoclips are recommended for achieving hemostasis in non-variceal type bleeding such as bleeding peptic ulcers, Mallory-Weiss tears, Dieulafoy's lesions, diverticular bleeding, and postpolyectomy bleeding [17–21].

As the name suggests, OTSC are deployed over the endoscope. Placement of OTSC requires clasping the edges of the hemorrhagic site and pulling them into the endoscope, effectively embedding them in the OTSC compartment (a cylindrical cap-like structure). OTSC can close bleeding sites of larger diameters than endoclips [22]. Despite this, OTSC are generally used as a second-line mechanical tool because they are more expensive and not always the most cost-effective option when compared to endoclips. OTSC can be used to treat rebleeding sites that were unsuccessfully managed by endoclips and are typically used to promote hemostasis of perforations and fistulas [14, 23–26]. Studies show that OTSC remain in situ up to 39 days longer (with an average of 25 days longer) than endoclips and result in decreased levels of recurrent bleeding [14, 27].

Some evidence suggests that clips are more efficacious than thermal therapy, especially for the treatment of ulcers. This is partly due to the way the clips result in hemostasis. Tamponade is promoted through compression of blood vessels and not through tissue damage, which is how thermal therapy works [28]. Meanwhile, other studies show that clips are less successful in achieving homeostasis of ulcers than thermal therapy [5]. Overall, more research is necessary to conclude which modality is more effective.

Endoscopic band ligation (EBL) is another mechanical tool that is used to compress the bleeding site and promote hemostasis (Fig. 10.4). The EBL is performed in a similar manner to OTSC, and rubber bands are used to compress the bleeding site instead of a cylindrical cap-like structure [29]. In contrast to clips, EBL is the preferred mechanical device used to treat variceal bleeding [30]. EBL is specifically recommended for treating esophageal varices due to decreased rebleeding rates and complications [31, 32]. The efficacy of EBL in treating non-variceal bleeding has

Fig. 10.4 Deployed band. (Copyright Boston Scientific Corporation. Courtesy of Boston Scientific)

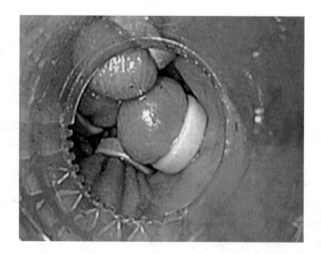

also been studied. With increasing research on the use of EBL to treat non-variceal bleeding, perceptions have changed regarding the efficacy of this technique. EBL can be also used in effectively managing Dieulafoy lesions, Mallory Weiss tears, and peptic ulcers [33–35].

Injection Therapy

Injection therapy for GI hemorrhage aims to promote hemostasis through the introduction of a variety of substances into the stigmata (Figs. 10.5 and 10.6). We will be focusing on three main injectable agents: epinephrine, tissue adhesives (or glue), and sclerosing agents, all of which are further discussed below.

Fig. 10.5 Needle. (Copyright Boston Scientific Corporation. Courtesy of Boston Scientific)

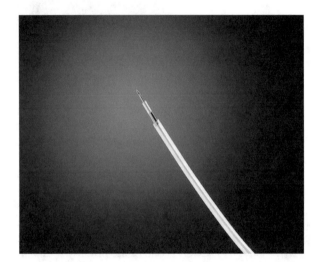

Fig. 10.6 Needle injection of an agent to promote hemostasis

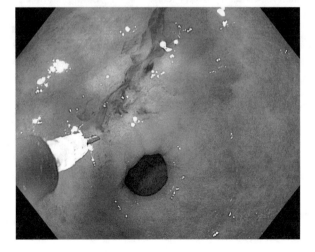

Fig. 10.7 White out effect on mucosa after epinephrine injection: it is important to realize that epinephrine is a temporary measure only and other therapeutic modalities are needed

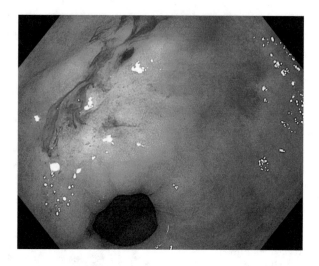

Epinephrine injections are administered around the source of bleeding to promote vasoconstriction, allowing for temporary hemostasis (Fig. 10.7). The volume of epinephrine injections ranges from 1 mL to 40 mL. Depending on the volume injected, epinephrine can produce different results. A larger dose produces a longer period of hemostasis and a decrease in the rate of rebleeding [36]. Advantages of epinephrine injections include straightforward application and temporary relief that clears the site of bleeding, allowing for better visibility of the stigmata. This is especially useful when following up the injection with mechanical or thermal therapy to achieve long-term hemostasis. Generally, one-time injections are rendered less efficacious than thermal and mechanical therapy. When paired with another treatment modality, injections are less likely to lead to rebleeding episodes [37–39].

Tissue adhesive injections (Glue) achieve initial hemostasis by causing temporary tissue injury. ECGI is one of the primary agents injected to promote thrombosis. ECGI is typically used in the management of gastric varices. Similar to epinephrine, it achieves short-term hemostasis [40]. Yet, recurrent bleeding post-treatment is common. Therefore, it is recommended to pair ECGI injections with another endoscopic treatment modality to achieve long-term hemostasis. An additional limitation is due to the tissue injury incurred from the injection; physicians can only administer minimal amounts of the ECGI [41]. Despite EBL being more efficacious than ECGI in treating esophageal varices, ECGI therapy is preferred over EBL to treat gastric varices due to its lower complication rate [31, 32, 42, 43].

Other injectable agents include *sclerosants*, which are not typically used during endoscopic therapy in the US. Injection of sclerosing agents results in tissue injury through endothelial damage, which leads to subsequent thrombosis and fibrosis of the area, resulting in hemostasis. Common sclerosing agents include saline, thrombin and fibrin sealant, fatty acid derivatives (ethanolamine oleate and sodium morrhuate), synthetic agents (sodium tetradecyl sulfate and polidocanol), and alcohols [44]. Saline has been shown to be less effective than epinephrine – leading to higher rebleeding rates [2]. Fibrin sealants show promising results in achieving primary hemostasis. Fibrin sealants promote coagulation through the facilitation of platelet-platelet aggregation. They have been shown to be more effective than polidocanol in preventing rebleeding events [45]. More research is needed to establish the efficacy of fibrin sealants in relation to other injectable agents and other therapeutic endoscopic modalities. Sclerosing agents are seen to be a preferred mode of treating esophageal varices, especially in developing and under resourced countries, where cost is a major barrier to care. Some case reports show that sclerotherapy has also been successful in managing non-variceal bleeding sites like Dieulafoy's lesions [44]. In terms of efficacy, there is a lot of conflicting research on which sclerosing agent is most successful. When choosing an agent, it is recommended that the physician take cost, risk for complications, and patient history into consideration. Overall, the current consensus is that injectable agents are more efficacious when used in combination therapy for ulcers, gastric varices, non-variceal bleeding, etc. [2, 37, 40].

Topical Therapy

Topical therapy is another modality used in treating hemorrhagic GI sites. Topical therapy comes in many forms, most notably as a procoagulant spray, *Hemospray*. Hemospray is an inorganic powder that is applied to the source of bleeding and causes coagulation through a couple of mechanisms (Fig. 10.8). Like mechanical agents, Hemospray facilitates a physical tamponade. Additionally, when the powder substance is dispensed, it adheres to the bleeding site and absorbs bleeding factors, creating a barrier over the source [46]. Advantages to this method of application include that it does not require much precision, it can cover large areas, and it is relatively safe to use because it does not create tissue injury.

Furthermore, the procoagulant spray is versatile and has been successfully used as a monotherapy in addition to its uses in combinatory therapy. Procoagulant spray can be used similarly to epinephrine injections where it promotes initial hemostasis to momentarily stop active bleeding [47]. Unlike epinephrine injections, procoagulant

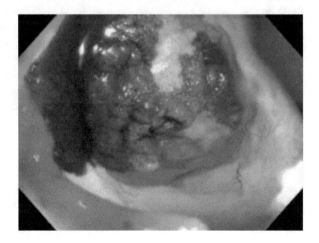

Fig. 10.8 This a picture of a small bowel tumor in the distal duodenum where active bleeding was stopped using Hemospray. Once stable, the patient underwent surgical resection

spray monotherapy has had success in achieving long-term hemostasis in patients with acute lesions that have low risks of recurrent bleeding. Disadvantages to this form of therapy include that it is relatively superficial, so it is limited to the types of lesions that it can treat and not recommended as the sole treatment of hemostasis of underlying vessels. For bleeding sites known for high recurrent rates, it is recommended that Hemospray is used in combination with another endoscopic intervention. Additionally, Hemospray presents technical challenges in how it is delivered, leading to the clogging of the endoscope [46]. Despite this, Hemospray has been demonstrated to have successful outcomes in controlling both non-variceal and variceal bleeding. Further applications of hemostatic powders include management of tumoral GI bleeds. Endoscopists are also using hemostatic spray as second-line intervention for individuals whose bleeding was unsuccessfully managed with conventional treatment (injection, thermal, or mechanical therapies) [48]. Overall, studies show that hemostatic spray is a viable modality to manage GI bleeding. As with many of the other therapeutic endoscopic modalities, more research is needed with larger experimental populations.

Combination Therapy

With lesions that have a high risk of rebleeding, it is common to use a combination of therapeutic endoscopic modalities to achieve homeostasis. A multimodal approach that pairs modalities that successfully achieve temporary hemostasis with interventions that promote long-term hemostasis is recommended for the management of peptic ulcers and actively bleeding sites [49]. For example, combining epinephrine injections, which promote immediate hemostasis, with endoclips can help the endoscopist gain better visibility of the bleeding site and decrease the chance of improper placement of the endoclip. In general, proper placement of the clips and deployment of bands is correlated with decreased chances of rebleeding. Research shows that when epinephrine injections are combined with another modality, they result in better outcomes than when used as a monotherapy [37–39]. Similarly, multimodal therapy including hemostatic powder and a conventional modality, has shown to be more efficacious than hemostatic powder alone in management of peptic ulcer bleeding [50]. However, when comparing thermal contact monotherapy with injection plus thermal contact dual therapy, there is no significant difference in patient outcomes [49]. Although there are limited studies evaluating dual endoscopy therapy, which includes a combination of thermal, mechanical, or sclerosing injections, vs. monotherapy efficacy, the present data indicates that both therapies are equally efficacious [49].

Complications of Endoscopic Therapy

Endoscopic therapy for GI bleeding has many benefits and is minimally invasive. Nevertheless, there are complications associated with endoscopic therapy. Complications can be due to procedural challenges – such as poor visualization, location of the lesion, and device limitations – and operational errors due to lack of experience. Although risks can be minimized by good technique, some complications cannot be escaped. As with any other procedure, risk of infection and trauma are high. Perforations and tissue injury are common complications, especially when using thermal therapy. Specifically, for severe cases, risk of recurrent bleeding is high. Therefore, with any patient, it is important to weigh the risks and benefits before performing treatment [51, 52].

Interventional Radiology Management of Gastrointestinal Bleeding

While the primary focus of this text is the treatment of occult GI bleeding, many of the techniques discussed may be utilized in the treatment of overt/acute GI bleeding. Similarly, many disease conditions, namely portal hypertensive conditions and systemic diseases, may result in both chronic occult and overt episodes of GI bleeding. Interventional radiology therapy of GI bleeding is most successful when a bleed can be localized usually via endoscopy or non-invasive imaging. Triple phase CT angiography (CTA) without oral contrast (noncontrast, arterial phase, and venous phase) may be obtained in any patient with occult GI bleeding. Referring providers should provide a clinical history of occult GI bleeding, to indicate a desire to rule out underlying vascular anomalies rather than active bleeding. Nuclear medicine tagged red blood cell scintigraphy ("bleeding scan") has added sensitivity with the ability to detect bleeding rates as low as 0.1 mL/min; however, image acquisition is time consuming, lacks anatomic detail, and fails to identify the bleeding source in up to 50% of patients. When physicians have failed to identify and manage the bleeding source through therapeutic endoscopic modalities, IR methods can be pursued. Treatment of occult arterial gastrointestinal bleeding is via angiography and embolization. Treatment of variceal hemorrhage requires different access methods, equipment, and techniques including portosystemic shunt creation (TIPS/DIPS) and/or balloon-occluded or plug-assisted retrograde transrenal obliteration of varices (BRTO/PARTO) [53, 54].

Arterial Bleed

Introduction

Angiography may be pursued in patients whose bleeding is not controlled endoscopically or when complete workup fails to identify a bleeding source (Fig. 10.9). Catheter directed angiography is less sensitive in detecting bleeding than computed tomographic angiography (CTA) or nuclear medicine scintigraphy, but offers the benefit of concomitant therapy, namely embolization. The goal of embolization is to provide a scaffold for thrombus formation to occlude the pathologic blood vessel, reducing arterial perfusion pressure and bleeding. Embolic materials include commonly used

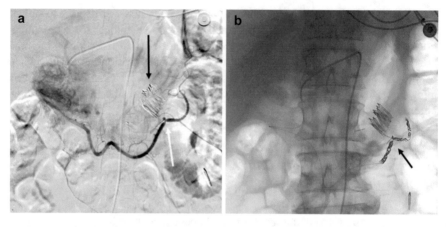

Fig. 10.9 (a) Selective arteriogram of the gastroepiploic artery reveals persistent pseudoaneurysm (*white arrow*) in the region of endoscoically placed clips over a suspected dieulafoy's lesion (*black arrow*) (b) Coil embolization was performed across the region of focal vascular abnormality (*black arrow*)

metallic coils and plugs, biologic and synthetic materials of varying shapes and sizes, and liquid glues or adhesives. These devices have varying biodegradability, onset, and visibility on fluoroscopy. Water or oil-based contrast media may be mixed with embolic agents to improve visibility on x-ray. Metallic embolic agents are generally permanent and will be visible on all of the patient's subsequent medical imaging.

Anatomy and Common Culprit Artery for Upper and Lower

The upper GI (UGI) tract is predominantly supplied by the celiac trunk. Superior mesenteric artery (SMA) interrogation is warranted if celiac interrogation does not reveal conventional anatomy. The lower GI (LGI) tract is supplied by the SMA, inferior mesenteric artery (IMA), and in cases of IMA occlusion, by the internal iliac arteries. Celiac artery interrogation may be necessary in rare instances of a replaced middle colic artery. Common culprit vessels in the UGI tract include the left gastric artery (fundal and gastroesophageal bleeding) and gastroduodenal artery (duodenal bleeding). LGI tract bleeding can be from a variety of sources and complete workup with non-invasive imaging and colonoscopy prior to angiography is highly recommended.

Access

The most common access site is via the right common femoral artery. This access point is usually palpable, offers a short distance to select the mesenteric vasculature, and offers the ability to tamponade access site bleeding with manual compression against the femoral head. Left radial artery access has emerged as an alternative to femoral arterial access, particularly in patients with increased risk of bleeding (high body mass index, chronic kidney disease, thrombocytopenia, inability to receive blood transfusion) or those with difficulty lying flat (low back pain, congestive heart failure, cognitive impairment) [55]. Radial access allows patients to sit up immediately following their procedure and is associated with increased patient satisfaction.

Prerequisite/Indications

The left gastric artery represents a special circumstance in UGI bleeding, as empiric embolization of endoscopically proven lesions is generally well tolerated due to the presence of multiple collateral vessels. Embolization for LGI bleeding is rarely empirical and recommended only upon confirmation of focal vascular anomaly or contrast extravasation due to the increased risk of bowel ischemia or delayed colonic ischemic stricture. Due to these risks, embolization for LGI bleeds may only be performed if selective catheterization is possible at the level of the mesenteric border of the colon. In the context of negative angiography and high clinical suspicion, provocative angiography may be considered to identify occult sources of bleeding localized by endoscopy or nuclear medicine scintigraphy. This approach requires an infusion of intra-arterial tissue plasminogen activator (tPA) or other thrombolytics to lyse suspected blood clots and "provoke" bleeding. Surgical consultation prior to considering this approach is prudent, as provoked bleeding may not be controllable and may necessitate emergent surgery. For this reason, provocative angiography is seldom employed [53, 56–59].

Technique

Coil embolization is the process of direct delivery of metallic coils to the area of vascular pathology (Fig. 10.10). Coils are sometimes referred to as mechanical embolic agents (in contrast with flow directed agents). Multiple coils are frequently utilized to create a "tight pack," amenable to thrombus formation. Embolic materials may be combined to increase the likelihood and speed of vessel thrombosis at the treating physician's discretion. If a catheter cannot be advanced close to the diseased vessel coil, embolization may still be performed across the branch vessel origin. When this approach is utilized, subsequent angiography of the Celiac, SMA, IMA, or internal iliac arteries must be performed to evaluate for collateral blood flow to the site of abnormality. In contrast to mechanical embolics, flow directed embolic agents such as N-butyl cyanoacrylate (NBCA), Onyx, spherical or irregular polyvinyl alcohol (PVA) particles, slurry or particle preparations of Gelfoam, or other spherical embolic agents, may be utilized to treat an entire vascular bed. This approach may be useful if there are multiple sources of bleeding or the cause of bleeding is determined to be an arteriovenous malformation or gastrointestinal

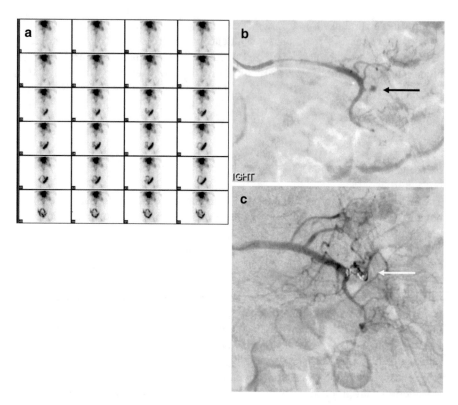

Fig. 10.10 (a) Selected images from tagged red blood cell scintigraphy show extravasation of radiotracer into small bowel in the left lower quadrant. (b) selective angiography of the jejunal artery reveals a pseudoaneurysm (*black arrow*). (c) coil embolization (*white arrow*) decreases filling of the pseudoaneurysm with preserved blood flow to distal small bowel

tumor. Liquid embolic agents, such as NBCA and Onyx, may be used in patients with uncorrected coagulopathy secondary to their ability to form a cast of the target vessel. Spherical embolic agents and drug-eluting beads are flow directed agents, which are advantageous in the treatment of an entire vascular bed [53]. Adequate diagnostic information regarding blood flow and experience preparing and using these agents is essential for safe deployment [53, 56–61].

Success Rate

Technical and clinical success of embolization for UGI bleeds is 93% and 67%, respectively [62]. The success rates for LGI bleeds are more varied by clinical context but average technical success is 88%, while average clinical success is 83% [63].

Complications

Arterial access for angiography is associated with risk of access site (groin) complications including hematoma (<3.1%), bleeding (<2.5%), and pain (<6.4%). Damage to the underlying artery resulting in pseudoaneurysm (<0.6%), retroperitoneal hematoma (<1%), AV fistula (<1%), or distal thromboembolism and limb ischemia (<0.4%), are rare complications, which warrant additional care and potentially subsequent procedures. All embolization procedures result in a degree of risk of subsequent bowel ischemia around 12%, which skews higher or lower based on the territory being treated and quality of collateral circulation [64]. Post procedure abdominal pain, passage of bloody stools, and occasionally fever and leukocytosis, may be encountered after embolization. The benefits of interventional radiology therapy relative to the risks should be discussed, but are generally recognized to have associated morbidity and mortality superior to surgical intervention [65].

Variceal Bleed

Introduction

Variceal hemorrhage (VH) is the leading cause of mortality in patients with portal hypertension. VH may present as occult bleeding, particularly secondary to ectopic varices, which are less amenable to endoscopic treatment [66].

Anatomy and Common Culprits

Esophageal varices (EV), gastric varices (GV), and gastroesophageal varices (GEV) make up the majority of endoscopically encountered culprits for bleeding. Ectopic varices are dilated mesoportal varices or portosystemic collaterals, which exist throughout the GI tract outside the gastroesophageal region. Ectopic varices are an underappreciated source of hemorrhage more common in extrahepatic (20–30%) versus intrahepatic portal hypertension (1–5%) [66].

Access

Clinical determination of the source of bleeding is important prior to interventional therapy of VH and access occurs via right internal jugular (RIJV) or right common femoral venous (RCFV) access rather than arterial access.

Prerequisites/Indications

Endoscopy is the preferred means of initial evaluation in patients with active or suspected VH. Since ectopic varices may be endoscopically occult, non-invasive cross-sectional imaging with portal venous or triple phase CT/CTA or contrast-enhanced MRI are recommended adjunctive testing. Patients with isolated or predominantly gastric varices may be amenable to treatment with BRTO and/or combination therapy with staged BRTO and TIPS or TIPS with antegrade transvenous obliteration or embolotherapy. Optimal management of VH requires multidisciplinary cooperation and thoughtful risk/benefit discussion with the patient prior to intervention.

Technique

TIPS RIJV is the conventional access method for TIPS. The left internal jugular vein may be utilized and is reported to offer more favorable angles for accessing the right hepatic vein, however, limited user experience may limit this benefit. Right hepatic vein access is preferred for its reliable positioning in the posterior liver parenchyma, which may be confirmed with lateral fluoroscopy. Reference to a preoperative CT or an intra-procedural wedged hepatic CO_2 venogram may be performed to confirm the relationship of the portal vein to the right hepatic vein. A non posterior location may suggest either selection of a middle hepatic vein or accessory right inferior hepatic vein, which in the cirrhotic liver may not have a consistent relationship with the portal vein and may increase the risk of extracapsular liver puncture and subsequent bleeding. Hockey stick shaped catheters and use of hydrophilic guidewires (Glidewire or Roadrunner) may facilitate right hepatic vein selection. Measurement of hepatic portal venous pressure gradient (HVPG) may be performed prior to and following the procedure to confirm adequate decompression for the indication (HVPG<12 mmHg is favored for treatment of varices). A needle is fired generally within the proximal 2–3 cm of a hepatic vein in the direction of the portal vein and slowly retracted under aspiration until portal venous blood is aspirated. Contrast injection through the needle confirms portal venous access. Coring (Colapinto) vs non-coring (Rosch-Uchida kits) needles allow for either advancing a wire through the access needle or over-sheathing and needle retraction to secure portal vein access. Dilatation of the parenchymal tract between the hepatic and portal veins with an angioplasty balloon is required to allow for sheath advancement into the portal vein and subsequent deployment of a bile-impermeable covered stent graft. Access to the portal venous system affords the opportunity for direct treatment of varices either via obliteration/sclerosis or embolotherapy. Portal venography prior to stent deployment illustrates flow dynamics of portal hypertension and the filling of varices and other porto-systemic shunts (Fig. 10.11).

Accessing the portal vein is generally considered to be the most technically challenging step of portosystemic shunt creation. Consequently, several advanced

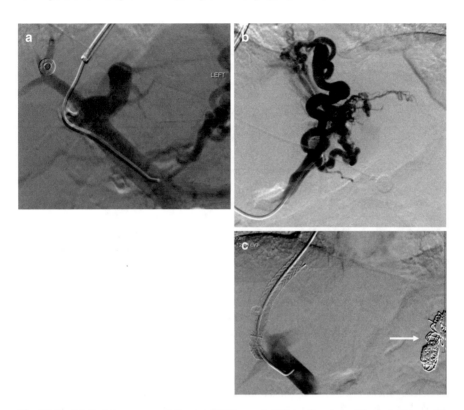

Fig. 10.11 (**a**) Portal venogram following TIPS reveals filling of gastroesophageal varices. (**b**) confirmed by selective injection of the coronary vein. (**c**) Varices are no longer filling following TIPS and coil embolization (*white arrow*)

techniques have been described in the literature to combat this challenge (Table 10.2) [67, 68]. In patients with non-opacification of the hepatic veins, as seen with Budd-Chiari syndrome, left internal jugular vein access may promote cannulation of a right or middle hepatic vein stump for wedged CO_2 portography. At the author's institution, percutaneous puncture of the liver targeting a snare in the IVC has been described as a means of creating an artificial tract through which CO_2 portography and subsequent portal vein localization may be performed. Either of these techniques carry increased risk of bleeding due to proximal puncture of the portal vein in the former case and liver capsule transgression in the latter.

Portal vein thrombosis is a rare situation which necessitates portal vein recanalization for successful shunt creation. Recanalization may proceed via transhepatic, transjugular, transmesenteric, trans-splenic, or combined surgical approaches. Wedged CO_2 portography and pre-procedural CT are again used to localize the main portal vein. Once access is obtained, a stiff, angled Glidewire and angiographic catheter are used to secure access and enable recanalization via either mechanical or Fogarty thrombectomy, catheter directed thrombolysis, or stenting.

Table 10.2 Complex portal vein access strategies

Problem	Technique	Special considerations
Hepatic vein occlusion	LIJ access and HV stump CO_2 portography	Increased bleeding risk
Hepatic vein occlusion	DIPS Transcaval puncture	Increased bleeding risk Special IVUS catheter is recommended
Intrahepatic tumor, cysts, poor IJ/SVC HV access	Pre-procedural CT localization, hybrid imaging	Increased radiation dose, increased procedure time, possibly increased bleeding risk, potential for malignant seeding
Inability to puncture portal vein despite multiple attempts	"Gun-sight" technique	Multiple punctures increase bleeding risk, increased radiation dose
Portal vein thrombus	Portal vein recanalization	Increased bleeding due to multiple punctures and/or procedures
Difficulty with portal vein localization	Marking hepatic artery with microcatheter Snare, basket, or wire deployment in portal vein via para-umbilical vein, direct varix access or trans-splenic puncture	Multiple access required, increased bleeding risk

Failure to localize the portal vein, despite wedged CO_2 portography and multiple puncture attempts, may be addressed with "gun-sight technique," described by Haskal et al. [68]. This technique involves placement of a snare within both the IVC and portal vein through access conventionally described via a recanalized para-umbilical vein, although trans-splenic puncture may enable similar snare deployment. As described, a large snare is deployed within the IVC and small snare within the portal vein, which are aligned on fluoroscopy allowing for needle puncture traversing both snares and through and through wire access. As with other advanced methods, bleeding risk is the primary concern given the need for additional punctures.

The presence of intrahepatic tumors, cysts, or no suitable hepatic vein access may necessitate transcaval shunt creation. Pre-procedural CT and/or hybrid imaging modalities (live fluoroscopy and either cone beam or pre-procedural CT) are essential to select an appropriate level for caval puncture in the direction of the portal vein. Portal access needles must be modified to assume an almost 90-degree angulation to allow for portal vein puncture, and caution to avoid capsule transgression is needed to minimize bleeding risk. The use of intravascular ultrasound (IVUS) to localize the portal vein from the IVC is the basis for the DIPS procedure described below.

Access to the portal vein may be obtained via a recanalized umbilical vein or via percutaneous trans-splenic puncture of a dilated splenic vein. These access routes allow for a snare to be deployed in a portal vein branch and targeted on fluoroscopy.

DIPS Direct intrahepatic portosystemic shunt arose as an advanced technique to portosystemic shunts directed at patients with absent jugular or SVC access to the hepatic veins, Budd-Chiari patients, and patients with pre-existing occluded TIPS. The portal vein is localized utilizing an intravascular ultrasound (IVUS) catheter positioned within the IVC via RCFV access. A modified needle is then fired into the portal vein under ultrasound guidance with the remaining steps identical to TIPS.

Balloon-occluded Retrograde Transvenous Obliteration (BRTO) and PARTO Unlike TIPS/DIPS, transvenous obliteration procedures are directed towards direct treatment of isolated gastric varices. These procedures do not alleviate and may exacerbate portal hypertension and associated sequelae (esophageal varices, ascites, pleural effusion, etc). A balloon or vascular plug is utilized to occlude the drainage of a gastrorenal or splenorenal shunt, prior to introduction of sclerosant to confine the sclerosant to varices (Fig. 10.12). The balloon is placed via a vascular access sheath and must be left inflated for up to 4 hours, after which the patient should have imaging to evaluate efficacy of variceal obliteration. Alternatively, coils and plugs may be utilized to permanently occlude shunt drainage, which eliminates the need for subsequent angiography, yielding a logistical improvement in patient management [69].

Success Rate

Combination of TIPS and embolotherapy is associated with statistically lower rebleeding rates when compared to TIPS alone in 5 of 8 studies performed between 2005 and 2014 [70]. Initial clinical success with TIPS is high (97–100%); however, rebleeding rates secondary to GEV's are as high as 20% and 20–40% for ectopic varices [59, 71]. DIPS is associated with a greater risk of extrahepatic puncture and bleeding relative to traditional TIPS, but has similar outcomes [72]. BRTO is successful in controlling bleeding from gastric varices in greater than 95% of patients and has significantly lower rates of hepatic encephalopathy when compared with TIPS (1% vs 30%). Efficacy of transvenous obliteration procedures for ectopic varices is not well established and requires further research [71].

Complications

TIPS is a generally safe procedure with a complication rate for experienced operators of 5% and a mortality rate of less than 2% in elective cases. Complications associated with right internal jugular vein access are rare with ultrasound guidance, but include carotid or subclavian artery puncture, pneumothorax, and injury to adjacent cervical structures. Guidewires advance into the right atrium or right ventricle may induce a cardiac arrhythmia which is typically transient and resolves with retraction of the offending catheter or guidewire. Rarely sustained arrhythmias may

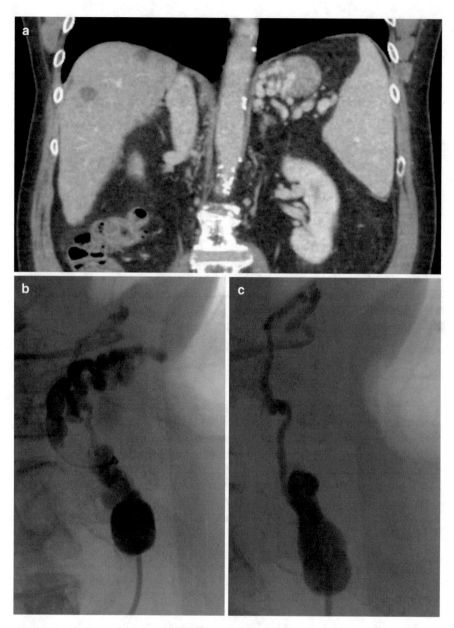

Fig. 10.12 (**a**) Coronal contrast enhanced CT shows filling of gastric varices. Additional images revealed the source as a prominent gastro-renal shunt. (**b**) Balloon assisted retrograde venogram of a gastrorenal shunt opacifying gastric varices. (**c**) Venogram following administration and indwelling of sodium tetradecyl sulfate foam and lipiodol shows reduced filling of gastric varices

be encountered including supraventricular or ventricular tachycardia. The most serious early complication associated with TIPS is intraperitoneal bleeding secondary to either extrahepatic portal vein puncture (2%) or extracapsular liver puncture (5%). Transgression of the liver capsule may allow for injury to extrahepatic organs such as bowel, kidney (1.5%), or gallbladder (10%) [73]. Intrahepatic biliary duct puncture (5%) is a complication of more commonly historically with the use of non-covered stent grafts [73]. Hemobilia related to biliary duct puncture or inadvertent hepatic arterial puncture (<1%) are rare but may require subsequent angiography embolization if there is suspicion of significant bleeding. Wedged hepatic venography, particularly with carbon dioxide can cause laceration of the liver parenchyma or liver capsule rupture if injections are performed too forcefully.

The most common early complication following TIPS is worsening of hepatic encephalopathy (20–50%), which is managed medically, but in less than 10% of cases may necessitate revision or occlusion of the portosystemic shunt. Additional complications ranging in incidence between 2–10% include hemobilia, portal vein thrombosis, stent migration/misplacement (<1%), infection/biliary peritonitis, nephropathy, and hemolysis [59, 74].

Complications of BRTO/PARTO are associated with exacerbation of the patient's existing portal hypertension and associated sequelae. The most notable of these is esophageal varices, which are expected to enlarge (30–68%) and potentially bleed (17–24%). Other complications include portal hypertensive gastropathy (5–13%), ascites (0–44%), and hydrothorax/pleural effusion (0–8%) [69].

Future IR Therapies

Embolization therapy for other indications, specifically bleeding secondary to hemorrhoids, is currently under investigation. Small case studies outside the United States have reported clinical success between 72–97% following either coil or coil and particle embolization of the superior rectal arteries. These treatment methods must first be validated, but in the future, they may offer an additional minimally invasive treatment strategy for GI bleeding secondary to hemorrhoids [75–77].

Surgical Management of Gastrointestinal Bleeding

For any patients with bleeding, the therapeutic protocol should include a thorough initial evaluation to classify the bleeding as occult, obscure, or overt, and then detect the source of bleeding through endoscopy and/or angiography. Resuscitation, medical therapy, and correction of coagulopathy are essential [78, 79]. Indications for surgical management of GI bleeds include inadequate resources for the management of GI bleeds, such as lack of skilled endoscopists, repeated hospitalization for GI bleeding, other indications for laparotomy, and, most importantly, failure of at least two attempts at endoscopic management [80–83]. The operative approach is dictated by the etiology of bleeding, the patient's hemodynamic status, whether the bleeding is obscure, and the location (known vs. unknown site of bleeding). With the advances in surgical techniques, most of the surgeries are now minimally invasive and done laparoscopically.

Upper GI Bleed

Peptic Ulcer Bleeding

The overall goals of surgery for peptic ulcer bleeding include control of bleeding, suppression of gastric acid secretion with or without an accompanying drainage procedure, eradication of *Helicobacter pylori* infection, and exclusion of cancer.

Surgical strategies that are used in clinical practice to control bleeding in the stomach secondary to peptic ulcer disease include:

- *excision of ulcers* in more proximal locations,
- distal *gastrectomy*, or
- simple *suture ligation* (a less morbid and preferred option).

Control of bleeding typically involves *over-sewing* of ulcers that occur in areas that are not easily amenable to resection, such as in the duodenum or the proximal stomach. Following a distal gastric resection, reconstruction can be done in two configurations: a gastroduodenostomy (***Billroth I reconstruction***) or a gastrojejunostomy (***Billroth II reconstruction***) [83]. A Billroth I reconstruction involves the creation of an anastomosis between the duodenum and the gastric remnant, while a Billroth II reconstruction consists of an anastomosis between the stomach and a jejunal loop. Based on the location and pathogenesis, gastric ulcers can be categorized into the five types. Type 1 ulcers occur in the body of the stomach, high along the lesser curvature near the incisura, and are associated with *H. pylori* infection. Type 2 ulcers usually occur in the pre-pyloric area and are often associated with duodenal ulcers. Type 3 ulcers occur in the antrum. Type 4 ulcers occur along the lesser curvature of the stomach near the gastroesophageal junction (GEJ). Type 5 ulcers are diffuse ulcerations of the gastric mucosa associated with nonsteroidal anti-inflammatory drug use. This classification of gastric ulcers not only reflects the pathogenesis but also determines the surgical management, which often includes a combination of the strategies discussed (Table 10.3).

Bleeding from a duodenal ulcer occurs when the ulcer posteriorly erodes into the gastroduodenal artery. This bleeding can be surgically controlled by simple suture ligation through an opening in the anterior duodenal wall (*anterior duodenotomy*). A generous Kocher maneuver is performed to mobilize the duodenum followed by an anterior duodenotomy over the first and second portions of the duodenum through the pylorus. Once the site of bleeding is exposed, direct digital pressure should be applied immediately, followed by placement of 3 to 4 U sutures around the bleeding ulcer using non-absorbable suture material. Finally, the duodenostomy should be closed in a transverse fashion.

Table 10.3 Summary of surgical management for GI bleeding

Source of GIB	Treatment options	Notes
Type 1 gastric ulcer	Distal gastrectomy (antrectomy) and Billroth I*	Type 1 gastric ulcers are higher on the lesser curvature and do not have elevated acid production
Type 2 gastric ulcer	Antrectomy and Billroth I/II and Vagotomy*	Associated with a duodenal ulcer and acid hypersecretion
Type 3 gastric ulcer	Antrectomy and Vagotomy*	Prepyloric ulcer. Acid overproduction
Type 4 gastric ulcer	No consensus on treatment. Subtotal gastric resection or distal gastrectomy often pursued	Near GEJ
Type 5 gastric ulcer	Packing of the stomach and subtotal gastrectomy	
Duodenal ulcer	1. Oversew + Truncal Vagotomy+ Pyloroplasty 2. Oversew + Truncal Vagotomy + Antrectomy 3. Oversew only**	
Mallory-Weiss tears	Over-sewing	
Dieulafoy lesions	Over-sewing	
Aorto-enteric fistulas	Graft explantation, extraanatomical bypass, enterotomy repair	
Hemobilia	Angiography	
Hemosuccus pancreaticus	Angiography	
Small bowel bleeding	Segmental resection	
Colonic bleeding	Segmental resection	
Bleeding esophageal varices	• Portocaval shunt • Splenorenal shunt • Esophagogastric devascularization and transection	
Sinistral hypertension	Splenectomy	

*For unstable patients, biopsy and oversew or wedge resection should be done instead.
**For unstable patients

After control of bleeding, it is important to initiate treatment to suppress gastric acid production. This can be effectively achieved with medications, and this strategy should be considered as first-line therapy in patients with bleeding peptic ulcers, who have not received prior treatment and are compliant with the regimen. Vagal denervation of the stomach effectively reduces acid secretion and contributes to duodenal ulcer healing. A *vagotomy* is achieved by severing the vagus nerve at three possible levels. Based on the level at which the nerve is cut, a vagotomy is classified into truncal, selective, or highly selective vagotomy. Truncal vagotomy involves transection of the vagus proximal to GEJ. Selective vagotomy involves transection of the vagus below the GEJ with preservation of the hepatic and celiac branches. Highly selective vagotomy involves transection of only those branches of the vagus that supply the stomach, with preservation of the hepatic, celiac, and antral branches. Emergency truncal vagotomy is necessary only for patients who have failed proton pump inhibitor (PPI) therapy or are allergic to PPIs. Selective vagotomy is time consuming and is not useful for the surgical management of peptic ulcer-induced bleeding [84]. Vagotomy induced acid suppression results in altered gastric emptying secondary to denervation of the pylorus and antral hypergastrinemia with gastrin cell hyperplasia. Highly selective vagotomy can effectively minimize hypergastrinemia and altered gastric emptying. However, highly selective vagotomy is associated with weaker acid suppression and a higher risk of ulcer recurrence.

Vagotomy should be accompanied by a *drainage procedure* as a counterregulatory mechanism for vagotomy induced delayed gastric emptying. A *Heineke-Mikulicz pyloroplasty* and *antrectomy* (removal of the pylorus) are examples of drainage procedures. The Heineke-Mikulicz pyloroplasty is a simple and rapid procedure. Antrectomy offers the advantage of including a bleeding ulcer in the resection and eliminates the parietal cells, resulting in greater acid suppression. However, performing an antrectomy is time consuming and is therefore not ideal in emergencies. Other complications of a vagotomy include dumping syndrome and post-vagotomy diarrhea.

In summary, surgical options for bleeding duodenal ulcers include the following:

- simple suture ligation through an anterior duodenotomy,
- suture ligation, antrectomy, and truncal vagotomy for stable patient's refractory to acid suppression therapy, or alternatively,
- suture ligation, vagotomy, and duodenoplasty.

Most of these procedures can be performed using minimally invasive technique; however, these techniques are not advisable in emergent situations.

Following gastric acid suppression, a urea breath test, fecal antigen test, or biopsy based tests should be performed for *H. pylori* testing, and antibiotics should be administered for eradication [85]. Lastly, cancer is ruled out by evaluation of biopsy specimens obtained from the edge and base of an ulcer [86].

Non-Peptic Ulcer Bleeding

Non-peptic ulcer bleeding includes bleeding from varices, tumors, Mallory-Weiss tears, Dieulafoy lesions, aorto-enteric fistulas, hemobilia, hemosuccus pancreaticus, as well as iatrogenic and traumatic injuries. Management of bleeding in such cases depends upon the specific lesion.

Bleeding from Mallory-Weiss tears is usually self-limited and rarely requires surgical intervention [87]. Dieulafoy lesions cause intermittent bleeding and are difficult to localize. In both cases, surgery when required, involves *over-sewing* of the lesions (the mucosa and the bleeding vessel, respectively) through a gastrotomy

[88]. Management of GIB is most challenging in patients with diffuse erosive gastritis refractory to medical management. Hemodynamic instability in patients necessitates packing of the stomach as a temporary measure, intra-arterial vasopressin injection, and ultimately subtotal or near-total gastrectomy [89–91]. In patients with benign or malignant GI tumors, partial gastric resection is often indicated [92].

Variceal Bleed

Sengstaken-Blakemore tube or self-expanding metal stent placement is useful to tamponade the bleeding site and stabilize patients with variceal bleeding that is refractory to multiple endoscopic treatments. This procedure provides adequate time for initiation of resuscitative measures, correction of coagulopathy, and optimization for further intervention [93]. Depending on the availability of surgeons with the required expertise, patients with active bleeding and acceptable surgical risks should be considered for portacaval (nonselective) shunt placement. For patients without active bleeding, a more selective distal splenorenal shunt should be considered. Complete esophagogastric devascularization and transection (the *Sugiura* procedure) may be performed as a last resort in patients in whom shunt placement is not possible. However, this approach is associated with a significantly high mortality rate [94].

Poor surgical candidates with variceal bleeding, who are otherwise stable, should undergo transjugular intrahepatic portosystemic shunt (TIPS) placement. However, careful patient selection is important because of serious complications, such as worsening encephalopathy associated with this procedure. Patients deemed appropriate candidates for the TIPS procedure should undergo evaluation for liver transplantation at a transplant center. For patients with noncirrhotic sinistral (left-sided) portal hypertension, the approach to treatment is different. Noncirrhotic sinistral portal hypertension results from occlusions in prehepatic structures, most commonly the splenic vein, which leads to the redirection of blood from the portal venous system to the systemic circulation, often causing isolated gastric varices. Pathological processes in the pancreas like pancreatitis, tumors, etc. can cause splenic vein obstruction. For patients with bleeding gastric varices secondary to noncirrhotic sinistral portal hypertension resulting from splenic vein thrombosis, *splenectomy* is curative and the treatment of choice [95].

Special Causes

Aorto-enteric fistula management necessarily involves surgical intervention owing to a breach in the integrity of the aortic wall and graft infection. Most patients undergo ligation of the aorta, and *explantation of the graft* with the placement of an *extra-anatomical bypass* (e.g., an axillary-to-femoral bypass). Alternatively, the infected aortic graft can be replaced with a femoral vein or cryopreserved aortic allograft. The enterotomy, which is commonly located in the third portion of the duodenum, should be resected with subsequent reconstruction [98].

Colonic Lower GI Bleed

Right or left hemicolectomy or any other segmental resection is recommended for patients with lower GIB that can be localized to the colon, provided the bleeding site can be accurately localized and/or embolized; blind total colectomy should be avoided. Depending on the size and spread, resection of an underlying tumor is often done through minimally invasive laparoscopic or laparotomic techniques. Both techniques have comparable outcomes, although laparoscopic resection lessens recovery time [96, 97].

Small Bowel Bleed

The small bowel should be suspected as the site of bleeding in patients with obscure GIB in whom mesenteric angiography, esophagogastroduodenoscopy, capsule endoscopy, colonoscopy, tagged red blood cell scan, enteroclysis, Meckel's scan, and enteroscopy are all non-diagnostic. The recommended course of action is to avoid exploratory procedures in patients in whom the source of bleeding cannot be confirmed. The most common source of bleeding in the small bowel is arteriovenous malformations (AVMs), which cannot be identified through visual inspection or palpation. Therefore, *intraoperative endoscopy* is essential in patients transferred to the operating room for management of obscure bleeding. The endoscopic procedure is performed to evaluate the small bowel lumen, and the surgeon feeds the small bowel on to the endoscope. The surgeon carefully manipulates the small bowel loops so that the endoscope can accurately capture views of most segments of the small bowel to evaluate as much of the small bowel lumen as possible. The combination of endoscopic luminal visualization, palpation of the bowel, and transillumination increases the rate of detection of AVMs, masses, or any mucosal defects. Endoscopic sclerotherapy, endoscopic coagulation, or resection of the affected small bowel segment can be performed following accurate localization of bleeding sites. Meckel's diverticulum and masses are more obvious pathologies, which are treated with segmental small bowel resection.

Conclusion

Gastrointestinal bleeding can be approached in a myriad of ways. Due to the variety of lesions, pathologies, and lack of large randomized control trials, there is no standardized treatment for GI bleeding. Therefore, management of the bleeding site is based on the location, type of lesion that is being treated, and available expertise. Generally, physicians tend to start with the least invasive therapies—endoscopic hemostasis—and then progress to more involved interventions such as embolization and minimally invasive surgery, and ultimately open surgery.

References

1. Millward SF. ACR Appropriateness Criteria on treatment of acute nonvariceal gastrointestinal tract bleeding. J Am Coll Radiol. 2008;5(4):550–4.
2. Laine L, Estrada R. Randomized trial of normal saline solution injection versus bipolar electrocoagulation for treatment of patients with high-risk bleeding ulcers: is local tamponade enough? Gastrointest Endosc. 2002;55(1):6–10.
3. Parsi MA, Schulman AR, Aslanian HR, Bhutani MS, Krishnan K, Lichtenstein DR, et al. Devices for endoscopic hemostasis of nonvariceal GI bleeding (with videos). VideoGIE: An Off Video J Am Soc Gastrointest Endosc. 2019;4(7):285–99.
4. Kovacs TO, Jensen DM. Endoscopic therapy for severe ulcer bleeding. Gastrointest Endosc Clin N Am. 2011;21(4):681–96.
5. Lin HJ, Hsieh YH, Tseng GY, Perng CL, Chang FY, Lee SD. A prospective, randomized trial of endoscopic hemoclip versus heater probe thermocoagulation for peptic ulcer bleeding. Am J Gastroenterol. 2002;97(9):2250–4.
6. Soon MS, Wu SS, Chen YY, Fan CS, Lin OS. Monopolar coagulation versus conventional endoscopic treatment for high-risk peptic ulcer bleeding: a prospective, randomized study. Gastrointest Endosc. 2003;58(3):323–9.
7. Nunoue T, Takenaka R, Hori K, Okazaki N, Hamada K, Baba Y, et al. A randomized trial of monopolar soft-mode coagulation versus heater probe thermocoagulation for peptic ulcer bleeding. J Clin Gastroenterol. 2015;49(6):472–6.
8. Toka B, Eminler AT, Karacaer C, Uslan MI, Koksal AS, Parlak E. Comparison of monopolar hemostatic forceps with soft coagulation versus hemoclip for peptic ulcer bleeding: a randomized trial (with video). Gastrointest Endosc. 2019;89(4):792–802.
9. Ginsberg GG, Barkun AN, Bosco JJ, Burdick JS, Isenberg GA, Nakao NL, et al. The argon plasma coagulator: February 2002. Gastrointest Endosc. 2002;55(7):807–10.
10. Eddi R, Depasquale JR. Radiofrequency ablation for the treatment of radiation proctitis: a case report and review of literature. Ther Adv Gastroenterol. 2013;6(1):69–76.
11. Mujtaba S, Chawla S, Diagnosis MJF. Management of non-variceal gastrointestinal hemorrhage: a review of current guidelines and future perspectives. J Clin Med. 2020;9(2):402.
12. Castela J, Mao de Ferro S, Ferreira S, Dias Pereira A. Management of severe radiation proctitis with radiofrequency ablation. GE Port J Gastroenterol. 2019;26(2):128–30.
13. Jensen DM, Machicado GA, Hirabayashi K. Randomized controlled study of 3 different types of hemoclips for hemostasis of bleeding canine acute gastric ulcers. Gastrointest Endosc. 2006;64(5):768–73.
14. Schmidt A, Golder S, Goetz M, Meining A, Lau J, von Delius S, et al. Over-the-scope clips are more effective than standard endoscopic therapy for patients with recurrent bleeding of peptic ulcers. Gastroenterology. 2018;155(3):674–86.e6.
15. Ji JS, Cho YS. Endoscopic band ligation: beyond prevention and management of gastroesophageal varices. World J Gastroenterol. 2013;19(27):4271–6.
16. Gralnek IM, Khamaysi I. Is the over-the-scope clip device a first-line or rescue therapy for patients at high risk for gastrointestinal bleeding? Clin Gastroenterol Hepatol. 2018;16(5):627–9.
17. Merrifield BF, Lautz D, Thompson CC. Endoscopic repair of gastric leaks after Roux-en-Y gastric bypass: a less invasive approach. Gastrointest Endosc. 2006;63(4):710–4.
18. Chung IK, Kim EJ, Lee MS, Kim HS, Park SH, Lee MH, et al. Bleeding Dieulafoy's lesions and the choice of endoscopic method: comparing the hemostatic efficacy of mechanical and injection methods. Gastrointest Endosc. 2000;52(6):721–4.
19. Huang SP, Wang HP, Lee YC, Lin CC, Yang CS, Wu MS, et al. Endoscopic hemoclip placement and epinephrine injection for Mallory-Weiss syndrome with active bleeding. Gastrointest Endosc. 2002;55(7):842–6.
20. Parra-Blanco A, Kaminaga N, Kojima T, Endo Y, Uragami N, Okawa N, et al. Hemoclipping for postpolypectomy and postbiopsy colonic bleeding. Gastrointest Endosc. 2000;51(1):37–41.

21. Sung JJ, Tsoi KK, Lai LH, Wu JC, Lau JY. Endoscopic clipping versus injection and thermo-coagulation in the treatment of non-variceal upper gastrointestinal bleeding: a meta-analysis. Gut. 2007;56(10):1364–73.
22. Baron TH, Wong Kee Song LM, Zielinski MD, Emura F, Fotoohi M, Kozarek RA. A comprehensive approach to the management of acute endoscopic perforations (with videos). Gastrointest Endosc. 2012;76(4):838–59.
23. Kichler A, Jang S. Endoscopic Hemostasis for non-variceal upper gastrointestinal bleeding: new frontiers. Clin Endosc. 2019;52(5):401–6.
24. Baron TH, Song LM, Ross A, Tokar JL, Irani S, Kozarek RA. Use of an over-the-scope clipping device: multicenter retrospective results of the first U.S. experience (with videos). Gastrointest Endosc. 2012;76(1):202–8.
25. Manta R, Galloro G, Mangiavillano B, Conigliaro R, Pasquale L, Arezzo A, et al. Over-the-scope clip (OTSC) represents an effective endoscopic treatment for acute GI bleeding after failure of conventional techniques. Surg Endosc. 2013;27(9):3162–4.
26. Wong Kee Song LM, Banerjee S, Barth BA, Bhat Y, Desilets D, Gottlieb KT, et al. Emerging technologies for endoscopic hemostasis. Gastrointest Endosc. 2012;75(5):933–7.
27. Jensen DM, Machicado GA. Hemoclipping of chronic canine ulcers: a randomized, prospective study of initial deployment success, clip retention rates, and ulcer healing. Gastrointest Endosc. 2009;70(5):969–75.
28. Chuttani R, Barkun A, Carpenter S, Chotiprasidhi P, Ginsberg GG, Hussain N, et al. Endoscopic clip application devices. Gastrointest Endosc. 2006;63(6):746–50.
29. Brock AS, Rockey DC. Mechanical hemostasis techniques in nonvariceal upper gastrointestinal bleeding. Gastrointest Endosc Clin N Am. 2015;25(3):523–33.
30. Alis H, Oner OZ, Kalayci MU, Dolay K, Kapan S, Soylu A, et al. Is endoscopic band ligation superior to injection therapy for Dieulafoy lesion? Surg Endosc. 2009;23(7):1465–9.
31. Zepeda-Gomez S, Marcon NE. Endoscopic band ligation for nonvariceal bleeding: a review. Can J Gastroenterol = J canadien de gastroenterologie. 2008;22(9):748–52.
32. Laine L, Cook D. Endoscopic ligation compared with sclerotherapy for treatment of esophageal variceal bleeding. A meta-analysis. Ann Intern Med. 1995;123(4):280–7.
33. Hurlstone DP. Successful endoscopic band ligation of duodenal Dieulafoy's lesions. Further large controlled studies are required. Scand J Gastroenterol. 2002;37(5):620.
34. Soetikno RM, Piper J, Montes H, Ukomadu C, Carr-Locke DL. Use of endoscopic band ligation to treat a Dieulafoy's lesion of the esophagus. Endoscopy. 2000;32(4):S15.
35. Krishnan A, Velayutham V, Satyanesan J, Eswaran S, Rajagopal S. Role of endoscopic band ligation in management of non-variceal upper gastrointestinal bleeding. Trop Gastroenterol: Off J Digest Dis Found. 2013;34(2):91–4.
36. Liou TC, Lin SC, Wang HY, Chang WH. Optimal injection volume of epinephrine for endoscopic treatment of peptic ulcer bleeding. World J Gastroenterol. 2006;12(19):3108–13.
37. Vergara M, Calvet X, Gisbert JP. Epinephrine injection versus epinephrine injection and a second endoscopic method in high risk bleeding ulcers. The Cochrane database of systematic reviews. 2007(2):Cd005584.
38. Calvet X, Vergara M, Brullet E, Gisbert JP, Campo R. Addition of a second endoscopic treatment following epinephrine injection improves outcome in high-risk bleeding ulcers. Gastroenterology. 2004;126(2):441–50.
39. Marmo R, Rotondano G, Piscopo R, Bianco MA, D'Angella R, Cipolletta L. Dual therapy versus monotherapy in the endoscopic treatment of high-risk bleeding ulcers: a meta-analysis of controlled trials. Am J Gastroenterol. 2007;102(2):279–89; quiz 469
40. Chandra S, Holm A, El Abiad RG, Gerke H. Endoscopic cyanoacrylate glue injection in management of gastric variceal bleeding: US tertiary care center experience. J Clin Exp Hepatol. 2018;8(2):181–7.
41. Kurek K, Baniukiewicz A, Swidnicka-Siergiejko A, Dabrowski A. Application of cyanoacrylate in difficult-to-arrest acute non-variceal gastrointestinal bleeding. Wideochirurgia i inne techniki maloinwazyjne = Videosurgery and other miniinvasive techniques. 2014;9(3):489–93.

42. Jutabha R, Jensen DM. Management of upper gastrointestinal bleeding in the patient with chronic liver disease. Med Clin North Am. 1996;80(5):1035–68.
43. Lo GH, Lai KH, Cheng JS, Chen MH, Chiang HTA. Prospective, randomized trial of butyl cyanoacrylate injection versus band ligation in the management of bleeding gastric varices. Hepatology (Baltimore, MD). 2001;33(5):1060–4.
44. Croffie J, Somogyi L, Chuttani R, DiSario J, Liu J, Mishkin D, et al. Sclerosing agents for use in GI endoscopy. Gastrointest Endosc. 2007;66(1):1–6.
45. Rutgeerts P, Rauws E, Wara P, Swain P, Hoos A, Solleder E, et al. Randomised trial of single and repeated fibrin glue compared with injection of polidocanol in treatment of bleeding peptic ulcer. Lancet (London, England). 1997;350(9079):692–6.
46. Barkun AN, Moosavi S, Martel M. Topical hemostatic agents: a systematic review with particular emphasis on endoscopic application in GI bleeding. Gastrointest Endosc. 2013;77(5):692–700.
47. Yau AH, Ou G, Galorport C, Amar J, Bressler B, Donnellan F, et al. Safety and efficacy of Hemospray(R) in upper gastrointestinal bleeding. Can J Gastroenterol Hepatol. 2014;28(2):72–6.
48. Pittayanon R, Rerknimitr R, Barkun A. Prognostic factors affecting outcomes in patients with malignant GI bleeding treated with a novel endoscopically delivered hemostatic powder. Gastrointest Endosc. 2018;87(4):994–1002.
49. Laine L, McQuaid KR. Endoscopic therapy for bleeding ulcers: an evidence-based approach based on meta-analyses of randomized controlled trials. Clin Gastroenterol Hepatol. 2009;7(1):33–47; quiz 1–2
50. Alzoubaidi D, Hussein M, Rusu R, Napier D, Dixon S, Rey JW, et al. Outcomes from an international multicenter registry of patients with acute gastrointestinal bleeding undergoing endoscopic treatment with Hemospray. Dig Endosc. 2020;32(1):96–105.
51. Paramasivam RK, Angsuwatcharakon P, Soontornmanokul T, Rerknimitr R. Management of endoscopic complications, in particular perforation. Dig Endosc. 2013;25(Suppl 2):132–6.
52. Palmer KR. Complications of gastrointestinal endoscopy. Gut. 2007;56(4):456–7.
53. Ramaswamy RS, Choi HW, Mouser HC, Narsinh KH, McCammack KC, Treesit T, et al. Role of interventional radiology in the management of acute gastrointestinal bleeding. World J Radiol. 2014;6(4):82–92.
54. Angle JF, Siddiqi NH, Wallace MJ, Kundu S, Stokes L, Wojak JC, et al. Quality improvement guidelines for percutaneous transcatheter embolization: Society of Interventional Radiology Standards of Practice Committee. J Vasc Interv Radiol. 2010;21(10):1479–86.
55. Guimaraes M, Lencioni R, Siskin G. Embolization therapy: principles and Clinical applications: Wolters Kluwer Health; 2014.
56. Moss AJ, Tuffaha H, Malik A. Lower GI bleeding: a review of current management, controversies and advances. Int J Color Dis. 2016;31(2):175–88.
57. Rollins ES, Picus D, Hicks ME, Darcy MD, Bower BL, Kleinhoffer MA. Angiography is useful in detecting the source of chronic gastrointestinal bleeding of obscure origin. AJR Am J Roentgenol. 1991;156(2):385–8.
58. Kim C. Provocative mesenteric angiography for diagnosis and treatment of occult gastrointestinal hemorrhage. Gastrointest Interv. 2018;7:150–4.
59. Kaufman JA, Lee MJ. Vascular and interventional radiology: the requisites: Elsevier Health Sciences; 2013.
60. Cherian MP, Mehta P, Kalyanpur TM, Hedgire SS, Narsinghpura KS. Arterial interventions in gastrointestinal bleeding. Semin Interv Radiol. 2009;26(3):184–96.
61. Loffroy R. Refractory acute upper gastrointestinal nonvariceal bleeding: should arterial embolization be the rule? J Clin Gastroenterol. 2015;49(3):258–9.
62. Loffroy R, Rao P, Ota S, De Lin M, Kwak BK, Geschwind JF. Embolization of acute nonvariceal upper gastrointestinal hemorrhage resistant to endoscopic treatment: results and predictors of recurrent bleeding. Cardiovasc Intervent Radiol. 2010;33(6):1088–100.

63. Darcy M. Treatment of lower gastrointestinal bleeding: vasopressin infusion versus emboliza-
    tion. J Vasc Interv Radiol. 2003;14(5):535–43.
64. d'Othée BJ, Surapaneni P, Rabkin D, Nasser I, Clouse M. Microcoil embolization for acute
    lower gastrointestinal bleeding. Cardiovasc Intervent Radiol. 2006;29(1):49–58.
65. Das R, Ahmed K, Athanasiou T, Morgan RA, Belli AM. Arterial closure devices versus manual
    compression for femoral haemostasis in interventional radiological procedures: a systematic
    review and meta-analysis. Cardiovasc Intervent Radiol. 2011;34(4):723–38.
66. Sharma B, Raina S, Sharma R. Bleeding ectopic varices as the first manifestation of portal
    hypertension. Case Rep Hepatol. 2014;2014:140959.
67. Ferral H, Bilbao JI. The difficult transjugular intrahepatic portosystemic shunt: alternative
    techniques and "tips" to successful shunt creation. Semin Interv Radiol. 2005;22(4):300–8.
68. Haskal ZJ, Duszak R Jr, Furth EE. Transjugular intrahepatic transcaval portosystemic shunt:
    the gun-sight approach. J Vasc Interv Radiol. 1996;7(1):139–42.
69. Saad WE, Sabri SS. Balloon-occluded retrograde transvenous obliteration (BRTO): technical
    results and outcomes. Semin Interv Radiol. 2011;28(3):333–8.
70. Lipnik AJ, Pandhi MB, Khabbaz RC, Gaba RC. Endovascular treatment for variceal hemor-
    rhage: TIPS, BRTO, and combined approaches. Semin Interv Radiol. 2018;35(3):169–84.
71. Saad WE. Vascular anatomy and the morphologic and hemodynamic classifications of gastric
    varices and spontaneous portosystemic shunts relevant to the BRTO procedure. Tech Vasc
    Interv Radiol. 2013;16(2):60–100.
72. Petersen B, Binkert C. Intravascular ultrasound-guided direct intrahepatic portacaval shunt:
    midterm follow-up. J Vasc Interv Radiol. 2004;15(9):927–38.
73. ACR. ACR-SIR-SPR practice parameter for the creation of a trans-jugular intrahepatic porto-
    systemic shunt (TIPS). ACR Comm Pract Parameters. 2014.
74. Gerbes AL, Gülberg V, Waggershauser T, Holl J, Reiser M. Transjugular intrahepatic portosys-
    temic shunt (TIPS) for variceal bleeding in portal hypertension: comparison of emergency and
    elective interventions. Dig Dis Sci. 1998;43(11):2463–9.
75. Vidal V, Sapoval M, Sielezneff Y, De Parades V, Tradi F, Louis G, et al. Emborrhoid: a new con-
    cept for the treatment of hemorrhoids with arterial embolization: the first 14 cases. Cardiovasc
    Intervent Radiol. 2015;38(1):72–8.
76. Tradi F, Louis G, Giorgi R, Mege D, Bartoli JM, Sielezneff I, et al. Embolization of the supe-
    rior rectal arteries for hemorrhoidal disease: prospective results in 25 patients. J Vasc Interv
    Radiol. 2018;29(6):884–92.e1.
77. Abd El Tawab K, Abdo Salem A, Khafagy R. New technique of embolization of the hemor-
    rhoidal arteries using embolization particles alone: retrospective results in 33 patients. Arab J
    Interv Radiol. 2020;4(1):27–31.
78. Laine L, Jensen DM. Management of patients with ulcer bleeding. Am J Gastroenterol.
    2012;107(3):345–60; quiz 61
79. Razzaghi A, Barkun AN. Platelet transfusion threshold in patients with upper gastrointestinal
    bleeding: a systematic review. J Clin Gastroenterol. 2012;46(6):482–6.
80. Prachayakul V, Aswakul P, Chantarojanasiri T, Leelakusolvong S. Factors influencing clini-
    cal outcomes of Histoacryl® glue injection-treated gastric variceal hemorrhage. World J
    Gastroenterol. 2013;19(15):2379–87.
81. Lee YJ, Min BR, Kim ES, Park KS, Cho KB, Jang BK, et al. Predictive factors of mortality
    within 30 days in patients with nonvariceal upper gastrointestinal bleeding. Korean J Intern
    Med. 2016;31(1):54–64.
82. Napolitano L. Refractory peptic ulcer disease. Gastroenterol Clin N Am. 2009;38(2):267–88.
83. Lee CW, Sarosi GA Jr. Emergency ulcer surgery. Surg Clin North Am. 2011;91(5):1001–13.
84. Lagoo J, Pappas TN, Perez A. A relic or still relevant: the narrowing role for vagotomy in the
    treatment of peptic ulcer disease. Am J Surg. 2014;207(1):120–6.
85. Chey WD, Leontiadis GI, Howden CW, Moss SF. ACG clinical guideline: treatment of helico-
    bacter pylori infection. Am J Gastroenterol. 2017;112(2):212–39.

86. Lv SX, Gan JH, Wang CC, Luo EP, Huang XP, Xie Y, et al. Biopsy from the base of gastric ulcer may find gastric cancer earlier. Med Hypotheses. 2011;76(2):249–50.
87. Sugawa C, Benishek D, Walt AJ. Mallory-Weiss syndrome. A study of 224 patients. Am J Surg. 1983;145(1):30–3.
88. Norton ID, Petersen BT, Sorbi D, Balm RK, Alexander GL, Gostout CJ. Management and long-term prognosis of Dieulafoy lesion. Gastrointest Endosc. 1999;50(6):762–7.
89. Brown DP. Gastric packing in the control of massive gastroduodenal hemorrhage. Am J Gastroenterol. 1970;54(1):49–51.
90. Cortese F, Colozzi S, Marcello R, Muttillo IA, Giacovazzo F, Nardi M, et al. Gastroduodenal major haemorrhages in critical patients: an original surgical technique. Ann Ital Chir. 2013;84(6):671–9.
91. White RI Jr, Harrington DP, Novak G, Miller FJ Jr, Giargiana FA Jr, Sheff RN. Pharmacologic control of hemorrhagic gastritis: clinical and experimental results. Radiology. 1974;111(3):549–57.
92. Abdel Khalek M, Joshi V, Kandil E. Robotic-assisted laparoscopic wedge resection of a gastric leiomyoma with intraoperative ultrasound localization. Minim Invasive Ther Allied Technol. 2011;20(6):360–4.
93. D'Amico G, Pagliaro L, Bosch J. The treatment of portal hypertension: a meta-analytic review. Hepatology (Baltimore, MD). 1995;22(1):332–54.
94. Yoshida H, Mamada Y, Taniai N, Yoshioka M, Hirakata A, Kawano Y, et al. Treatment modalities for bleeding esophagogastric varices. J Nippon Med Sch. 2012;79(1):19–30.
95. Evans GR, Yellin AE, Weaver FA, Stain SC. Sinistral (left-sided) portal hypertension. Am Surg. 1990;56(12):758–63.
96. Bonjer HJ, Hop WC, Nelson H, Sargent DJ, Lacy AM, Castells A, et al. Laparoscopically assisted vs open colectomy for colon cancer: a meta-analysis. Arch Surg. 2007;142(3):298–303.
97. Nelson H, Sargent DJ, Wieand HS, Fleshman J, Anvari M, Stryker SJ, et al. A comparison of laparoscopically assisted and open colectomy for colon cancer. N Engl J Med. 2004;350(20):2050–9.
98. Chopra A, Cieciura L, Modrall JG, Valentine RJ, Chung J. Twenty-year experience with Aorto-enteric fistula repair: gastrointestinal complications predict mortality. J Am Coll Surg. 2017;225(1):9–18.

Part IV
Special Populations

Chapter 11
Pediatric population

Jeremy P. Middleton and Craig A. McKinney

Intro

The pediatric mantra "children are not just small adults" certainly holds true for the evaluation and management of occult gastrointestinal bleeding. Unlike the adult population in which fecal immunochemical testing or guaiac based hemoccult testing are commonly performed to detect occult bleeding as part of routine colorectal cancer surveillance algorithms, evaluation for occult bleeding in children is most often triggered by findings of unexplained and/or refractory anemia. Although the differential diagnosis of occult gastrointestinal blood loss in children has similarities to adult causes, there are several pediatric specific processes that vary based on the age of the child. While occult bleeding in adults raises concern for potential gastrointestinal malignancies, these are extraordinarily rare in pediatrics. In contrast, problems such as allergic colitis (cow milk protein allergy), anatomic abnormalities (juvenile polyps, Meckel's diverticulum, vascular malformations, anastomotic ulcers and intestinal duplications), and inflammatory etiologies (Crohn's disease) are more prevalent in infant, school aged, and adolescent populations respectively. Furthermore, there are particular pediatric specific implications in the diagnostic and therapeutic approach, particularly in infant and preschool aged children. These include limitations interpreting fecal occult blood testing as well as challenges with endoscopic evaluation. Patient age and size present potential barriers when obtaining small bowel evaluation with capsule endoscopy or enteroscopy. Addressing the causes of occult gastrointestinal bleeding with therapeutic endoscopy can also be more challenging since there are fewer endoscopic tools available because of the smaller working channel on 5.2 mm endoscopes.

J. P. Middleton (✉) · C. A. McKinney
Division of Pediatric Gastroenterology, Hepatology and Nutrition, University of Virginia
Children's Hospital, Charlottesville, VA, USA
e-mail: jpm8k@virginia.edu; cam7hy@virginia.edu

© The Author(s), under exclusive license to Springer Nature
Switzerland AG 2021
M. Tadros, G. Y. Wu (eds.), *Management of Occult GI Bleeding*, Clinical
Gastroenterology, https://doi.org/10.1007/978-3-030-71468-0_11

Epidemiology/Etiology

It is difficult to ascertain the epidemiology of occult gastrointestinal bleeding in pediatrics given its occult nature, underrecognition, and diagnostic limitations. In general, the epidemiology of all pediatric gastrointestinal bleeding, both occult and overt bleeding, is poorly elucidated in the current literature [1, 2]. While overt gastrointestinal bleeds have more obvious clinical signs of hematemesis, melena, etc. the suspicion for occult bleeding relies on more subtle findings of pallor and iron deficiency anemia in combination with fecal occult blood testing.

The potential etiologies which formulate the differential diagnosis of occult bleeding in pediatrics are unique to that of their adult counterparts. In approaching pediatric occult gastrointestinal bleeding, clinicians must take into account the patient's age as well as the presenting symptoms and physical exam. Dividing populations up into infant/preschool, school aged, and adolescent can be helpful in approaching potential causes of gastrointestinal bleeding in children (Table 11.1). Overall, children show a greater likelihood of having anatomic abnormalities such

Table 11.1 Etiology of occult gastrointestinal bleeding by age

	Infant/preschool	School aged	Adolescent

Inflammatory	Allergic
	  Cow milk protein
	  allergy (allergic colitis)
	Eosinophilic
	  gastrointestinal disease
	Celiac sprue
	Gastritis/esophagitis
		Celiac sprue
		Very early onset IBD
		Gastritis/esophagitis
		Eosinophilic
		  gastrointestinal disease
		Lymphonodular
		  hyperplasia
			Inflammatory bowel
			disease
			Celiac sprue
			Gastritis/esophagitis
			Eosinophilic
			  gastrointestinal disease
			Lymphonodular
			  hyperplasia

Anatomic	Juvenile polyps
	Meckel's diverticulum
	Gastrointestinal
	  duplications
	Anastomotic ulcers
		Juvenile polyps
		Meckel's diverticulum
		Gastrointestinal
		  duplications
		Anastomotic ulcers
			Meckel's diverticulum
			Juvenile polyps
			Gastrointestinal
			  duplications
			Anastomotic ulcers

Vascular	Telangiectasia
	Hemangiomas
	Vasculitis (Henoch
	  Schönlein Purpura)
		Telangiectasia
		Hemangiomas
		Angiodysplasia
		Vasculitis (Henoch
		  Schönlein Purpura)
			Telangiectasia
			Hemangiomas
			Angiodysplasia
			Vasculitis (Henoch
			  Schönlein Purpura)

Hepatobiliary	N/A	Esophageal/rectal
		varices
		  Portal vein thrombosis
		  Cirrhosis
			Esophageal/rectal
			varices
			  Portal vein thrombosis
			  Cirrhosis

Infectious	Hookworm Strongyloides/Ascaris	Hookworm Strongyloides/Ascaris	Hookworm Strongyloides/Ascaris
Malignancy	N/A	Gastrointestinal stromal tumors (GIST)	Gastrointestinal stromal tumors (GIST)
Miscellaneous	Coagulation disorders Non-accidental trauma	Coagulation disorders Non-accidental trauma	Coagulation disorders Non-accidental trauma

as small intestinal polyps, Meckel's diverticulum, intestinal duplications, vascular malformations, as well as inflammatory etiology such as Crohn's disease compared to their adult counterparts.

Inflammatory

Allergic

Cow milk protein allergy (CMPA), also referred to as food protein induced colitis/ enterocolitis, is a non-IgE mediated food protein induced allergic inflammatory disorder that has a diverse spectrum of clinical manifestations. These range from nonspecific symptoms such as abdominal pain, fussiness, poor weight gain, regurgitation, emesis, and loose stools to more striking symptoms such as growth failure, hematochezia, acidosis, and enterocolitis syndrome [3, 4]. Gastrointestinal blood loss is more often occult, though can progress to more fulminant proctocolitis with overtly bloody stools. Cow milk protein allergy presents in infants with the peak onset at around 4–6 months of age. Its overall incidence is estimated to be quite high at nearly 2–3% of infants out of a general population cohort [3], and is even higher in some select populations including premature infants. The natural course of this disorder is gradual resolution over the first 2 years of life and in normally growing children with no other symptoms besides occult blood loss, families can continue an unrestricted diet with close outpatient monitoring. While histopathology reveals a predominately eosinophilic infiltrate [4, 5], the diagnosis of CMPA is typically a clinical diagnosis and endoscopy/colonoscopy is not routinely recommended. Rather CMPA can be presumed based off of compatible clinical history, exclusion of other potential etiologies, and symptomatic response when breastfeeding mothers restrict their diet or infants are transitioned to a partially hydrolyzed or elemental formula. While the majority of infants will have clinical response and resolution of bleeding with transition to a partially hydrolyzed formula, a small percentage will require an elemental formula [6]. CMPA is the most common etiology for occult gastrointestinal blood loss in the first year of life. Attempts to comport the diagnosis with positive fecal occult blood test are limited by its poor specificity in this age range and thus the diagnosis of CMPA largely remains a clinical diagnosis based on symptom constellation and clinical response to dietary exclusion [7].

Celiac

Celiac disease is an immune-mediated enteropathy driven by gluten sensitivity and it is highly prevalent with estimated rates of pediatric Celiac disease ranging from 1:300 to as many as 1:80 children. The classic presentation of abdominal distention, diarrhea, and weight loss/growth failure is more common in childhood celiac disease than in adults [8]. However, with increased availability and widespread use of serologic testing, there has been a shift in how children with celiac disease present with one study describing the classic symptomatology decreasing from 67% to 19% [9]. They attributed this to increased detection of atypical cases in older children and adolescents which led to a dramatic corresponding shift in the average age of diagnosis from approximately 2 years of age to 9 years of age during that same time span [9, 10]. While the presentation of refractory iron deficiency anemia has long been well described in adult celiac patients, it was only more recently confirmed as a common initial manifestation in children. One pediatric cohort study demonstrated that upwards of 25% with refractory iron deficiency anemia had positive celiac serologies and another noted that more than 25% of children with untreated celiac disease had a positive fecal occult blood test [11, 12]. This yielded recommendations for early celiac serologic screening in the setting of iron deficiency anemia and concern for occult bleeding in order to make more timely diagnosis, minimize celiac associated complications, and avoid repeated courses of iron supplementation [8].

Inflammatory Bowel Disease

With an incidence of 10 per 100,000 children, there are approximately 70,000 children with inflammatory bowel disease (IBD) in the United States. Although children frequently present with abdominal pain, diarrhea, and weight loss, a small percentage of children have symptoms associated with anemia alone. Unexplained iron deficiency anemia with gastrointestinal bleeding, particularly in school aged and adolescent patients, must raise concern for IBD. While in younger children with occult GI bleeding the possibility of IBD must be entertained, very early onset inflammatory bowel disease defined as onset of symptoms prior to 6 years of age is quite rare. Chronic occult blood loss and iron deficiency are a common presentation for inflammatory bowel disease in the pediatric population, with 67–76% of children with IBD having anemia at the time of diagnosis [13]. Interestingly, 70% of school age children with IBD present with anemia compared to 42% in adolescents and 40% in adults [14]. Diagnosis of children with suspected inflammatory bowel disease frequently relies on laboratory testing, though fecal occult blood testing has been suggested as a screening tool. In one study of 335 children undergoing testing for IBD, combining screening laboratory studies with fecal occult blood testing and perianal examination increased the sensitivity of diagnosing IBD from 80.5% to 97.6% [15].

Helicobacter Pylori

Helicobacter pylori infection in children is a frequent cause of upper abdominal pain, nausea and dyspepsia. Although noninvasive screening for H pylori exist, national guidelines still recommend endoscopic evaluation to evaluate for infection [16]. Indeed nodular antral gastritis is a nearly pathognomonic finding for childhood H pylori infection and is seen more commonly in children than in their adult counterparts [17]. Lymphoid follicle hypertrophy and thickening of the gastric mucosa folds were also seen more commonly in the pediatric population, while gastric mucosal atrophy, intestinal metaplasia and dysplasia occurred less frequently in children. Because H pylori has been associated with duodenal ulcers and chronic gastritis, children can have both positive fecal occult blood tests and iron deficiency anemia with an active H pylori infection. Several meta-analyses have confirmed that the association between unexplained iron deficiency anemia and H pylori infection is also seen in pediatrics [18, 19]. Diagnostic testing for H. pylori infection should be considered in children with refractory iron-deficiency anemia. Indeed, one small study evaluating adolescents with unexplained iron deficiency anemia found that the most common endoscopic finding was antral gastritis. With almost 40% of their cohort population having histopathologic findings consistent with H pylori infection, this prompted guidelines to recommend targeted biopsies for H pylori on upper endoscopy for the indication of iron deficiency anemia [16, 18, 19].

Anatomic

Juvenile polyps are the most common cause for painless lower gastrointestinal bleeding in children [20, 21]. Frequently, bleeding associated with colonic polyps is overt bright red blood per rectum, but presentation is variable based on polyp location and can be more insidious in nature. Juvenile polyps are hamartomatous growths that are commonly seen in children with peak age on incidence from 2 to 4 years of age. Large retrospective cohort indicates that the incidence of colorectal polyp across all pediatric colonoscopies is approximately 6% irrespective of indication, but increases to 12% for indication of lower gastrointestinal bleeding [21]. Younger age, male sex, and non-white race were all significantly associated with polyp detection. However, it appears that the likelihood of polyp detection may be significantly higher in certain populations as smaller cohort studies have found incidence rates that range as high as 42–57% based on population characteristics [22, 23]. In children and adolescents, 85–90% of polyps are juvenile (hamartomas) polyps with the remainder made up of hyperplastic/inflammatory polyps and adenomas. The vast majority of patients (80–95%) will have a single isolated polyp detected with the bulk of these located in the left colon [22]. One study characterizing distribution of juvenile polyps noted that 68% were isolated to rectum, 20%

to the rectosigmoid, and 12% in the descending colon [21, 23]. While single iso-lated polyps are predominant, the presence of multiple polyps, particularly in the setting of positive family history or polyp location outside the colon should raise concern for genetic polyposis syndromes prompting consideration for further diag-nostic evaluation. Small bowel polyps in particular can represent an obscure cause for occult bleeding that may not be readily identifiable with standard esophagogas-troduodenoscopy and ileocolonoscopy.

A number of other anatomic variants can manifest with gastrointestinal bleeding early in childhood. These includes Meckel's diverticulum which is a small out-pouching that represents the most prevalent congenital abnormality of the gastroin-testinal tract. It is a remnant of the omphalomesenteric duct and has associated ectopic gastric or pancreatic tissue in estimated 44% and 37% of cases respectively [24]. While most characteristically it presents with overt episodes of painless gas-trointestinal bleeding it has been described in cases of insidious chronic bleeding and may also represents an incidental finding in completely asymptomatic individu-als. It is classically known for its "rule of 2's" in which estimated fraction of 2% of the population has this small diverticulum with typical length of approximately 2 inches and location roughly 2 feet from the ileocecal valve. The peak age of inci-dence is prior to 2 years of age and frequently the diverticulum expresses ectopic gastric tissue which predisposes to bleeding. While Meckel's is most commonly described it is possible to get duplication cysts in a number of locations throughout the gastrointestinal tract and if gastric ectopic tissue is present so too is the potential risk for bleeding. Technetium-99 m pertechnetate imaging offered high diagnostic yield in detecting Meckel's or other diverticulum which express ectopic gastric mucosa [24, 25].

Chronic occult bleeding and anemia are well described long term complica-tions associated with ulcer formation at intestinal anastomoses. Ileocolonic anas-tomotic sites in infants with history of necrotizing enterocolitis are commonly described to have delayed complications such as ulcer formation (Fig. 11.1a). One

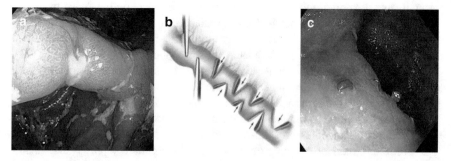

Fig. 11.1 Anastomotic ulceration. (**a**) Ulceration at ileocolonic anastomosis. (**b**) Serial transverse enteroplasty [26]. (**c**) Staple line erythema as a complication of serial transverse enteroplasty (STEP) bowel lengthening procedure

study described symptomatic ulceration at previous ileocolonic anastomosis in six children who had underwent ileocecal resection for necrotizing enterocolitis with mean onset of symptoms over 5 years after initial successful surgical management. The etiology for these inflammatory ulcerations is unclear but anecdotally they are refractory to treatment with anti-inflammatory medications and have high recurrence rate following surgical revision [27]. Ileocolonic anastomoses seem particularly vulnerable to anastomotic ulcer bleeding and multiple studies demonstrate the timing can be markedly delayed with one study showing the interval between surgery and detection of anastomotic ulcer ranged from 15 months to over 2 decades. In this study where a small cohort of patients with ileocolonic anastomotic ulcer bleeds underwent surgical revision, the majority failed to demonstrate clinical improvement with ulcer recurrence at the new anastomotic site [28]. Additionally, staple line associated ulcerations in patients with intestinal failure who have undergone serial transverse enteroplasty procedure (STEP) for bowel lengthening is a well described phenomenon that leads to chronic refractory occult gastrointestinal bleeding (Fig. 11.1b, c) [29].

Vascular

Multisystem vascular disorders and vascular anomalies including angiodysplasia, telangiectasia, hemangiomas, and more rare vasculocutaneous syndromes such as blue rubber bleb nevus syndrome can lead to chronic occult gastrointestinal blood loss (Table 11.2) [2]. Additionally, genetic polyposis syndromes are often associated with occult bleeding. These commonly present in childhood and careful physical exam and history can be helpful in raising suspicion for such vascular lesions and polyposis syndromes. Skin findings such as telangiectasias, blue nodules, hemangiomas, or pigmented macules (lentigines) raise suspicion for multisystem vascular disorders such as hereditary hemorrhagic telangiectasia, blue rubber bleb nevus syndrome as well as polyposis disorders, such as Peutz-Jeghers syndrome and juvenile polyposis syndrome (Fig. 11.2) [2, 30].

Table 11.2 History and cutaneous findings associated with multisystem vascular and polypsosis syndromes

Cutaneous manifestation, historical clues	Diagnosis/vascular lesion
Oral lentigines, pigmented macules	Peutz-jeghers (Hamartomatous polyps)
Epistaxis, cutaneous telangiectasia's, and positive family history	Osler-Weber-Rendu or hereditary hemorrhagic telangiectasia
Cutaneous hemangiomas	Infantile visceral hemangiomas
Multifocal nodular blue venous malformations	Blue rubber bleb nevus syndrome
Purpuric rash, abdominal pain, hematuria	Henoch Schonlein Purpura (IgA mediated vasculitis, intestinal purpura)
	Juvenile polyposis syndrome

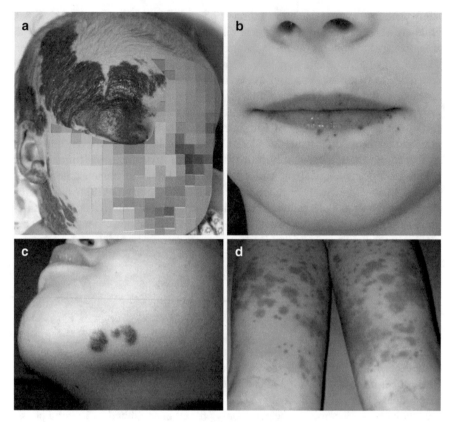

Fig. 11.2 (**a**) Segmental hemangioma seen in PHACES Syndrome [31]. (**b**) Oral lentigines associated with Peutz-Jegher Syndrome. (**c**) Blue vascular lesions in Blue Rubber Bleb Nevus Syndrome [32]. (**d**) Palpable purpura of Henoch-Schönlein Purpura [33]

Hepatobiliary

Esophageal varices and portal hypertensive gastropathy related to chronic liver disease can present with occult gastrointestinal bleeding (Fig. 11.3). Overall, chronic liver disease presenting with portal hypertensive sequelae is relatively uncommon in the pediatric population. However, variceal bleeding from portal hypertension caused by cirrhosis from chronic liver disease or portal vein thrombosis may occur. Prematurity and history of umbilical vein catheterization as well as hypercoagulable disorders are notable risk factors for portal vein thrombosis. Smoldering chronic hepatitis from Wilson disease, alpha-1 antitrypsin, or autoimmune hepatitis leading to cirrhosis infrequently presents as unexplained anemia from varices or portal gastropathy.

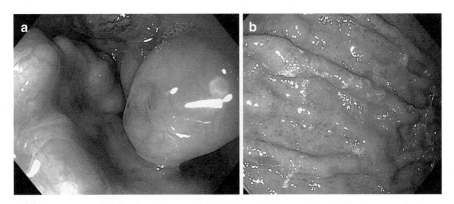

Fig. 11.3 Sequelae of portal hypertension in children. (**a**) Esophageal varices from portal vein thrombosis (**b**) portal gastropathy from autoimmune hepatitis

Infectious

Although chronic helminthic infections in the United States and other developed nations are relatively uncommon given sanitation efforts and safe water supply, parasitic infection still must be considered in the evaluation of occult gastrointestinal bleeding. This particularly should be a concern in the setting of growth failure. Careful history to elucidate risk factors such as immigrant status and history of recent international travel should direct attention towards ova and parasite testing as part of the evaluation of chronic bleeding. Hookworm, Strongyloides, and Ascaris are the most common helminthic infections to manifest with occult bleeding.

Malignancy

In contrast to the adults where occult bleeding may portent colorectal carcinomas, gastrointestinal malignancies are exceedingly rare in children. Secondary malignancies with intestinal metastasis are more common than primary tumors. Of those primary gastrointestinal tumors, gastrointestinal stromal tumors are the most common though still quite rare with an estimated incidence of 0.02 cases per million children [34]. Juvenile polyposis syndromes place individuals at increased risk for development of intestinal malignancy, but most of these carcinomas manifest beyond the second decade of life.

Diagnostic Considerations

In adult populations screening for fecal occult blood with stool guaiac based and immunohistochemical screening methods is commonplace to evaluate for occult gastrointestinal blood loss and plays a huge role in surveillance for early detection of colonic malignancies. However, widespread use in pediatrics is more limited particularly in infants and younger children. Multiple studies have demonstrated that stool guaiac has poor specificity in the infant population [7, 35, 36]. One study looked at fecal occult blood tests in all hospitalized infants, irrespective of the etiology for their admission, and found that approximately 22% of infants had at least one positive hemoccult result during their inpatient stay [35]. A more recent study trying to determine the role of fecal occult blood testing in screening for cow milk protein allergy found that their asymptomatic control populations of healthy infants at standard well checks had positive stool guaiac rates of 34% despite the absence of any gastrointestinal symptoms [7]. Given its marked poor specificity, fecal occult blood testing in the infant population is not recommended and must be interpreted with caution as it may lead to excessive diagnostic workup, treatment, and unnecessary formula changes. The exact mechanism to explain this high positive stool guaiac test rate is poorly elucidated at this point, but is speculated to represent a degree of immaturity of barrier function and immunity in the gut.

Endoscopy

Chronic occult gastrointestinal bleeding may occur anywhere in the gastrointestinal tract from the oral cavity to the anus. In most cases, the site can be identified by upper endoscopy and ileocolonoscopy. Esophagogastroduodenoscopy and colonoscopy are the first line diagnostic tools for detection of occult gastrointestinal bleeding. However, while the yield of endoscopy for detection of overt gastrointestinal bleeding is well defined, the yield of esophagogastroduodenoscopy and colonoscopy for evaluation of occult gastrointestinal bleeding and iron deficiency anemia is less clearly delineated in the pediatric literature.

Insidious blood loss from the gastrointestinal tract has been identified as one of the most frequent causes of iron deficiency anemia in older children and adolescents. Two retrospective studies examining the yield of esophagogastroduodenoscopy for evaluation of unexplained chronic iron deficiency anemia and gastrointestinal bleeding suggested that the diagnostic yield was 53% and 57% respectively [18, 37]. In the cohort of patients with unexplained chronic iron deficiency anemia the most common endoscopic abnormalities described were antral gastritis followed by duodenal ulcers [18]. However, the remaining cases of obscure gastrointestinal bleeding in which occult bleeding is not localized with endoscopy or small bowel radiological imaging is referred to as obscure-occult bleeding and these patients benefit from further small bowel evaluation for the source of bleeding [1]. A separate study evaluating diagnostic yield of colonoscopy for various indications found a yield of approximately 66% which was second only to the etiology of overt lower gastrointestinal bleeding [38].

Once endoscopic abnormalities are detected the ability to provide therapeutic intervention can have pediatric size specific obstacles. Particularly in neonates and young infants, smaller caliber endoscopes are necessary which often have a narrow diameter and smaller working channel which can restrict options for therapeutic intervention of bleeding. Commercially available gastroscopes for infants commonly have an outer diameter of approximately 5.5 mm and a working channel diameter of approximately 2.0 mm. When no source of bleeding is found on EGD and colonoscopy, bleeding from the jejunum or proximal ileum is usually the culprit. Evaluation of the small bowel is technically challenging at baseline in all populations, but certainly pediatric size can play a role in complicating evaluation of small bowel disease.

Wireless Capsule Endoscopy

Wireless capsule endoscopy (WCE) is a minimally invasive technique for the evaluation of small bowel pathology and obscure gastrointestinal bleeding (Fig. 11.4). It was first employed in the pediatric population in 2004 for use in adolescent patients

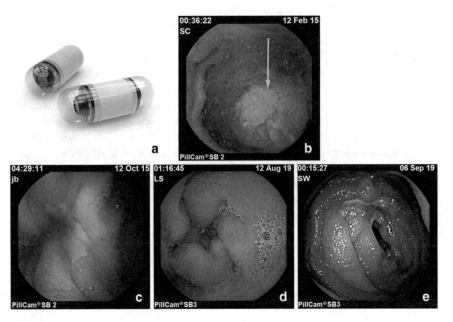

Fig. 11.4 (**a**) Wireless capsule endoscopy [39]. (**b**) Small bowel polyp (**c**) Small bowel aphthous ulcer (**d**) Small bowel ulceration from eosinophilic gastroenteritis (**e**) Small bowel Crohn's disease

10–18 years of age and was later expanded to use in children greater than 2 years of age in 2009. Over the past decade it has steadily gained traction as the primary modality for assessing small bowel disease involvement. While an early case series was concerning for a relatively high adverse event rate from capsule retention and capsule failure requiring endoscopic or surgical retrieval, these have not been realized in larger scale studies that demonstrate an excellent safety profile [40–42]. Even in populations with established Crohn's disease where risk of stricture is the greatest, wireless capsule endoscopy has been found to have an excellent safety profile with minimal risk of retention [41, 42]. To assuage concerns regarding potential capsule retention, passage of a dissolvable patency capsule is typically recommended to exclude an unrecognized stricture prior to video capsule swallowing or deployment.

The diagnostic yield for WCE in pediatrics is estimated to be as high as 61% across all indications. However, its yield appears to be greatest in evaluation of polyposis syndromes and established Crohn's disease with rates of detection of positive findings in 75% and 65% for these populations respectively. While in comparison, yield in detection of a small bowel source of obscure gastrointestinal bleeding and iron deficiency anemia ranges from 27% to 42% [41, 43, 44]. While WCE has gained traction in the assessment of small bowel disease, certain limitations and pediatric implications still apply. Tolerability of capsule swallowing remains a pediatric specific barrier as the typical video capsule measures 26 × 11 mm and thus remains an obstacle for ingestion in young children. One study evaluating tolerability of video capsule endoscopy in school aged children identified age, height, and prior experience with capsule swallowing as the best predictors and determinants of swallowability. If children are unable to swallow the pill, endoscopic deployment is typically completed at the time of EGD. However, placement at the completion of upper endoscopic evaluation with biopsy can complicate interpretation given the creation of biopsy related bleeding as possible artifact in the small bowel that must be distinguished and differentiated by the interpreter from true small bowel pathology. WCE is most commonly employed for the evaluation of chronic gastrointestinal bleeding in the setting of Crohn's disease with known normal upper and lower endoscopy findings. Further limitations of WCE are similar to that in adults in that it does not allow for direct tissue sampling, leads to imprecise localization of bleeding, and inability to therapeutically intervene. WCE is a novel, noninvasive, and useful tool for the investigation of the small intestine in children. It is superior and more sensitive than other conventional endoscopic and radiologic investigations in the assessment of the small bowel and should be routinely employed as a diagnostic tool in the work-up of obscure gastrointestinal bleeding.

Small Bowel Enteroscopy

Balloon assisted enteroscopy to assess for a small bowel source of bleeding has been used sparingly in the pediatric population largely due to limited experience and lack of expertise in performing enteroscopy in small children. However, case reports have described the success of single balloon assisted anterograde enteroscopy and retrograde enteroscopy in patients as young as 3.7 years and 1.6 years respectively and with lowest body size down to 12.9 and 10.8 kg respectively [45, 46]. While anterograde and retrograde techniques are both employed, anal route retrograde enteroscopy has been associated with shorter procedure duration for achieving diagnosis. The overall diagnostic yield for small bowel lesions using double balloon enteroscopy ranges from 48% to 70% depending on patient population, indication, and inter-center variation [46–49]. Enteroscopy findings in the setting of occult bleeding include most commonly polyps, mucosal ulcers and erosions, and more rarely angiomas, angiodysplasia, and other vascular anomalies. Head to head studies have demonstrated similar diagnostic yield between WCE evaluation and double balloon enteroscopy but note that enteroscopy is advantageous in that it facilitates the possibility of endotherapeutic intervention to address abnormal mucosal findings. Studies have shown up to 46.5% success rate in completion of therapeutic intervention with small bowel enteroscopy. Many experts purport the usage of MR-enterography and capsule endoscopy as complementary in tools in the diagnostic work-up to better identify candidates appropriate for enteroscopy. One study evaluating an algorithmic approach of WCE evaluation prior to enteroscopy found that capsule endoscopy enhances the diagnostic and therapeutic yield of enteroscopy to 95% and 82% respectively. Although the procedure is technically challenging, few major complications have been reported and are primarily associated with therapeutic interventions [48]. Ultimately, few centers have sufficient patient volume and technical expertise to perform routine enteroscopy in young children, and thus it has not become a mainstay in the evaluation of small bowel pathology.

Radiology Evaluation

Diagnosis of lower gastrointestinal bleeding (LGIB) represents a significant diagnostic and therapeutic challenge and the utilization of radiologic cross sectional imaging is often helpful. While CT enterography (CTE) has been utilized in adults with occult LGIB, its use in children has been primarily limited to evaluation of extent of disease for patients with inflammatory bowel disease. Although, one study suggests CTE may have value in localizing the source of LGIB prior to surgical or endoscopic intervention [50]. However, the benefit of earlier lesion identification prior to endoscopy evaluation must be weighed against the radiation exposure and patient discomfort due to bowel distention associated with enterography. In addition to cross sectional imaging, nuclear medicine technetium-labeled tagged red blood cell scans have also been utilized to locate occult GI bleeding. Although typically thoughts of more often in individuals with larger lower GI bleeds since there is a threshold of active bleeding necessary to detect the bleeding, reports that as little at 0.1 ml/min is needed to detect a bleed [51]. Although little data is available on tagged red blood cell scans in children, a 2008 study of 22 patients with GI bleeding demonstrated a diagnostic yield of almost 40% with this study [52].

Conclusion

Occult gastrointestinal bleeding is a relatively uncommon problem in the pediatric population but fecal occult blood testing should be considered in children with unexplained anemia. There are more differences than similarities in the causes of occult gastrointestinal bleeding in children compared to adults. Careful consideration of the child's age, history and physical exam is important when deciding on the most appropriate diagnostic test for occult gastrointestinal bleeding. Evaluation with endoscopy, wireless capsule endoscopy and radiographic imaging is similar to that of adults but can be more challenging primarily due to size limitations in young children.

References

1. Pai AK, Fox VL. Gastrointestinal bleeding and management. Pediatr Clin N Am. 2017;64(3):543–61.
2. Romano C, Oliva S, Martellossi S, Miele E, Arrigo S, Graziani MG, et al. Pediatric gastrointestinal bleeding: perspectives from the Italian Society of Pediatric Gastroenterology. World J Gastroenterol. 2017;23(8):1328–37.
3. Schrander JJ, van den Bogart JP, Forget PP, Schrander-Stumpel CT, Kuijten RH, Kester AD. Cow's milk protein intolerance in infants under 1 year of age: a prospective epidemiological study. Eur J Pediatr. 1993;152(8):640–4.
4. Cervantes-Bustamante R, Pedrero-Olivares I, Toro-Monjaraz EM, Murillo-Márquez P, Ramírez-Mayans JA, Montijo-Barrios E, et al. Histopathologic findings in children diagnosed with cow's milk protein allergy. Rev Gastroenterol Mex. 2015;80(2):130–4.
5. Lozinsky AC, de Morais MB. Eosinophilic colitis in infants. J Pediatr. 2014;90(1):16–21.
6. Nowak-Węgrzyn A, Chehade M, Groetch ME, Spergel JM, Wood RA, Allen K, et al. International consensus guidelines for the diagnosis and management of food protein-induced enterocolitis syndrome: Executive summary-Workgroup Report of the Adverse Reactions to Foods Committee, American Academy of Allergy, Asthma & Immunology. J Allergy Clin Immunol. 2017;139(4):1111–1126.e4.
7. Concha S, Cabalín C, Iturriaga C, Pérez-Mateluna G, Gomez C, Cifuentes L, et al. Diagnostic validity of fecal occult blood test in infants with food protein-induced allergic proctocolitis. Rev Chil Pediatr. 2018;89(5):630–7.
8. Hill I, Dirks M, Liptak G. Guideline for the diagnosis and treatment of celiac disease in children: recommendations of the North American Society for Pediatric Gastroenterology, Hepatology, and Nutrition. J Pediatr Gastroenterol Nutr. 2005;40(1):1–19.
9. McGowan KE, Castiglione DA, Butzner JD. The changing face of childhood celiac disease in North America: impact of serological testing. Pediatrics. 2009;124(6):1572–8.
10. Rodrigo-Sáez L, Fuentes-Álvarez D, Pérez-Martínez I, Alvarez-Mieres N, Niño-García P, de-Francisco-García R, et al. Differences between pediatric and adult celiac disease. Rev Espanola Enfermedades Dig Organo Of Soc Espanola Patol Dig. 2011;103(5):238–44.
11. Shahriari M, Honar N, Yousefi A, Javaherizadeh H. Association of potential celiac disease and refractory iron deficiency anemia in children and adolescents. Arq Gastroenterol. 2018;55(1):78–81.
12. Shamir R, Levine A, Yalon-Hacohen M, Shapiro R, Zahavi I, Rosenbach Y, et al. Faecal occult blood in children with coeliac disease. Eur J Pediatr. 2000;159(11):832–4.

13. Aljomah G, Baker SS, Schmidt K, Alkhouri R, Kozielski R, Zhu L, et al. Anemia in pediatric inflammatory bowel disease. J Pediatr Gastroenterol Nutr. 2018;67(3):351–5.

14. de Carvalho FSG, de Medeiros IA, Antunes H. Prevalence of iron deficiency anemia and iron deficiency in a pediatric population with inflammatory bowel disease. Scand J Gastroenterol. 2017;52(10):1099–103.

15. Moran CJ, Kaplan JL, Winter HS, Masiakos PT. Occult blood and perianal examination: value added in pediatric inflammatory bowel disease screening. J Pediatr Gastroenterol Nutr. 2015;61(1):52–5.

16. Koletzko S, Jones NL, Goodman KJ, Gold B, Rowland M, Cadranel S, et al. Evidence-based guidelines from ESPGHAN and NASPGHAN for Helicobacter pylori infection in children. J Pediatr Gastroenterol Nutr. 2011;53(2):230–43.

17. Meining A, Behrens R, Lehn N, Bayerdörffer E, Stolte M. Different expression of Helicobacter pylori gastritis in children: evidence for a specific pediatric disease? Helicobacter. 1996;1(2):92–7.

18. Gulen H, Kasirga E, Yildirim SA, Kader S, Sahin G, Ayhan S. Diagnostic yield of upper gastrointestinal endoscopy in the evaluation of iron deficiency anemia in older children and adolescents. Pediatr Hematol Oncol. 2011;28(8):694–701.

19. Iwańczak BM, Buchner AM, Iwańczak F. Clinical differences of Helicobacter pylori infection in children. Adv Clin Exp Med Off Organ Wroclaw Med Univ. 2017;26(7):1131–6.

20. Perisic VN. Colorectal polyps: an important cause of rectal bleeding. Arch Dis Child. 1987;62(2):188–9.

21. Thakkar K, Alsarraj A, Fong E, Holub JL, Gilger MA, El Serag HB. Prevalence of colorectal polyps in pediatric colonoscopy. Dig Dis Sci. 2012;57(4):1050–5.

22. Silbermintz A, Matar M, Assa A, Zevit N, Glassberg YM, Shamir R. Endoscopic findings in children with isolated lower gastrointestinal bleeding. Clin Endosc. 2019;52(3):258–61.

23. El-Shabrawi MHF, El Din ZE, Isa M, Kamal N, Hassanin F, El-Koofy N, et al. Colorectal polyps: a frequently-missed cause of rectal bleeding in Egyptian children. Ann Trop Paediatr. 2011;31(3):213–8.

24. Lin X-K, Huang X-Z, Bao X-Z, Zheng N, Xia Q-Z, Chen C. Clinical characteristics of Meckel diverticulum in children: a retrospective review of a 15-year single-center experience. Medicine (Baltimore). 2017;96(32):e7760.

25. Chen Q, Gao Z, Zhang L, Zhang Y, Pan T, Cai D, et al. Multifaceted behavior of Meckel's diverticulum in children. J Pediatr Surg. 2018;53(4):676–81.

26. Bianchi A. The Pediatric Short Bowel State: Practical Concepts Toward Enteral Autonomy. In: Lima M. (eds) Pediatric Digestive Surgery. Springer, Cham: 2017.

27. Sondheimer JM, Sokol RJ, Narkewicz MR, Tyson RW. Anastomotic ulceration: a late complication of ileocolonic anastomosis. J Pediatr. 1995;127(2):225–30.

28. Chari ST, Keate RF. Ileocolonic anastomotic ulcers: a case series and review of the literature. Am J Gastroenterol. 2000;95(5):1239–43.

29. Gibbons TE, Casteel HB, Vaughan JF, Dassinger MS. Staple line ulcers: a cause of chronic GI bleeding following STEP procedure. J Pediatr Surg. 2013;48(6):E1–3.

30. Lybecker MB, Stawowy M, Clausen N. Blue rubber bleb naevus syndrome: a rare cause of chronic occult blood loss and iron deficiency anaemia. BMJ Case Rep. 2016;20:2016.

31. Gupta D, Rosbe K. PHACE Syndrome. In: Perkins J, Balakrishnan K. (eds) Evidence-Based Management of Head and Neck Vascular Anomalies. Springer, Cham: 2018.

32. Ma JE, Hand JL. Blue Rubber Bleb Nevus Syndrome. In: Perkins J, Balakrishnan K. (eds) Evidence-Based Management of Head and Neck Vascular Anomalies. Springer, Cham: 2018.

33. Falcini F. Henoch-Schönlein Purpura. In: Matucci-Cerinic M, Furst D, Fiorentino D. (eds) Skin Manifestations in Rheumatic Disease. Springer, New York, NY: 2014.

34. Quiroz HJ, Willobee BA, Sussman MS, Fox BR, Thorson CM, Sola JE, et al. Pediatric gastrointestinal stromal tumors-a review of diagnostic modalities. Transl Gastroenterol Hepatol. 2018;3:54.

35. Gralton KS. The incidence of guiac positive stools in newborns and infants. Pediatr Nurs. 1999;25(3):306–8.
36. Pinheiro JMB, Clark DA, Benjamin KG. A critical analysis of the routine testing of newborn stools for occult blood and reducing substances. Adv Neonatal Care Off J Natl Assoc Neonatal Nurses. 2003;3(3):133–8.
37. Sheiko MA, Feinstein JA, Capocelli KE, Kramer RE. Diagnostic yield of EGD in children: a retrospective single-center study of 1000 cases. Gastrointest Endosc. 2013;78(1):47–54.e1.
38. Wu C-T, Chen C-A, Yang Y-J. Characteristics and diagnostic yield of pediatric colonoscopy in Taiwan. Pediatr Neonatol. 2015;56(5):334–8.
39. Peter S. Pill-sized camera for capsule endoscopy isolated on white. 3D rendering. Stock illustration ID: 1065935069. Shutterstock. Standard license.
40. Moy L, Levine J. Wireless capsule endoscopy in the pediatric age group: experience and complications. J Pediatr Gastroenterol Nutr. 2007;44(4):516–20.
41. Cohen SA, Ephrath H, Lewis JD, Klevens A, Bergwerk A, Liu S, et al. Pediatric capsule endoscopy: review of the small bowel and patency capsules. J Pediatr Gastroenterol Nutr. 2012;54(3):409–13.
42. Antao B, Bishop J, Shawis R, Thomson M. Clinical application and diagnostic yield of wireless capsule endoscopy in children. J Laparoendosc Adv Surg Tech A. 2007;17(3):364–70.
43. Dupont-Lucas C, Bellaïche M, Mouterde O, Bernard O, Besnard M, Campeotto F, et al. Capsule endoscopy in children: which are the best indications? Arch Pediatr Organe Off Soc Francaise Pediatr. 2010;17(9):1264–72.
44. Oliva S, Cohen SA, Di Nardo G, Gualdi G, Cucchiara S, Casciani E. Capsule endoscopy in pediatrics: a 10-years journey. World J Gastroenterol. 2014;20(44):16603–8.
45. Kramer RE, Brumbaugh DE, Soden JS, Capocelli KE, Hoffenberg EJ. First successful antegrade single-balloon enteroscopy in a 3-year-old with occult GI bleeding. Gastrointest Endosc. 2009;70(3):546–9.
46. Hagiwara S-I, Kudo T, Kakuta F, Inoue M, Yokoyama K, Umetsu S, et al. Clinical safety and utility of pediatric balloon-assisted enteroscopy: a multicenter prospective study in Japan. J Pediatr Gastroenterol Nutr. 2019;68(3):306–10.
47. Oliva S, Pennazio M, Cohen SA, Aloi M, Barabino A, Hassan C, et al. Capsule endoscopy followed by single balloon enteroscopy in children with obscure gastrointestinal bleeding: a combined approach. Dig Liver Dis Off J Ital Soc Gastroenterol Ital Assoc Study Liver. 2015;47(2):125–30.
48. Nishimura N, Yamamoto H, Yano T, Hayashi Y, Arashiro M, Miyata T, et al. Safety and efficacy of double-balloon enteroscopy in pediatric patients. Gastrointest Endosc. 2010;71(2):287–94.
49. Urs AN, Martinelli M, Rao P, Thomson MA. Diagnostic and therapeutic utility of double-balloon enteroscopy in children. J Pediatr Gastroenterol Nutr. 2014;58(2):204–12.
50. Davis JS, Ryan ML, Fields JM, Neville HL, Perez EA, Sola JE. Use of CT enterography for the diagnosis of lower gastrointestinal bleeding in pediatric patients. J Pediatr Surg. 2013;48(3):681–4.
51. Howarth DM. The role of nuclear medicine in the detection of acute gastrointestinal bleeding. Semin Nucl Med. 2006;36(2):133–46.
52. Lee J, Lai M-W, Chen C-C, Chen S-Y, Chao H-C, Chan S-C, et al. Red blood cell scintigraphy in children with acute massive gastrointestinal bleeding. Pediatr Int Off J Jpn Pediatr Soc. 2008;50(2):199–203.

Chapter 12
Premenopausal Women

Alicia Wiczulis and Katherine Kashinsky

Anemia in a menstruating woman may be falsely attributed to heavy periods, and an opportunity to recognize an occult gastrointestinal bleed could be missed.

A woman of reproductive age who reports abnormal menstrual bleeding deserves further evaluation. Her concerns may include a change in her typical bleeding pattern or an increase in blood loss. Her evaluation begins with a careful history, and her provider should have a basic understanding of what constitutes normal bleeding and when further testing or referral is warranted.

Normal Menses

A normal menstrual cycle requires complex coordination between multiple systems: neural, endocrine, hematologic, and other pathways interact to maintain this fundamental part of the reproductive system. Any insult to this process, including stress, weight change, illness, or medications, may upset this balance and change an individual's typical pattern.

Normal menstrual flow usually lasts about 5 days, and the normal cycle duration (including bleeding days) is 21–35 days.

Some women never establish normal menses and may report abnormal bleeding since menarche. These women may have an underlying bleeding disorder, such as von Willebrand disease (VWD), and a longstanding history of heavy menses. Those patients will likely report other symptoms, such as frequent nosebleeds, that can help steer a provider toward the correct diagnosis.

A. Wiczulis (✉) · K. Kashinsky
Albany Medical Center, Albany, NY, USA
e-mail: wiczula@amc.edu; kashink@amc.edu

© The Author(s), under exclusive license to Springer Nature Switzerland AG 2021
M. Tadros, G. Y. Wu (eds.), *Management of Occult GI Bleeding*, Clinical Gastroenterology, https://doi.org/10.1007/978-3-030-71468-0_12

Some women may not realize that their menses are abnormal, especially if they have always been heavy, so it is important to quantify the amount of blood lost in a standardized fashion. Conversely, some women may report heavy bleeding, when in fact, the amount of blood lost is within the normal range.

Bleeding Interval

Typical menstrual cycles occur at a regular frequency anywhere from 24 to 38 days in duration. Bleeding usually occurs for 4.5–8 days. More than 9 days may be considered abnormal [1].

Certain types of contraceptives may cause irregular bleeding outside of normal menstruation. This is especially true in the first 1–3 months of use. Thirty percent of women using a combined estrogen-progestin pill, a patch, or the ring may see unscheduled bleeding during the first month; 25% with progestin only contraceptives during the first year; and with the copper-IUD [2].

Anovulatory bleeding is defined as uterine bleeding that does not result in response to ovulation.

In adolescents up to 18 years old, anovulatory bleeding may occur due to an immature or dysregulated hypothalamic-pituitary-ovarian axis. This is not considered pathologic in nature.

In patients aged 40+ until menopause, anovulatory may be due to a physiologic decline in ovarian function. However, a range of pathologies may also cause anovulatory bleeding, and therefore should not be ruled out in favor of physiologic decline [3].

Quantifying Bleeding

During menses, the average amount of blood lost is 34 ml ± 2.4 ml per month. The amount is generally consistent in an individual patient from onset of menarche to menopause, so significant changes in the amount lost may indicate other factors at play [4].

Heavy menstrual bleeding (HMB) lasts longer than 7 days or exceeds 80 ml per period. Women with HMB may develop iron deficiency anemia, which can be profound. On average, 1.0 mg of iron is lost per 60 ml of blood during menses. The critical loss at which iron deficiency may occur is around 1.2–1.6 mg of iron, which is about 72–96 ml of blood. It must be noted however, that the exact amount needed to cause an anemic state depends on dietary intake and absorption as well as overall state of health of the patient [4].

Our ability to quantify menstrual blood loss is limited in the clinical setting. While the average woman doesn't know the volume of blood lost with menses, she can usually report the number of sanitary products she uses on a typical day of bleeding. The provider may ask what products she is using (see below), how often she changes them, and whether they are saturated when they are changed. The provider should also ask whether the patient passes blood clots or bleeds through clothing or bedding [5].

There are many different sanitary products available to women, including pads, tampons, menstrual cups, and absorbent underwear. Some products have different levels of absorbency or come in different sizes to accommodate different volumes of flow. The approximate volumes held by different products are outlined in Table 12.1.

The most commonly used sanitary products are tampons and pads. Sanitary pads vary widely in their absorbency, which can make it difficult to quantify blood loss. If a woman changes the type or brand of pad she is using, she may report needing to change it more or less frequently, when in fact, her bleeding is unchanged [6].

Patients must not just be asked how many times per day that they change their product, they must also be asked why. Some women may change them on a schedule whereas others may only change them when they're fully saturated [6]. A sample set of questions is included in Table 12.2.

Table 12.1 The maximum volumes held by various sanitary products based on data from the FDA and various product listings by brands

Sanitary product	Volume (ml)
Pads	
Liner	–
Regular	–
Maxi pad	–
Tampons	
Light	<5.5
Regular	5.5–8.5
Super	8.5–11.5
Menstrual cups	
Slim/small	17–22
Regular	30
Large	32
Underwear	10–15

Table 12.2 Suggested questions to characterize uterine bleeding [6]

When was the first day of your last menstrual period and several previous menstrual periods?
Is there a possibility that you could be pregnant?
How heavy is your bleeding?
Do you pass blood clots?

Abnormal Uterine Bleeding

Terminology

The classification system for abnormal bleeding was updated in 2011 by the International Federation of Gynecology and Obstetrics (FIGO), and this new nomenclature has been adopted by the American College of Obstetricians and Gynecologists (ACOG) [3].

Although the previous system for classifying abnormal bleeding has been replaced, familiarity with the old terms may be useful when reviewing patient records or older publications, shown in Table 12.3 below.

Additionally, the older phrase *dysfunctional uterine bleeding* (DUB) has been replaced by the term *abnormal uterine bleeding* (AUB), which includes *heavy menstrual bleeding* (HMB) and *intermenstrual bleeding* (IMB). HMB and IMB may occur alone or together in an individual patient. The term DUB should no longer be used, but it may still be seen in patient records [3].

The FIGO classification system was created to improve standardization and specificity when describing AUB in reproductive-aged women. The system does not apply to pregnant women or postmenopausal women. The new classification system incorporates bleeding pattern and etiology, and it is referred to by the acronym PALM-COEIN (polyp, adenomyosis, leiomyoma, malignancy and hyperplasia, coagulopathy, ovulatory dysfunction, endometrial, iatrogenic, and not yet classified) [7].

PALM-COEIN

In the PALM-COEIN system (Fig. 12.1), PALM represents structural causes of AUB (polyps, adenomyosis, leiomyoma, malignancy and hyperplasia), and COEIN represents nonstructural causes (coagulopathy, ovulatory dysfunction, endometrial, iatrogenic, and not yet classified). Understanding the fundamentals of this classification system can provide some guidance to providers when they begin to evaluate a patient with AUB [7].

Table 12.3 Preferred terminology per ACOG recommendations to characterize bleeding and pain complaints [1]

Polymenorrhea	Cycle lasting less than 21 days
Oligomenorrhea	Cycle lasting longer than 35 days
Menorrhagia	Menstrual blood loss greater than 80 ml
Metrorrhagia	Bleeding between periods
Menometrorrhagia	Heavy menstrual bleeding with intermenstrual bleeding

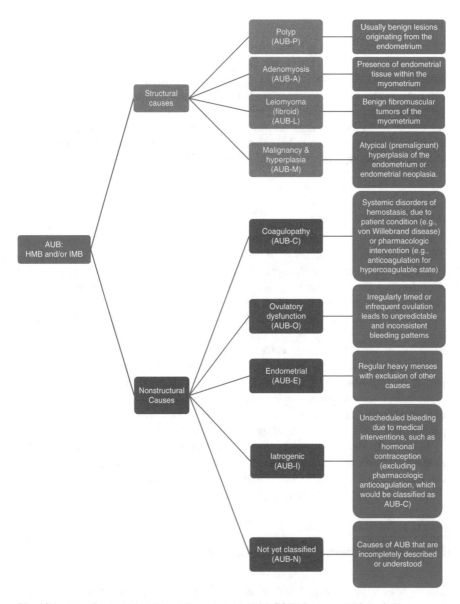

Fig. 12.1 Classification of AUB based on current PALM-COEIN system. [Adapted, 7]

Pregnancy

The possibility of pregnancy should always be considered in sexually active women. Pregnancy and miscarriage can lead to a change in a woman's bleeding pattern, and these diagnoses can be easily excluded with a point-of-care urine test. Failure to promptly diagnose pregnancy may occur in women who report a history of irregular menses or infertility. All contraceptive methods have the potential to fail; even surgical sterilization, so a sexually active woman who reports using contraception can still become pregnant, even if that likelihood is low.

AUB Etiology by Age

The most common causes for AUB vary at different stages of the reproductive lifespan. While anovulation and coagulation defects account for a greater proportion of AUB in adolescents, older reproductive-aged women experience more AUB from pregnancy and sexually transmitted infections [8].

As women age, the incidence of uterine fibroids, polyps, and adenomyosis all increase, and as women approach menopause, ovulation becomes less frequent, so anovulation once again accounts for a significant amount of AUB cases.

The risk of gynecologic malignancy also increases with age, and cancer in any part of the reproductive tract can lead to vaginal bleeding. Globally, cervical cancer is the most common gynecologic malignancy and the leading cause of death from gynecologic cancer. Its incidence is highest in regions without effective screening programs, especially in less developed countries [9].

In more developed countries, uterine cancer (most of which occurs in the endometrium) is the most common gynecologic malignancy. Because endometrial cancer leads to AUB, many of these women present for care early enough that the diagnosis is made at an early stage, when outcomes tend to be better.

Endometrial Hyperplasia and Cancer

Endometrial hyperplasia describes a range of histopathologic changes to the uterine lining. The World Health Organization classified endometrial hyperplasia into two broad categories:

- Hyperplasia without atypia, which contains low levels of mutations and normal glandular structure. These structures may be simple or complex. This type of pathology has only a 1–3% chance of becoming an invasive carcinoma.
- Atypical Hyperplasia/Endometrioid Intraepithelial Neoplasia, whereby there are mutations and structural changes that are typical for invasive carcinoma. These patients are at a very high risk of developing endometrial cancer [10].

There are multiple risk factors for endometrial hyperplasia in women, most notably unopposed estrogen stimulation of the endometrium, which causes increased cell proliferation and growth. Without progesterone to stimulate shedding of the endometrium, the unopposed estrogen can lead to changes in the tissue causing hyperplasia. This can come from exogenous estrogen exposure as with use of estrogen agonists, obesity, early menarche or late menopause, or nullparity.

There are several different forms of endometrial cancer, but 80% are endometrioid adenocarcinoma. This type is graded on a scale of 1–3 based on the level of differentiation of the tissue and it develops from endometrial hyperplasia [11]. As with hyperplasia, endometrial cancer is dependent on estrogen stimulation for growth. Other forms include papillary serous carcinomas, clear cell carcinoma, mixed cell type, and carcinosarcomas [12].

Both hyperplasia and cancer can cause increased or prolonged bleeding during menstruation or off-cycle in premenopausal women. As the disease progresses, patients may present with pressure or pain in the uterus, enlargement of the uterus and increased girth of the abdomen, bloating, or early satiety [8].

Lynch Syndrome

Lynch Syndrome, formerly called Hereditary Nonpolyposis Colorectal Cancer (HNPCC), is an autosomal dominant hereditary mutation in DNA mismatch proteins that leads to a high risk of certain types of cancer, including colorectal, endometrial, ovarian, and breast cancer [13]. Thus, patients with a family history of this disease should be screened and properly counseled [14].

The most common extracolonic manifestation of Lynch syndrome is endometrial cancer, and the mean age at diagnosis (46–54 years) is about 10 years sooner than in the general population. Because this age range overlaps with perimenopause in many women, AUB may be attributed to anovulation, which may delay diagnosis [15].

Women known to be affected by Lynch syndrome should undergo increased surveillance for endometrial cancer via annual endometrial sampling beginning at age 30–35 or 5–10 years prior to the earliest age of first diagnosis of Lynch-associated cancer of any kind in the family [15].

Initial Evaluation of AUB

Figure 12.2 illustrate management steps for AUB. Taking a thorough history can elicit a sound differential in many women with AUB. This can lead to an expedited diagnosis while minimizing superfluous tests, and initial studies should be based on the patient's history and physical exam.

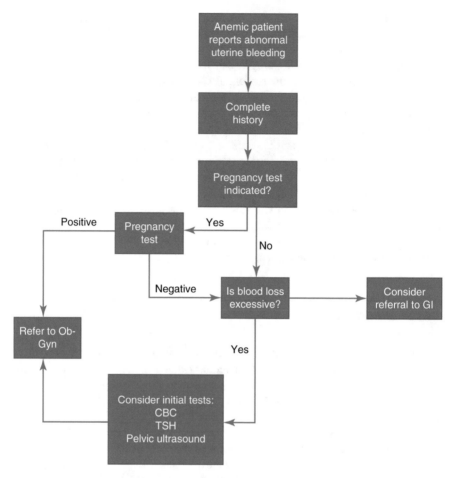

Fig. 12.2 Algorithm for initial work up including labs and imaging studies. [Adapted, 1]

Basic labs to consider:

- Pregnancy test
- Complete blood count (CBC)
- Thyroid-stimulating hormone (TSH)
- Gonorrhea and chlamydia screening
- Pap smear*
- Coagulation studies*
- Prolactin*

If indicated by history

Pelvic ultrasound, including transvaginal evaluation, is the gold standard for imaging the pelvic organs, and it should be considered as part of an initial workup. A CT of the abdomen and pelvis may identify abnormalities in the uterus or ovaries, but ultrasound may still be necessary to better characterize the findings [8].

References

1. Kaunitz A. Approach to abnormal uterine bleeding in nonpregnant reproductive-age women. Barbieri R, Levine D, Eckler K, editors. UpToDate. May 2019.
2. Edelman A. Evaluation and management of unscheduled bleeding in women using contraception. Kaneshiro B, Schreiber C, editors. UpToDate.
3. Practice Bulletin No. 128. Obstet Gynecol. 2012;120(1):197–206. https://doi.org/10.1097/aog.0b013e318262e320.
4. Hallberg L, Högdahl A-M, Nilsson L, Rybo G. Menstrual blood loss and iron deficiency. Acta Med Scand. 1966;180(5):639–50.
5. Warner P, Critchley H, Lumsden MA, Campbell-Brown M, Douglas A, Murray G. Menorrhagia I: measured blood loss, clinical features, and outcome in women with heavy periods: a survey with follow-up data. Am J Obstet Gynecol. 2004;190(5):1216–23.
6. Warrilow GM, Kirkham CM, Ismail KM, et al. Quantification of menstrual blood loss. Obstet Gynaecol. 2004;6(2):88–98.
7. Munro MG, Critchley HO, Broder MS, Fraser IS. FIGO classification system (PALM-COEIN) for causes of abnormal uterine bleeding in nongravid women of reproductive age. Int J Gynecol Obstet. 2011;113(1):3–13.
8. Hoffman B, Schorge J, Bradshaw K, Halvorson L, Schaffer J, Corton M. Williams gynecology. 3rd ed. New York: McGraw-Hill; 2016.
9. Torre L, Islami F, Siegel R, Ward E, Jemal A. Global cancer in women: burden and trends. Cancer Epidemiol Biomark Prev. 2017;26(4):444–57.
10. Emons G, Beckmann MW, Schmidt D, Mallmann P, New WHO. Classification of endometrial hyperplasias. Geburtshilfe Frauenheilkd. 2015;75(2):135–6.
11. Bloom SL, Dashe JS, Hoffman BL. Chapter 5: Implantation and placental development. In: Cunningham FG, Leveno KJ, editors. Williams obstetrics. 25th ed. New York: McGraw-Hill; 2018.
12. Onstad MA, Pakish JB. Chapter 32: Tumors of the uterine corpus. In: Lu KH, editor. The MD Anderson manual of medical oncology. New York, NY: McGraw-Hill. 2016.
13. Temkin SM, Gregory T, Kohn EC, Duska L. Chapter 41: Gynecology. In: Schwartz's principles of surgery. 11th ed. New York: McGraw-Hill; 2019.
14. Hampel H, Frankel WL, Martin E, Arnold M. Screening for the lynch syndrome (hereditary nonpolyposis colorectal cancer). N Engl J Med. 2005;352:1851–60.
15. Lindor NM, Petersen GM, Hadley DW, et al. Recommendations for the care of individuals with an inherited predisposition to lynch syndrome. JAMA. 2006;296(12):1507–17.

Chapter 13
Geriatric Population

Rebecca J. Stetzer, Julian Remouns, and Ali Hani Al-Tarbsheh

Introduction

Evaluation of occult bleeding in older adults warrants special consideration due to changes in likely etiology along with the balance of potential risks of the procedures used to evaluate bleeding to the potential benefit of diagnosing the source of the bleeding. The likelihood of serious life-limiting conditions increases with age, but so does the potential for complications from evaluation and treatment. It is essential to evaluate patients' comorbidities, frailty status, and care priorities before deciding on the approach to evaluation of occult blood in the older adult.

Common Causes of Occult GI Bleeding in Older Adults

Upper Gastrointestinal Tract

Peptic Ulcer Disease, Esophagitis and Gastritis

Similar to the general adult population, peptic ulcer disease (PUD) is the most common cause of upper gastrointestinal bleeding (UGIB) in the geriatric population [1, 2]. PUD with associated esophagitis, gastritis and duodenitis accounts for up to 70% of UGIB cases in elderly patients and is responsible for 60–90% of hospitalizations for UGIB [3–5]. The increasing incidence of GI tract inflammation and PUD is due in part to the widespread use of nonsteroidal anti-inflammatory drugs

R. J. Stetzer (✉) · J. Remouns · A. H. Al-Tarbsheh
Albany Medical College, Albany, NY, USA
e-mail: remounj@amc.edu; altarba@amc.edu

© The Author(s), under exclusive license to Springer Nature
Switzerland AG 2021
M. Tadros, G. Y. Wu (eds.), *Management of Occult GI Bleeding*, Clinical
Gastroenterology, https://doi.org/10.1007/978-3-030-71468-0_13

225

(NSAIDs) and aspirin, particularly in older adults. With the consumption of daily aspirin for cardiac health in addition to chronic NSAID use for musculoskeletal pathologies, older adults are at a higher risk of mortality almost four times that of NSAID non-users.

Varices

Esophageal and gastric varices are another source of UGIB that may present with occult findings. Although overt hematemesis is a common symptom of variceal hemorrhages, a small or slow bleed may not be visualized by a patient with emesis or alternatively, the patient may present without emesis. Population-based studies found that variceal disease was found in up to 21% of older adults over the age of 65 years [4]. While portal hypertension-related bleeds are more commonly seen in patients younger than 60 years, older patients with chronic liver disease are at high risk for the development of varices and subsequent hemorrhage [1]. Without such history, the incidence of esophageal varices is actually quite low in elderly.

Angioectasia

Angioectasia, the degeneration of normal vasculature, are the most common vascular aberration of the GI tract. Risk increases with age [2], with studies reporting incidence of approximately 25% in those age 60–70 and 70% in people over 70 years of age. Incidence in older adults with UGIB range from 4% to 11%. Bleeding is typically occult, recurrent and presents as iron deficiency anemia.

Lower Gastrointestinal Tract

Diverticular Hemorrhage

Bleeding from colon diverticula is the main cause of lower GI bleeding (LGIB) in adults accounting for almost half of all cases [6]. The presence of diverticuli increases with age with studies showing a prevalence of less than 5% in patients under 40 years of age, 30% over 50, 60% over 80 and 65% over 85 years of age.

Most patients with diverticulosis are symptomatic and approximately 3–15% have clinically significant bleeding, typically presenting with painless hematochezia [7]. Mortality rates may be up to 10% of all elderly patients with signs of diverticular hemorrhage. Patients at highest risk of bleeding include those with aspirin and NSAID use, anticoagulation, hypertension, and constipation. Bleeding spontaneously resolves in about two-thirds of patients but may recur in up to 40% within 4 years [5, 7].

Colitis

Colitis can result from a variety of different etiologies and may be difficult to determine based on clinical presentation and endoscopic findings. In the elderly population, ischemic and infectious colitis are more common than inflammatory bowel disease (IBD) with ischemic colitis as the cause of LGIB in up to 19% of patients.

Ischemia of the colon typically affects the splenic flexure and rectosigmoid colon, the "watershed" areas of the colon. High risk patients are those with cardiovascular disease, cardiac thromboembolism, and acute hypotension. Other risk factors include hypercoagulable states, vasculitis and medications. The high occurrence of colonic atherosclerosis in older adults makes its significance difficult to determine. The typical presenting symptom of ischemic colitis is crampy abdominal pain. Bleeding occurs from reperfusion injury after the ischemic event has resolved so occult bleed may be an initial sign of progression [5, 7].

Infectious colitis patients will present with signs and symptoms of infection but may have occult bleeding as a herald event signifying an insidious course of infection. Elderly population is at increased risk for infectious colitis and mortality increases with age. Common pathogens include Campylobacter, Salmonella, Shigella, and certain strains of E. coli. E. coli O157:H7 can cause acute thrombotic thrombocytopenic purpura. Clostridium difficile causes bleeding in less than 10% of cases but should be on the differential as well. LGIB in patients with AIDS-related thrombocytopenia and opportunistic infections with CMV, HSV, and HHV-8 carry over a 25% mortality rate [5, 7].

The second peak in incidence for inflammatory bowel disease (IBD) following a bimodal age distribution occurs between 60 and 70 years of age and approximately 15% of patients with IBD develop symptoms in this age group. Of those patients, only 1.2–6% of patients present with acute LGIB. There are limited studies that evaluate occult bleeds and IBD diagnosis and given the broad differential for colitis in the older adult population, it is often difficult to definitively diagnose IBD [5, 7].

Neoplasm

Multiple studies have shown that a significant proportion of upper GI neoplasms present with bleeding as the initial symptom. The majority of patients who are found to have UGIB due to neoplasm present with severe signs of bleeding including frank hematochezia, melena or symptoms of anemia [8, 9]. Additionally, neoplasms have been found to be the cause of up to 20% of cases of LGIB in older adults. While hematochezia may be present, such bleeds are commonly occult, particularly tumors of the ascending colon [5, 7]. In the setting of weight loss or obstructive symptoms, patients with signs of occult blood loss, high suspicion for malignancy is warranted.

Other Causes

As in UGIB, vascular anomalies, predominantly vascular ectasias may be the source of occult bleeding of the lower GI tract. Vascular ectasias account for 3–15% of patients with LGIB. The same risk factors associated with upper GI tract ectasias apply to the lower GI tract.

In a patient with a history of recent lower endoscopy, post polypectomy bleeding may be considered [10]. If the patient has been using chronic NSAIDs, in addition to being at higher risk of aforementioned source of bleeds, NSAIDs can be an etiology of occult hemorrhage. Anorectal pathologies such as hemorrhoids, rectal ulcers, radiation proctopathy can also be a source of occult bleeding although these causes do not characteristically result enough loss to lead to anemia [7].

Due to increased vulnerabilities in older patients, the decision about employing these procedures necessitates analysis of risks and benefits.

Evaluation of the Positive Fecal Occult Blood Test

The preferred method of evaluation of a positive fecal occult blood test is through direct visualization via endoscopy. While evaluation may lead to an etiology of the bleeding and subsequent targeted management, the procedure itself exposes the patient to risks that may cause even more harm. Over 25% of patients over the age of 65 have more than five comorbid medical conditions. While comorbid conditions can increase the risk and severity of GI bleeds from sources like ulcers or neoplasms, it can also reduce the benefit from treatment in older patients. It has been shown that there is lower survival rates after initial diagnosis, poorer survival after chemotherapy and increased duration of hospitalizations in older, sicker patients [11]. Given the higher rate of medical comorbidities and propensity of polypharmacy in elderly patients, the impact of the patient's medical conditions should be weighed against the need for endoscopy. Before proceeding with evaluation, one must address the question of whether or not evaluation and treatment of the occult bleed will improve quality of life and/or survival.

Procedure-Specific Considerations

Adequate sedation is one of the most important factors for a successful endoscopy. Age-related effects on the body put the geriatric population at higher risk for adverse effects from sedation. Physiologic changes such as decreased arterial oxygenation,

delayed or blunted cardiorespiratory stimulation in response to the body's requirements, increased risk of aspiration, and reduced hepatic and renal clearance mechanisms are factors that make the choice of sedation more difficult when managing an
older adult [12, 13]. For these reasons, guidelines recommend using fewer sedative
agents at lower doses and infusion rates. Endoscopies without sedation are not commonly performed in the United States, but are an option for higher risk patients
[11–13].

The major procedural complication of endoscopy, particularly colonoscopy, is
perforation. Bowel perforation can be a surgical emergency and puts the patient at
significant risk of life-threatening infection. Older patients have a 30% higher risk
of experiencing a perforation during colonoscopy when compared to sigimodos-
copy [14]. This is due to the higher prevalence of diverticulosis, tortuosity of the
intestines, inadequate bowel preparation and post-surgical adhesions or strictures,
which threaten the integrity of the tissue as well as making the procedure more
technically challenging [12, 13, 15, 16]. Furthermore, there is a higher risk of mortality associated with perforation [14]. Other complications include bleeding, diverticulitis, acute cardiopulmonary events, and other serious illness directly related to
the endoscopy procedure [17].

According to multiple population-based studies, the largest barrier to evaluating
GI bleed in older adults was inability to complete the colonoscopy. Strictures and
severe diverticular disease contribute to such difficulty but the predominant cause of
incomplete evaluation is poor bowel preparation [18]. In a systematic review, the
colonoscopy success rate was found to be directly related to the quality of colonic
preparation in patients over 80 years of age [15]. There are multiple reasons for
poorer bowel preparation in older populations compared to younger adults that are
both physiologic and non-physiologic. Altered gastrointestinal motility, altered
anatomy from previous surgeries, medication-related constipation and higher incidence of obstipation are major physiologic culprits in the patient's inability to successfully complete a bowel regimen. Outside factors such as decreased understanding
of instructions, functional limitations, greater burden of comorbid conditions are
significant as well [11]. Due to the potentially fatal effects of sodium phosphate and
magnesium-based solutions for colonoscopy preparation such as hyperphosphatemia, hypernatremia, hypokalemia, hypermagnesemia, these substances are discour-
aged from use, particularly in older patients who are more likely to have comorbid
cardiac, renal or hepatic issues [16]. The superior safety profiles of polyethylene
glycol-based solutions make it the first-line colonoscopy preparation. While PEG-
based solutions are preferred, the large volume of fluid consumption required is
often difficult to achieve, even when dosing is split [11, 12, 16].

Pre-procedure Considerations

Comorbid medical conditions, cognitive function and functional status have been
shown to have significant impact on the risk of both adverse events and negative
long-term outcomes older adults [11, 12]. If concerns are identified during

pre-procedure assessment, they will need to be evaluated and optimized. Furthermore, whenever there is a question of benefit, the proposed procedure should be discussed with the patient's primary care provider prior to scheduling.

The history and physical can identify specific conditions that pose particular risk or may require specific accommodations or approaches. Cardiac and pulmonary disease needs optimization and assessment of tolerance of anesthesia as would be done prior to any surgical procedure. The presence of implanted cardiac devices should be noted as they have the potential for electromagnetic interference if electro cautery must be used, and thus warrant continuous cardiac monitoring during the procedure [13]. As always, careful medication review is important and the necessity of continuing or discontinuing daily medications such as antiplatelet, anticoagulant or anti-hypertensive agents evaluated [12]. People with Parkinson's disease have increased anesthesia-associated risks due to autonomic dysfunction, respiratory dysfunction and medication interactions [19]; consultation with an anesthesiologist would be recommended in these cases. Furthermore, exposure to anesthesia increases the risk of additional cognitive decline in those with mild cognitive impairment or dementia [20], necessitating risk-specific counseling.

Even if the patient's comorbid conditions do not specifically affect the procedure, the body has a decreased ability to compensate for and recover from stresses. These comorbidities, combined with normal physiologic changes of aging, create a state of *homeostenosis*, or decreased physiologic reserve [21]. This renders patients at higher risk for complications from even low-risk procedures. Thus, it is essential to assess the patient's degree of homeostenosis prior to proceeding. This can be done by evaluating frailty and cognitive status.

Frailty Evaluation

Frailty is a syndrome of weakness, fatigue and vulnerability that is common with aging, and usually multifactorial in etiology. The presence of frailty has been shown to be predictive of falls, worsening mobility, ADL disability, hospitalization, and death. It provides important information about functional status and longevity [22, 23]. In the perioperative setting, the presence of frailty has been shown to independently predict postoperative complications, length of stay, likelihood of discharge to subacute nursing facilities, and mortality at 30 days and 6 months [24]. When evaluating patients for endoscopy and colonoscopy, risks can be estimated by considering it a minor surgery, as some anesthesia is used and anticoagulants and antiplatelet agents need to be held for biopsies to be taken. Assessing the patient's frailty status can help put presenting symptoms and potential work up in perspective, which can be helpful to patients and providers alike. A frailty screening initiative studied in VA setting found communication of frailty scores with surgeons, anesthesiologists, and critical care providers resulted in care plan modification and goals of care discussion with palliative care consultants with mortality reduction demonstrated at 30, 180 and 365 days [25].

The question then becomes how to best measure frailty. This is a challenge: there are dozens of different published scores, with varying approaches and data used to define the syndrome, and only a few evaluated in a surgical setting. Perhaps best well known is the Fried score, which measures specific criteria for unintentional weight loss, self-reported exhaustion, weakness, slow walking speed, and low physical activity [22]. However, the details and time needed for the Fried and most scores can seem prohibitive for use in a gastroenterology office consult. The scale that is perhaps most accessible during a time-constrained office visit is the Clinical Frailty Scale.

The Clinical Frailty Scale assesses patients on a 9-point scale ranging from fit to severely frail. It requires an understanding of the patient's daily activity level. This can be assessed with a few questions, which also help to assess goals and priorities. Although it has not been evaluated specifically in a surgical setting, the Clinical Frailty Scale has been validated against the very detailed Canadian Study of Health and Aging 70-item Frailty Index [26]. Most importantly, it helps the provider factor in the patient's vulnerability when making evaluation and treatment recommendations. Please see Fig. 13.1 for details.

The 9-point Clinical Frailty Scale (CFS) was adapted from the 7-point scale used in the Canadian Study of Health and Aging (CMAJ 2005;173:489–495) and has been reprinted with permission of Geriatric Medicine Research, Dalhousie University, Halifax, Nova Scotia [26].

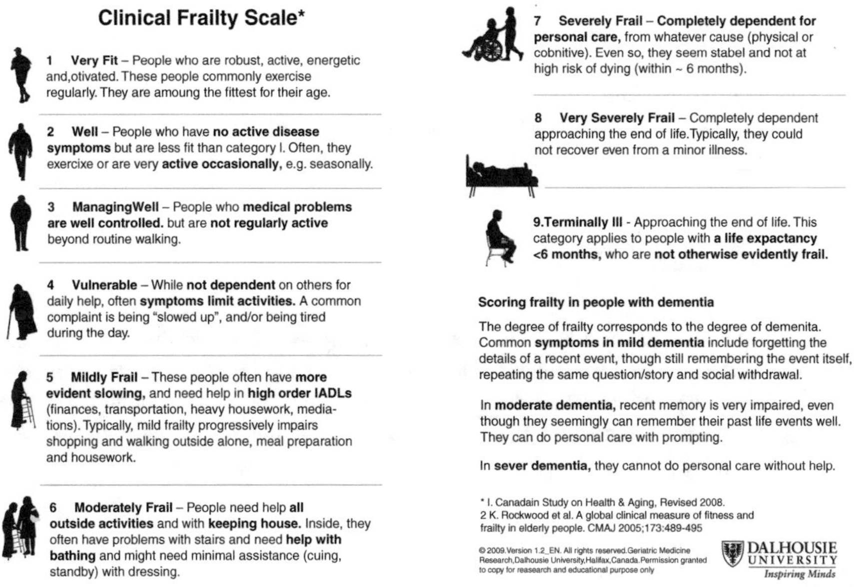

Clinical Frailty Scale*

1 **Very Fit** – People who are robust, active, energetic and,otivated. These people commonly exercise regularly. They are amoung the fittest for their age.

2 **Well** – People who have **no active disease symptoms** but are less fit than category I. Often, they exercixe or are very **active occasionally**, e.g. seasonally.

3 **ManagingWell** – People who **medical problems are well controlled.** but are **not regularly active** beyond routine walking.

4 **Vulnerable** – While **not dependent** on others for daily help, often **symptoms limit activities.** A common complaint is being "slowed up", and/or being tired during the day.

5 **Mildly Frail** – These people often have **more evident slowing,** and need help in **high order IADLs** (finances, transportation, heavy housework, media-tions). Typically, mild frailty progressively impairs shopping and walking outside alone, meal preparation and housework.

6 **Moderately Frail** – People need help **all outside activities** and with **keeping house.** Inside, they often have problems with stairs and need **help with bathing** and might need minimal assistance (cuing, standby) with dressing.

7 **Severely Frail – Completely dependent for personal care,** from whatever cause (physical or cobnitive). Even so, they seem stabel and not at high risk of dying (within ~ 6 months).

8 **Very Severely Frail** – Completely dependent approaching the end of life. Typically, they could not recover even from a minor illness.

9.**Terminally Ill** - Approaching the end of life. This category applies to people with **a life expactancy <6 months,** who are **not** otherwise evidently frail.

Scoring frailty in people with dementia

The degree of frailty corresponds to the degree of demenita. Common **symptoms in mild dementia** include forgetting the details of a recent event, though still remembering the event itself, repeating the same question/story and social withdrawal.

In **moderate dementia,** recent memory is very impaired, even though they seemingly can remember their past life events well. They can do personal care with prompting.

In **sever dementia,** they cannot do personal care without help.

* I. Canadain Study on Health & Aging, Revised 2008.
2 K. Rockwood et al. A global clinical measure of fitness and frailty in elderly people. CMAJ 2005;173:489-495

© 2009.Version 1.2_EN. All rights reserved.Geriatric Medicine Research,Dalhousie University,Halifax,Canada.Permission granted to copy for reasearch and educational purpose only

DALHOUSIE UNIVERSITY
Inspiring Minds

Fig. 13.1 Clinical Frailty Scale

Cognitive Status

Some frailty scales incorporate cognitive evaluation, but this is not true for all of them, including the Clinical Frailty Scale. It is important to evaluate this independently. Cognitive evaluation provides insight about the patient's baseline functioning, ability to understand discussion of the medical issues and ability to follow instructions. Fortunately, there is a quick and simple cognitive screening tool that is relatively uninfluenced by level of education or language, the Mini-Cog [27]. The Mini-Cog has three steps: 3-word registration, clock drawing, and 3-word recall. It is scored on a scale of 0–5 based on number of words recalled and accuracy of the clock. If abnormal, attention should be given to complexity of discussion and instructions, with consideration for inclusion of a caregiver or healthcare proxy. The patient should also be referred for further evaluation. The Mini-Cog can be found in the end of this chapter and accessed at https://mini-cog.com/mini-cog-instrument/standardized-mini-cog-instrument/.

Life Expectancy

The presence of frailty and cognitive impairment informs estimation of life expectancy. Although not a precise science, there are a number of prediction tools that have been studied and can offer a prediction using many of the same factors involved in frailty evaluation. These can be accessed at ePrognosis (https://eprognosis.ucsf.edu/bubbleview.php), where the tool best suited to the question at hand can be selected (ie community-dwelling versus nursing home patients, 1-year versus 10-year life expectancy. Having an understanding of the patient's frailty, cognitive status and life expectancy will help guide realistic goal-setting for patients and families.

Patient-Centered Care

The term patient-centered care can seem confusing – one would think *all* medical care is centered around the patient. This term refers to the medical team approaching the patient's problem rather than their diagnosis. The patient's problem includes not just the medical issues, but the context of physical and emotional comfort, personal and family preferences, and socioeconomic status [28].

Collaborative Goal Setting

Patient-centered care begins with exploring what health outcomes are most important. For some, this may be longevity or surviving to a specific family event. For others the priority may be maintaining independence or mobility, avoiding pain, or minimizing time at the doctor's office. Within the context of the patient's health-priority outcomes the clinician must then evaluate the presentation of problem, potential causes, potential outcomes of evaluation and treatment against the natural history of the disease. Questions to ask include: Is the anemia severe or mild? Is the patient frail or robust? Are there comorbidities that increase the risk of endoscopy? With these considerations in mind, the provider can provide evaluation options, and together with the patient (and loved ones) create a plan. Part of the provider's job is to help guide goal-setting so that the patient and family have realistic and achievable outcomes [29].

Deciding When to Adhere to Guidelines and When to Stray

One of the challenges in treating older adult is that the disease-specific guidelines or usual procedures may not be the best fit for our patients due to comorbidities or frailty. Decision-making is less complex for those on either end of the scale. For those with a 10-year or greater life expectancy who have few comorbid conditions and are not frail, it is reasonable to proceed with disease-based guidelines insomuch as they are aligned with patient preferences. For those with a 2-year or less life expectancy or advanced end-stage disease it is usually best to de-escalate care and focus on palliative symptom management [30].

The group in-between, with shortened life expectancy, multiple chronic conditions, and impaired functional status, poses a particular challenge. It is this group that is the focus of the Patient Priorities Care efforts to align decision-making with each individual's health care priorities [31]. Clinicians must acknowledge and communicate the patient's health trajectory, tradeoffs to proceeding or stopping evaluation, and the uncertainty inherent to either decision [32]. The key to making this happen is communication among patient, family, and medical team. It is essential to involve the primary care giver and any physician the patient has identified as a trusted source of counsel and guidance. We have observed that patients are more comfortable and confident when they come in to see a physician who can tell them their team has discussed what is happening and have agreed on their recommendation. Please see Fig. 13.2.

Before proceeding with any interventions, health care proxy established and advanced directives documented. Assessment of medical decision-making capacity should be completed as well.

Medical Decision-Making Capacity Evaluation

Before concluding and acting upon plan the provider needs to be sure that the patient fully understands what has been discussed and decided upon. The patient should be able to describe the medical problem, engage in a discussion about the treatment options including risks, benefits, and alternatives and clearly indicate a treatment

Patient-Centered Approach to Evaluation
of Occult Bleeding in Olde r Adults[25,32,33]

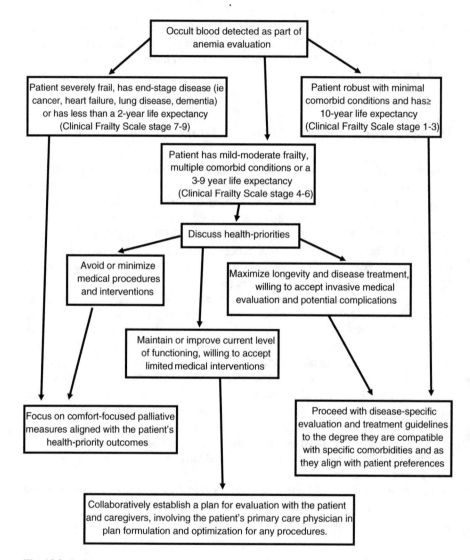

Fig. 13.2 Patient-centered approach to evaluation of occult bleeding in older adults

choice. If the patient does not appear to have capacity it is necessary to obtain consent from the health care proxy as well while ensuring that the patient is not excluded from the conversation or consent process [33]. If the patient's medical decision-making capacity is not clear, consult with the primary care physician and possibly, a mental health specialist.

Conclusion

Both increasing age and the presence of chronic medical conditions impact the approach to evaluation of fecal occult blood. Opening conversations with patients about their health priorities will allow discovery of goals, hopes and fears. This understanding gives medical providers a framework within which to consider potential etiologies, evaluation approaches, comorbid conditions, frailty and cognitive status. Combined with input from the patient's loved ones and primary care provider, this promotes a patient-centered approach to care in what can be challenging cases to manage.

References

1. Hearnshaw SA, Logan RFA, Lowe D, Travis SPL, Murphy MF, Palmer KR. Acute upper gastrointestinal bleeding in the UK: patient characteristics, diagnoses and outcomes in the 2007 UK audit. Gut. 2011;60(10):1327–35.
2. Jóhann P, Hreinsson EK, Gudmundsson S, Björnsson ES. Upper gastrointestinal bleeding: incidence, etiology and outcomes in a population-based setting. Scand J Gastroenterol. 2013;48(4):439–47.
3. Stéphane Nahon ON, Hagège H, Cassan P, Pariente A, Combes R, Kerjean A, Doumet S, Cocq-Vezilier P, Tielman G, Paupard T, Janicki E, Bernardini D, Antoni M, Haioun J, Pillon D, Bretagnolle P. Favorable prognosis of upper-gastrointestinal bleeding in 1041 older patients: results of a prospective multicenter study. Clin Gastroenterol Hepatol. 2008;6(8):886–92.
4. Marco Vincenzo Lenti LP, Cococcia S, Cortesi L, Miceli E, Dominioni CC, Pisati M, Mengoli C, Perticone F, Nobili A, Di Sabatino A, Corazza GR. Mortality rate and risk factors for gastrointestinal bleeding in elderly patients. Eur J Intern Med. 2019;61:54–61.
5. Dharmarajan TS. Gastrointestinal bleeding in older adults. Pract Gastroenterol. 2006:13.
6. Weizman AV, Nguyen GC. Diverticular disease: epidemiology and management. Can J Gastroenterol. 2011;25(7):385–9.
7. Pasha SF, Shergill A, Acosta RD, Chandrasekhara V, Chathadi KV, Early D, Evans JA, Fisher D, Fonkalsrud L, Hwang JH, Khashab MA, Lightdale JR, Muthusamy VR, Saltzman JR, Cash BD. The role of endoscopy in the patient with lower GI bleeding. Gastrointest Endosc. 2014;79(6):875–85.
8. Sami SS, Al-Araji S, Ragunath K. Review article: gastrointestinal angiodysplasia – pathogenesis, diagnosis and management. Aliment Pharmacol Ther. 2014;39(1):15–34.
9. Rockey RASC. Gastrointestinal bleeding due to gastrointestinal tract malignancy: natural history, management, and outcomes. Dig Dis Sci. 2017;62(2):491–501.
10. Warren JL, Mariotto AB, Meekins A, Topor M, Brown ML, Ransohoff DF. Adverse events after outpatient colonoscopy in the medicare population. Ann Intern Med. 2009;150(12):849–57.
11. Velayos F, Day LW. Colorectal cancer screening and surveillance in the elderly: updates and controversies. Gut Liver. 2015;9(2):143–51.

12. Early DS, Acosta RD, Chandrasekhara V, Chathadi KV, Decker GA, Evans JA, Fanelli RD, Fisher DA, Foley KQ, Fonkalsrud L, Hwang JH, Jue T, Khashab MA, Lightdale JR, Muthusamy VR, Pasha SF, Saltzman JR, Sharaf R, Shergill AK, Cash BD. Modifications in endoscopic practice for the elderly. Gastrointest Endosc. 2013;78(3):1–7.
13. Travis ACM, Pievsky D, Saltzman JR. Endoscopy in the elderly. Am J Gastroenterol. 2012;107(10):1495–501.
14. Gatto NM, Frucht H, Sundararajan V, Jacobson JS, Grann VR, Neugut AI. Risk of perforation after colonoscopy and sigmoidoscopy: a population-based study. J Natl Cancer Inst. 2003;95(3):230–6.
15. Jafri SM, Monkemuller K, Lukens FJ. Endoscopy in the elderly: a review of the efficacy and safety of colonoscopy, esophagogastroduodenoscopy, and endoscopic retrograde cholangio-pancreatography. J Clin Gastroenterol. 2010;44(3):161–6.
16. Lin OS. Performing colonoscopy in elderly and very elderly patients: risks, costs and benefits. World J Gastrointest Endosc. 2014;6(6):220–6.
17. Levin TR, Zhao W, Conell C, Seeff LC, Manninen DL, Shapiro JA, Schulman J. Complications of Colonoscopy in an Integrated health Care Delivery System. Ann Intern Med. 2006; 145:880–6.
18. Yoong KK, Heymann T. Colonoscopy in the very old: why bother? Postgrad Med J. 2004;81(953):196–7.
19. Safiya I Shaikh HV. Parkinson's disease and anaesthesia. Indian J Anaesth. 2011;55(3):228–34.
20. Patel D, Lunn A, Smith AD, Lehmann DJ, Dorrington KL. Cognitive decline in the elderly after surgery and anaesthesia: results from the Oxford Project to Investigate Memory and Ageing (OPTIMA) cohort. Anaesthesia. 2016;71(10):1144–52.
21. Halter JB, Studenski S, High KP, Asthana S, Woolard N, Ritchie CS, Supiano MA. Chapter 45: Aging and homeostatic regulation. In: Hazzard's geriatric medicine and gerontology. 7th ed; 2016. p. 2096.
22. Fried LP, Walston J, Newman AB, Hirsch C, Gottdiener J, Seeman T, Tracy R, Kop WJ, Burke G, McBurnie MA, Cardiovascular Health Study Collaborative Research Group. Frailty in older adults: evidence for a phenotype. J Gerontol A Biol Sci Med Sci. 2001;56(3):146–56.
23. Shamliyan T, Talley K, Ramakrishnan R, Kane RL. Association of frailty with survival: a systematic literature review. Ageing Res Rev. 2013;12(2):719.
24. Partridge JS, Harari D, Dhesi JK. Frailty in the older surgical patient: a review. Age Ageing. 2012;41(2):142–7.
25. Hall DE, Arya S, Schmid KK, Carlson MA, Lavedan P, Bailey TL, Purviance G, Bockman T, Lynch TG, Johanning JM. Association of a frailty screening initiative with postoperative survival at 30, 180, and 365 days. JAMA Surg. 2017;152(3):233–40.
26. Rockwood K, Song X, MacKnight C, Bergman H, Hogan DB, McDowell I, Mitnitski A. A global clinical measure of fitness and frailty in elderly people. CMAJ. 2005;173(5):489–95.
27. Borson S, Scanlan J, Watanabe J, Tu SP, Lessig M. Improving identification of cognitive impairment in primary care. Int J Geriatr Psychiatry. 2006;21(4):349–55.
28. What Is Patient-Centered Care? (nejm.org) NEJM Catalyst Brief Article. January 1, 2017. Accessed at catalyst.nejm.org/doi/full/10.1056/CAT.17.0559 on March 12, 2021.
29. Aanand D, Naik M, Martin LA, Moye J, Karel MJ. Health values and treatment goals of older, multimorbid adults facing life-threatening illness. J Am Geriatr Soc. 2016;64(3):625–31.
30. Tinetti, ME. Integrating patient-centered goals into the care of older persons: patient priority care. AGS Scientific Meeting, Portland, OR: 2019.
31. Tinetti ME, Esterson J, Ferris R, Posner P, Blaum CS. Patient priority-directed decision making and care for older adults with multiple chronic conditions. Clin Geriatr Med. 2016;32(2):261–75.
32. Tinetti M, Dindo L, Smith CD, Blaum C, Costello D, Ouellet G, Rosen J, Hernandez-Bigos K, Geda M, Naik A. Challenges and strategies in patients' health priorities-aligned decision-making for older adults with multiple chronic conditions. PLoS One. 2019;14(6):e0218249.
33. Appelbaum PS. Assessment of patients' competence to consent to treatment. N Engl J Med. 2007;357:1834.

Chapter 14
Patients with Native Cardiovascular Disease and Implantable Cardiac Devices

Mark Hanscom and Deepika Devuni

Introduction

The association between cardiovascular disease and gastrointestinal bleeding has been well described. Gastrointestinal bleeding can occur with most cardiovascular conditions, including aortic stenosis, aortic regurgitation, mitral valve stenosis, mitral valve regurgitation, and hypertrophic cardiomyopathy. The most well reported association is between gastrointestinal bleeding and aortic stenosis, a condition called Heyde's syndrome. Like other forms of gastrointestinal bleeding, management of bleeding with cardiovascular disease centers around initial resuscitation, source identification, and subsequent hemostasis. More specific to bleeding associated with cardiovascular disease, management must also take into consideration the presence of pre-existing coagulopathies. In addition to the fact that most cardiac patients are on aspirin or other anti-platelet or anti-coagulant agents, most cardiac patients also suffer from an acquired bleeding disorder mediated by the loss of von Willebrand factor (VWF) multimers, a condition called acquired von Willebrand syndrome (AVWS). Overall, gastrointestinal bleeding associated with cardiovascular disease tends to be recurrent and resistant to endoscopic treatment alone, necessitating more aggressive pharmacologic and surgical interventions for sustained control.

M. Hanscom · D. Devuni (✉)
Division of Gastroenterology, University of Massachusetts Medical School,
Worcester, MA, USA
e-mail: mark.hanscom@umassmemorial.org; Deepika.devuni@umassmemorial.org

© The Author(s), under exclusive license to Springer Nature   237
Switzerland AG 2021
M. Tadros, G. Y. Wu (eds.), *Management of Occult GI Bleeding*, Clinical
Gastroenterology, https://doi.org/10.1007/978-3-030-71468-0_14

Aortic Stenosis

The association between calcific aortic stenosis and gastrointestinal bleeding was first described by Dr. Edward Heyde in 1958 [1]. His observations prompted further reports of similar patients with both aortic stenosis and idiopathic gastrointestinal bleeding [2–4]. The culprit lesion in these patients remained unidentified until advancements in imaging and histopathology came to recognize it as the small, tufted, red lesion known now as the angioectasia [5, 6]. The constellation of findings comprising aortic stenosis and gastrointestinal bleeding from angioectasias has since come to be called Heyde's syndrome after its eponymous first describer.

The diagnosis of Heyde's syndrome has been controversial since its first description in 1958. Initial reports based the diagnosis of aortic stenosis on less objective criteria such as auscultation and other exam findings, and critics have raised concerns about methodological deficiencies in these studies [7, 8]. The overall reported prevalence rates of aortic stenosis in patients with angioectasias range from 0% to 41% [9]. However, more recent studies using echocardiographic confirmation of aortic stenosis have suggested prevalence rates in the range of 0–1.6% [10, 11]. In patients with pre-existing aortic stenosis, the rates of gastrointestinal bleeding range from 2% to 20% [12]. Despite these criticisms, the diagnosis of Heyde's syndrome has remained durable, in part because of the elucidation of an explanatory mechanism and demonstrated treatment strategies.

Pathogenesis

Multiple mechanisms have been proposed to explain the gastrointestinal bleeding seen in patients with aortic stenosis and angioectasias. Initial proposals included the presence of a common connective tissue disorder, mucosal ischemia from low cardiac output, mucosal damage from cholesterol emboli, and mucosal damage and vasodilatation from decreased tissue perfusion [13]. The true mechanism appears to be multifactorial, resulting from a combination of increased angioectasia formation and an acquired predisposition to bleeding from the loss of hemostatic von Willebrand factor multimers.

The formation of angioectasias is believed to result from poor perfusion and chronic obstruction of submucosal veins. In patients with cardiac, vascular, or pulmonary disease, decreased perfusion to local gastrointestinal tissue leads to hypo-oxygenation. In response, gastrointestinal smooth muscle contracts in an attempt to compensate, causing an obstruction where the innervating vessels interface. This obstruction then leads to increased intravascular pressure and subsequent dilatation of the veins, venules, and capillaries. The vessels and capillaries become tortuous and form an arteriovenous communication, or angioectasia. There terms angiodysplasia and arteriovenous malformation (AVM) are often used synonymously with angioectasia. Further ischemia or mechanical trauma to these lesions can then lead to gastrointestinal bleeding [5, 6].

Patients with aortic stenosis are also at increased risk of bleeding from an acquired bleeding disorder. Upwards of 80% of patients with severe aortic stenosis have been demonstrated to have loss of the high molecular weight variant of von Willebrand factor, a protein implicated in both hemostasis and angiogenesis [14]. High molecular weight multimers of VWF are created in the organelles of endothelial cells and platelets, before being secreted into plasma in order to contribute to hemostasis. HMW multimers are of particular importance in areas of turbulent blood flow, such as AVMs, which require the high molecular weight multimers for appropriate hemostasis [15, 16]. Once secreted into the plasma, multimers of von Willebrand factor undergo proteolysis at the hands of the enzyme ADAMTS13. In patients with aortic stenosis, the high shear stress imparted upon von Willebrand factor as it traverses the stenotic valve leads to conformational changes in the protein and exposure of additional binding sites. These previously protected binding sites are targeted and cleaved by ADAMTS13, resulting in accelerated degradation of the von Willebrand factor multimers. The end result is an increase in the destruction of high molecular weight multimers of von Willebrand factor and an acquired coagulopathy called acquired von Willebrand syndrome 2A (AVWS-2A).

Together, the combination of increased angioectasia formation and an acquired bleeding disorder from loss of hemostatic high molecular weight VWF multimers is thought to explain the increased risk of gastrointestinal bleeding seen in patients with Heyde's syndrome [15–18].

Diagnosis

Gastrointestinal bleeding in Heyde's syndromes can manifest as overt bleeding with melena or hematochezia or obscure bleeding with anemia or guaiac positive stools. The characteristic bleeding lesion in Heyde's syndrome is the angioectasia. Most patients will present with multiple angioectasias, with a few patients having more than 10 on initial evaluation. The most common location of bleeding lesions is in the jejunum, comprising up to 36% of all cases. The next most common locations are the duodenum and ileum, respectively [19].

The characteristic lab abnormality in Heyde's syndrome is the loss of HMW VWF. However, standard lab testing for the presence of von Willebrand disease is often normal, as the defect is specific to the HMW multimers. If available, a point-of-care platelet function analyzer can detect the presence of the bleeding disorder, although this is not specific for AVWS-2A [12, 14].

Standard guidelines should be followed in the approach to the patient with gastrointestinal bleeding [20]. Following resuscitation, endoscopy is the standard of care for its diagnostic and therapeutic capabilities. The initial endoscopic evaluation comprises upper endoscopy and colonoscopy. If the initial exam does not identify a source of bleeding, second look endoscopy can be considered depending on the clinical presentation. Given the high rate of small bowel lesions, second look examination with push enteroscopy might have the added benefit of improved diagnostic yield. In cases of obscure bleeding, VCE is a first-line procedure for evaluation of the small bowel, followed by deep enteroscopy and, in rare cases, intra-operative enteroscopy, if needed [20].

The identification of angioectasias on endoscopy can be difficult. Lesions can often be missed or misidentified as endoscope trauma, tube trauma, artifact, or gastritis. Furthermore, the vascular nature of angioectasias means that alterations in blood flow, such as from intra-procedural narcotics or anesthesia, can influence their size and visibility. The use of naloxone has been suggested as a tool to enhance the appearance of angioectasias and improve detection during endoscopic evaluation [21].

Treatment and Prevention

Treatment of gastrointestinal bleeding associated with cardiac valvular disease can be challenging. The difficulties arise, in part, from the multifocal and recurrent nature of bleeding in these patients. Most patients with angioectasias will have multiple lesions across multiple sites. Over 60% of patients will have multiple upper gastrointestinal lesions, and in up to 50% of patients with an upper gastrointestinal tract lesion, there will be a concurrent colonic lesion as well [22].

In the acute setting, undifferentiated bleeding should be approached according to established societal guidelines, with attention paid first to patient resuscitation and stabilization [20, 23]. Medication lists should be reviewed for blood thinning agents and stopped if it is safe to do so. Coagulopathies should be reversed if present. In general, AVWS-2A does not respond to desmopressin or transfusion of clotting factors. However, it is reasonable to administer at least a test dose of desmopressin to identify the rare patient who will respond [24]. Proton pump inhibitors, while of questionable effectiveness, are still commonly administered.

Endoscopic intervention is both safe and effective in Heyde's syndrome. The most commonly used endoscopic intervention is APC [19]. Thermal cauterization has also been demonstrated to be safe and effective, and in studies has been demonstrated to reduce the number of blood transfusions needed in treated patients [25]. Close to half of patients will require eventual additional endoscopic procedures for full control, with an average number of procedures of 1.94 per patient [25]. Surgical resection, while the historic treatment of choice, is no longer considered first-line and has not been demonstrated to be superior to endoscopic therapy alone [26].

Following initial hemostasis, prevention must then be considered. The rate of rebleeding in Heyde's syndrome is high, with rebleeding occurring in up to 33–50% of patients, often from other lesions in the gastrointestinal tract [27]. Iron supplementation is popular, and in patients who suffer from iron-deficiency anemia despite oral supplementation, intravenous infusions should be administered [19, 27]. Other pharmacologic treatments to prevent recurrent bleeding in Heyde's syndrome include octreotide, thalidomide, and hormones. Octreotide does not cure the culprit lesion, but has been shown to reduce bleeding and the need for blood transfusions [28]. Octreotide also benefits from being well tolerated. Hormone treatment, on the other hand, has not been shown to be effective. In 1 RCT of 72 patients randomized to ethinylestradiol and norethisterone or placebo, there was no difference in the number of bleeding episodes or number of transfusions [29]. Furthermore, adverse events were significantly higher in the treatment group, with the most common adverse event being metrorrhagia, affecting 29% of patients. Other worrisome complications of hormone therapy include pulmonary embolism and stroke. Thalidomide has gained interest because of its anti-neoangiogenesis properties through the inhibition of VEGF. It has been demonstrated to reduce bleeding episodes, hospital admissions, hospital readmissions, hospital admission duration, and number of blood transfusions in patients with refractory bleeding. However, its use has been limited by its high rate of adverse events, which approach 72% and include fatigue, dizziness, and abdominal discomfort [30]. More rare but serious side effects include thrombosis, peripheral neuropathy, and childbirth defects. Despite its reported efficacy in international studies, thalidomide has not been widely adopted in part because of these side effects.

The most durable treatment for gastrointestinal bleeding in Heyde's syndrome is aortic valve replacement (AVR). AVR offers the best chance for long-term resolution of bleeding and should be offered to patients who are surgical candidates [31]. The overall success rate of AVR in stopping further bleeding is 93% [32]. AVR has been demonstrated to not just resolve further bleeding, but also increase VWF multimers and in doing so correct the underlying coagulopathy [33, 34]. Vincentelli and colleagues, for example, reported that in 92% of patients with Heyde's syndrome and AVWS-2A who underwent AVR, *all* had their VWF abnormalities corrected on the first post-operative morning [15]. The reduction in bleeding episodes post-AVR appears durable up to at least 12 months out post-operatively [35].

Both surgical and transcatheter aortic valve replacement have demonstrated benefit in resolving bleeding and returning HMW VWF to normal levels. However, when possible, use of a bioprosthetic valve has still been advocated for in order to minimize the need for oral anticoagulation post-operatively [35–37].

Aortic and Mitral Regurgitation

There is more limited data on the association between regurgitant valvular disease and gastrointestinal bleeding. There are case series reporting the loss of VWF multimers and AVWS in patients with aortic regurgitation from various causes [12]. The overall prevalence of gastrointestinal bleeding in severe aortic regurgitation without co-existing aortic stenosis is 9% [38]. The degree of bleeding disorder, as determined by abnormal VWF, appears to be less than that seen in aortic stenosis.

The association between mitral regurgitation and gastrointestinal bleeding has been better described. Several case series have described the constellation of mitral regurgitation, bleeding, loss of HMW VWF multimers, and AVWS which corrected after surgical repair of the mitral valve [12]. The presence of AVWS in patients with MR increases with more severe valve disease, reaching up to 85% in patients with severe MR. In patients with mild and moderate MR, the presence of AVWS is 8% and 64%, respectively. The rate of gastrointestinal bleeding in patients with MR is 17%, of which 89% of cases have severe MR [12, 39].

Hypertrophic Cardiomyopathy

Gastrointestinal bleeding has been well described in patients with HCM. Despite a structurally normal valve, subvalvular obstruction creates an environment of turbulent blood flow in the outflow tract that resembles that seen with aortic stenosis and Heyde's syndrome. Abnormal VWF multimers and Heyde's syndrome-like bleeding have both been reported [12]. The degree of abnormality is related to the severity of outflow obstruction, and can be corrected with septal reduction therapy, as with septal myectomy or ablation [12, 14, 27].

Summary

Gastrointestinal bleeding has been well associated with cardiovascular disease. While the most well-known association is with aortic stenosis, it also occurs with other valvular diseases including aortic regurgitation, mitral regurgitation, and HCM. The pathogenesis in each case is centered on an acquired bleeding disorder resulting from the loss of HMW multimers of VWF as blood courses past the abnormal valve. Clinical presentation varies, and an ultimate diagnosis can be difficult, but evaluation should proceed according to standard guidelines with the exception of consideration of early small bowel investigation. Once identified, gastrointestinal bleeding is often remedied with correction of the underlying valvular problem. In patients who are not surgical candidates, various pharmacologic options have been studied with iron-supplementation and octreotide being among the best tolerated.

Implantable Cardiac Devices

The evolution of cardiac assist devices has introduced new problems for the practicing gastroenterologist, including complications related to a range of prosthetic devices, spanning from simple prosthetic and mechanical cardiac replacement valves to entire implantable pumps such as the Impella or intra-aortic balloon pump.

These devices have all been associated with significant rates of gastrointestinal bleeding. In recent times, the introduction of the left ventricular assist device, or LVAD, has seen even higher post-operative rates of gastrointestinal bleeding. Given the expansion of cardiac assist devices in clinical care, it is important for the gastro-enterologist to be comfortable and capable in the management of bleeding in patients with these devices.

Left Ventricular Assist Devices (LVADs)

LVADs are surgically implanted mechanical pumps that provide circulatory support to patients with end stage heart failure. Initial iterations of the LVAD used a pulsa-tile flow mechanism that mimicked natural cardiac physiology. More recent itera-tions have evolved to use a non-pulsatile flow or continuous flow mechanism. Compared to their predecessors, the continuous flow devices are smaller, easier to implement, and more durable, leading to their widespread adoption [40]. LVADs have demonstrated improved quality of life and increased survival in patients with end stage heart failure, leading to a proliferation in their use over the past decade [41]. LVADs can be used now as both a bridge to transplantation or as a destination treatment in patients who are not transplant candidates but desire life-prolonging treatment.

One of the most common complications following LVAD implantation is gastro-intestinal bleeding. The incidence of gastrointestinal bleeding in the newer continu-ous flow LVADs is ten times that of their older pulsatile flow counterparts [40]. Additional risk factors for gastrointestinal bleeding include patient age, an elevated creatinine, an elevated INR, a low platelet count, right ventricular dysfunction, and a post-LVAD ejection fraction >30% [40, 42–44]. The incidence of gastrointestinal bleeding is estimated between 20% and 61% [43–46]. Most bleeding occurs late after implantation at an average onset of 159 days after implantation [47]. Recurrent bleeding is common with estimates ranging from 9% to 43% and as high as 71% [40, 43, 44].

Pathogenesis

The mechanism behind bleeding in patients with LVADs is multifactorial, involving anticoagulant use, alterations in hemodynamics, and loss of von Willebrand factor multimers [40]. Most patients following LVAD implantation will be placed on anti-coagulation. However, the rates of bleeding seen following LVAD implantation exceed those expected with anticoagulation alone by more than fourfold [48].

Implantation with continuous flow LVADs also disrupts normal cardiovascular hemodynamics through loss of the physiologic pulsatile flow [40]. Instead, LVADs result in an environment similar to that seen in aortic stenosis, with a narrow pulse pressure, reduced aortic valve opening, and high shear stress. Similar to aortic stenosis, there is loss of high molecular weight multimers of VWF associated with LVADs from increased shear forces and subsequent multimer degradation. This same loss of VWF multimers is not seen in patients following heart transplantation. The loss of VWF multimers contributes to an acquired bleeding disorder and an increased predisposition to bleeding [49, 50]. LVAD implantation has also been associated with impaired platelet aggregation [51].

Diagnosis

The most common presentation of gastrointestinal bleeding in patients with LVADs is overt upper gastrointestinal bleeding. Half of patients will present with melena and another 7% of patients will present with hematemesis. Lower gastrointestinal bleeding with hematochezia is relatively rare and occurs in 13% of cases. Most patients present from the outpatient setting as hemodynamic instability is uncommon [47].

The diagnostic approach to gastrointestinal bleeding in patients with LVADs is similar to the approach in the general population. Following resuscitation, endoscopic evaluation is the standard of care [40]. Endoscopy will identify the bleeding lesion in 60–90% of cases [52, 53]. EGD is the best first test with a diagnostic yield approaching 50%. If no bleeding lesion is found, colonoscopy should then be pursued, followed with deep enteroscopy. One alternative to this conventional approach to endoscopy favors early enteroscopy. Early small bowel evaluation with device-assisted enteroscopy has been associated with decreased number of transfusions, decreased number of days to treatment, and decreased number of diagnostic tests [54]. Initial evaluation with push enteroscopy might be an effective compromise and has been advocated for by some practitioners [40]. Colonoscopies, on the other hand, are likely overused [52]. Multiple procedures are often required before a definitive diagnosis is reached, and the average patient will undergo 3.3 procedures during the course of his investigation [52].

If small bowel evaluation is pursued, video capsule endoscopy is an important adjunct to device-assisted enteroscopy. VCE allows the endoscopist to localize the site of bleeding, plan his approach, and provide targeted treatment. VCE has been demonstrated to be both safe and effective in patients with LVADs. In patients with obscure gastrointestinal bleeding, the diagnostic yield of VCE ranges up to 80–100%. The most common finding is intraluminal blood and the most common location is the jejunum [55, 56]. While there have been concerns related to LVAD interference with capsule image acquisition, this can be minimized by positioning the device leads as far away as possible from the capsule recorder. In over 100 studies of VCE in patients with implantable electromedical devices, including pacemakers, ICDs, and LVADs, VCE did not result in disturbance of the cardiac devices function [57].

Treatment and Prevention

Standard guidelines for the management of gastrointestinal bleeding should be followed in the initial approach to bleeding in patients with LVADs. The initial approach includes establishing appropriate peripheral access, adequate resuscitation with intravenous fluids and packed red blood cell transfusion, acid suppression in cases of suspected upper gastrointestinal bleeding, and ongoing hemodynamic monitoring. Reversal agents, such as phytonadione, FFP, and concentrated VWF can be used but must be done so with caution and in consideration of the risk of pump thrombosis. It can be prudent to consult with a Cardiologist before reversal if safety is in question.

Once the patient has been well resuscitated, endoscopy is the initial treatment of choice. The most common bleeding lesion in LVAD-associated bleeding is the peptic ulcer, being identified in over 30% of cases. Behind peptic ulcers, vascular malformations (27%), colitis (7%), and polyps (5%) are the next most commonly identified lesions [47]. Endoscopic intervention of high-risk lesions results in successful hemostasis in 90% or more of cases [52, 53]. Multiple modalities have demonstrated success in LVAD-associated bleeding including argon plasma coagulation, contact coagulation, and mechanical clips, with no one technique demonstrating superiority over the others. Both moderate and deep sedation have been demonstrated to be safe in the setting of endoscopy [40].

Rebleeding is frequent and can occur in up to half of cases but often remains amenable to endoscopic intervention [53]. The median time to rebleeding is 7 days and half of patients will bleed from a separate site than the initial target of hemostasis. In cases of refractory bleeding, lowering the speed of the LVAD to increase pulsatility might help to reduce bleeding. However, concerns related to the risk of thrombosis has limited its widespread adoption outside of certain centers [58]. Endovascular embolization remains another treatment option for bleeding resistant to endoscopic intervention [59].

Once initial endoscopic hemostasis has been achieved, attention is turned to the prevention of recurrent bleeding. Pharmacologic treatments are similar to those used for the prevention of angioectasia-related bleeding, and include octreotide, thalidomide, and danazol. Octreotide alone has not been demonstrated to reduce the rate of recurrent bleeding, the need for blood transfusions, or the need for further endoscopic procedures outside of small case reports [60, 61]. However, there was a favorable trend in the direction of these reductions. Thalidomide has been used in case reports in the treatment of refractory gastrointestinal bleeding. However, its use is limited by severe adverse events and regulations surrounding its prescription [62]. There has been one successful case report describing the use of danazol in the prevention of gastrointestinal bleeding [63]. Omega-3 acids have been demonstrated to increase days free from gastrointestinal bleeding in limited reports [64].

The decision of what to do with anticoagulation is difficult and without uniform guidance. Management of anticoagulation must include consideration of both the risks of gastrointestinal bleeding and the risks of pump thrombosis. Some centers have moved to lower international ratio targets in patients with LVADs and experimented with a target of 1.8–2.2 down from 2 to 3. Further studies with longer follow up are needed before the lower target range can be universally recommended [65].

The most durable treatment is cardiac transplant. Similar to sclerotic aortic valvular disease, the gastrointestinal bleeding seen in association with LVADs resolves with correction of the underlying flow problem. Cardiac transplant and removal of the device has been shown to prevent further episodes of bleeding [40].

Aortic Valve Prothesis

The lifetime of an aortic valve prosthesis is between 7 and 20 years. Prosthetic failure can occur as a result of thrombosis, calcification and obstruction, leaflet tear, and paravalvular leakage [12, 14]. Failure of the prosthetic valve leads to recurrent aortic stenosis or regurgitation and resumption of the previous pathophysiology. Overall, gastrointestinal complications comprise close to 40% of bleeding complications in patients who undergo transcatheter aortic valve replacement. The rate of late major bleeding seen after transcatheter aortic valve replacement is 5.9% and occurs at a median time of 132 days [67]. The presence of a moderate or severe paravalvular leak is an independent predictor of bleeding complications. Other risk factors include baseline anemia, atrial fibrillation or flutter, and greater left ventricular mass. Compared to normal valves, abnormal valves have higher rates of abnormal VWF multimers. The abnormal VWF multimers correct in patients with minimal to no paravalvular regurgitation compared to those with moderate to severe regurgitation, and intraprocedure measurement of abnormal VWF multimers using PFA have been used to predict later valve dysfunction.

Mitral Valve Prosthesis

Mitral valve protheses are associated with gastrointestinal bleeding in cases with abnormal valve function. For example, both gastrointestinal bleeding and abnormal VWF multimers have been described with mitral paravalvular leak [12, 14]. Compared to normal valves after replacement or repair, dysfunctional valves are associated with abnormal VWF and have an incidence of gastrointestinal bleeding of 26%. In most cases, the bleeding originates from an angioectasia [12, 14]. Both gastrointestinal bleeding and abnormal VWF multimers correct after surgical repair of the abnormal valve.

Other Cardiac Assist Devices

Other implantable cardiac devices associated with increased rates of gastrointestinal bleeding include the Impella and intra-aortic balloon pump. The rates of gastrointestinal bleeding in these devices can reach upwards of 31% and is driven by a similar shear-stress acquired bleeding disorder [66].

Summary

Gastrointestinal bleeding is a common complication associated with implantable cardiac devices. The LVAD, in particular, has been associated with bleeding in over half of cases, and gastrointestinal bleeding is also seen with protheses and other ICDs. Like with native cardiovascular disease, the pathogenesis is centered around an acquired bleeding disorder resulting from destruction of HMW multimers of VWF that degrade from shear stress as blood courses past the foreign device. Clinical presentation varies, and resuscitation and investigation is similar to other sources of gastrointestinal bleeding with the exception of consideration of early small bowel investigation. In patients with a correctable problem – such as a paravalvular leak – correction can result in hemostasis. In patients with an LVAD who are transplant candidates, heart transplantation is among the most durable treatment option. In other patients who are not operative candidates, recurrent bleeding is common, and prevention is multifactorial including device settings, anticoagulation adjustment, and various pharmacologic agents.

References

1. Heyde E. Gastrointestinal bleeding in aortic stenosis. N Engl J Med. 1958;259:196.
2. Williams RC. Aortic stenosis and unexplained gastrointestinal bleeding. Arch Intern Med. 1961;108:859–63.
3. Boss EG, Rosenbaum JM. Bleeding from the right colon associated with aortic stenosis. Am J Dig Dis. 1971;16(3):269–75.
4. Cody MC, O'Donovan TP, Hughes RW. Idiopathic gastrointestinal bleeding and aortic stenosis. Am J Dig Dis. 1974;19(5):393–8.
5. Rogers BH. Endoscopic diagnosis and therapy of mucosal vascular abnormalities of the gastrointestinal tract occurring in elderly patients and associated with cardiac, vascular, and pulmonary disease. Gastrointest Endosc. 1980;26(4):134–8.
6. Boley SJ, Sprayregen S, Sammartano RJ, Adams A, Kleinhaus S. The pathophysiologic basis for the angiographic signs of vascular ectasias of the colon. Radiology. 1977;125(3):615–21.
7. Gostout CJ. Angiodysplasia and aortic valve disease: let's close the book on this association. Gastrointest Endosc. 1995;42(5):491–3.

8. Imperiale TF, Ransohoff DF. Aortic stenosis, idiopathic gastrointestinal bleeding, and angio-dysplasia: is there an association? A methodologic critique of the literature. Gastroenterology. 1988;95(6):1670–6.

9. Perry PA, Atkins BZ, Amsterdam EA. Gastrointestinal bleeding, aortic stenosis, and the hiding culprit. Am J Med. 2015;128(8):e5–6.

10. Bhutani MS, Gupta SC, Markert RJ, Barde CJ, Donese R, Gopalswamy N. A prospective controlled evaluation of endoscopic detection of angiodysplasia and its association with aortic valve disease. Gastrointest Endosc. 1995;42(5):398–402.

11. Oneglia C, Sabatini T, Rusconi C, Gardini A, Paterlini A, Buffoli F, et al. Prevalence of aortic valve stenosis in patients affected by gastrointestinal angiodysplasia. Eur J Med. 1993;2(2):75–8.

12. Blackshear JL. Heyde syndrome: aortic stenosis and beyond. Clin Geriatr Med. 2019;35(3):369–79.

13. Saad RA, Lwaleed BA, Kazmi RS. Gastrointestinal bleeding and aortic stenosis (Heyde syndrome): the role of aortic valve replacement. J Card Surg. 2013;28(4):414–6.

14. Blackshear JL. Gastrointestinal bleeding in native and prosthetic valve disease. Curr Treat Options Cardiovasc Med. 2018;20(1):6.

15. Vincentelli A, Susen S, Le Tourneau T, Six I, Fabre O, Juthier F, et al. Acquired von Willebrand syndrome in aortic stenosis. N Engl J Med. 2003;349(4):343–9.

16. Veyradier A, Balian A, Wolf M, Giraud V, Montembault S, Obert B, et al. Abnormal von Willebrand factor in bleeding angiodysplasias of the digestive tract. Gastroenterology. 2001;120(2):346–53.

17. Sadler JE. Aortic stenosis, von Willebrand factor, and bleeding. N Engl J Med. 2003;349(4):323–5.

18. Sucker C. The Heyde syndrome: proposal for a unifying concept explaining the association of aortic valve stenosis, gastrointestinal angiodysplasia and bleeding. Int J Cardiol. 2007;115(1):77–8.

19. Grooteman KV, van Geenen EJM, Drenth JPH. High variation in treatment strategies for gastrointestinal angiodysplasias. Eur J Gastroenterol Hepatol. 2016;28(9):1082–6.

20. Gerson LB, Fidler JL, Cave DR, Leighton JA. ACG clinical guideline: diagnosis and management of small bowel bleeding. Am J Gastroenterol. 2015;110(9):1265–87; quiz 1288.

21. Brandt LJ, Spinnell MK. Ability of naloxone to enhance the colonoscopic appearance of normal colon vasculature and colon vascular ectasias. Gastrointest Endosc. 1999;49(1):79–83.

22. Clouse RE, Costigan DJ, Mills BA, Zuckerman GR. Angiodysplasia as a cause of upper gastrointestinal bleeding. Arch Intern Med. 1985;145(3):458–61.

23. Laine L, Jensen DM. Management of patients with ulcer bleeding. Am J Gastroenterol. 2012;107(3):345–60; quiz 361.

24. Sadler JE, Budde U, Eikenboom JCJ, Favaloro EJ, Hill FGH, Holmberg L, et al. Update on the pathophysiology and classification of von Willebrand disease: a report of the subcommittee on von Willebrand factor. J Thromb Haemost. 2006;4(10):2103–14.

25. Askin MP, Lewis BS. Push enteroscopic cauterization: long-term follow-up of 83 patients with bleeding small intestinal angiodysplasia. Gastrointest Endosc. 1996;43(6):580–3.

26. Hutcheon DF, Kabelin J, Bulkley GB, Smith GW. Effect of therapy on bleeding rates in gastrointestinal angiodysplasia. Am Surg. 1987;53(1):6–9.

27. Warkentin TE, Moore JC, Anand SS, Lonn EM, Morgan DG. Gastrointestinal bleeding, angiodysplasia, cardiovascular disease, and acquired von Willebrand syndrome. Transfus Med Rev. 2003;17(4):272–86.

28. Jackson CS, Gerson LB. Management of gastrointestinal angiodysplastic lesions (GIADs): a systematic review and meta-analysis. Am J Gastroenterol. 2014;109(4):474–83; quiz 484.

29. Junquera F, Feu F, Papo M, Videla S, Armengol JR, Bordas JM, et al. A multicenter, randomized, clinical trial of hormonal therapy in the prevention of rebleeding from gastrointestinal angiodysplasia. Gastroenterology. 2001;121(5):1073–9.

30. Ge Z-Z, Chen H-M, Gao Y-J, Liu W-Z, Xu C-H, Tan H-H, et al. Efficacy of thalidomide for refractory gastrointestinal bleeding from vascular malformation. Gastroenterology. 2011;141(5):1629–37.e1-4.
31. Pate GE, Chandavimol M, Naiman SC, Webb JG. Heyde's syndrome: a review. J Heart Valve Dis. 2004;13(5):701–12.
32. King RM, Pluth JR, Giuliani ER. The association of unexplained gastrointestinal bleeding with calcific aortic stenosis. Ann Thorac Surg. 1987;44(5):514–6.
33. Yoshida K, Tobe S, Kawata M, Yamaguchi M. Acquired and reversible von Willebrand disease with high shear stress aortic valve stenosis. Ann Thorac Surg. 2006;81(2):490–4.
34. Solomon C, Budde U, Schneppenheim S, Czaja E, Hagl C, Schoechl H, et al. Acquired type 2A von Willebrand syndrome caused by aortic valve disease corrects during valve surgery. Br J Anaesth. 2011;106(4):494–500.
35. Thompson JL, Schaff HV, Dearani JA, Park SJ, Sundt TM, Suri RM, et al. Risk of recurrent gastrointestinal bleeding after aortic valve replacement in patients with Heyde syndrome. J Thorac Cardiovasc Surg. 2012;144(1):112–6.
36. Godino C, Lauretta L, Pavon AG, Mangieri A, Viani G, Chieffo A, et al. Heyde's syndrome incidence and outcome in patients undergoing transcatheter aortic valve implantation. J Am Coll Cardiol. 2013;61(6):687–9.
37. Iyengar A, Sanaiha Y, Aguayo E, Seo Y-J, Dobaria V, Toppen W, et al. Comparison of frequency of late gastrointestinal bleeding with transcatheter versus surgical aortic valve replacement. Am J Cardiol. 2018;122(10):1727–31.
38. Blackshear JL, McRee CW, Safford RE, Pollak PM, Stark ME, Thomas CS, et al. von Willebrand factor abnormalities and Heyde syndrome in dysfunctional heart valve prostheses. JAMA Cardiol. 2016;1(2):198–204.
39. Blackshear JL, Wysokinska EM, Safford RE, Thomas CS, Shapiro BP, Ung S, et al. Shear stress-associated acquired von Willebrand syndrome in patients with mitral regurgitation. J Thromb Haemost. 2014;12(12):1966–74.
40. Cushing K, Kushnir V. Gastrointestinal bleeding following LVAD placement from top to bottom. Dig Dis Sci. 2016;61(6):1440–7.
41. Slaughter MS, Rogers JG, Milano CA, Russell SD, Conte JV, Feldman D, et al. Advanced heart failure treated with continuous-flow left ventricular assist device. N Engl J Med. 2009;361(23):2241–51.
42. Aggarwal A, Pant R, Kumar S, Sharma P, Gallagher C, Tatooles AJ, et al. Incidence and management of gastrointestinal bleeding with continuous flow assist devices. Ann Thorac Surg. 2012;93(5):1534–40.
43. Draper KV, Huang RJ, Gerson LB. GI bleeding in patients with continuous-flow left ventricular assist devices: a systematic review and meta-analysis. Gastrointest Endosc. 2014;80(3):435–46.e1.
44. Jabbar HR, Abbas A, Ahmed M, Klodell CT, Chang M, Dai Y, et al. The incidence, predictors and outcomes of gastrointestinal bleeding in patients with left ventricular assist device (LVAD). Dig Dis Sci. 2015;60(12):3697–706.
45. Islam S, Cevik C, Madonna R, Frandah W, Islam E, Islam S, et al. Left ventricular assist devices and gastrointestinal bleeding: a narrative review of case reports and case series. Clin Cardiol. 2013;36(4):190–200.
46. Marsano J, Desai J, Chang S, Chau M, Pochapin M, Gurvits GE. Characteristics of gastrointestinal bleeding after placement of continuous-flow left ventricular assist device: a case series. Dig Dis Sci. 2015;60(6):1859–67.
47. Kushnir VM, Sharma S, Ewald GA, Seccombe J, Novak E, Wang I-W, et al. Evaluation of GI bleeding after implantation of left ventricular assist device. Gastrointest Endosc. 2012;75(5):973–9.
48. Shrode CW, Draper KV, Huang RJ, Kennedy JLW, Godsey AC, Morrison CC, et al. Significantly higher rates of gastrointestinal bleeding and thromboembolic events with left ventricular assist devices. Clin Gastroenterol Hepatol. 2014;12(9):1461–7.

49. Geisen U, Heilmann C, Beyersdorf F, Benk C, Berchtold-Herz M, Schlensak C, et al. Non-surgical bleeding in patients with ventricular assist devices could be explained by acquired von Willebrand disease. Eur J Cardiothorac Surg. 2008;33(4):679–84.
50. Uriel N, Pak S-W, Jorde UP, Jude B, Susen S, Vincentelli A, et al. Acquired von Willebrand syndrome after continuous-flow mechanical device support contributes to a high prevalence of bleeding during long-term support and at the time of transplantation. J Am Coll Cardiol. 2010;56(15):1207–13.
51. Klovaite J, Gustafsson F, Mortensen SA, Sander K, Nielsen LB. Severely impaired von Willebrand factor-dependent platelet aggregation in patients with a continuous-flow left ventricular assist device (HeartMate II). J Am Coll Cardiol. 2009;53(23):2162–7.
52. Elmunzer BJ, Elmunzer BJ, Padhya KT, Lewis JJ, Rangnekar AS, Saini SD, et al. Endoscopic findings and clinical outcomes in ventricular assist device recipients with gastrointestinal bleeding. Dig Dis Sci. 2011;56(11):3241–6.
53. Meyer MM, Young SD, Sun B, Azzouz M, Firstenberg MS. Endoscopic evaluation and management of gastrointestinal bleeding in patients with ventricular assist devices. Gastroenterol Res Pract. 2012;2012:630483.
54. Sarosiek K, Bogar L, Conn MI, O'Hare B, Hirose H, Cavarocchi NC. An old problem with a new therapy: gastrointestinal bleeding in ventricular assist device patients and deep overtube-assisted enteroscopy. ASAIO J. 2013;59(4):384–9.
55. Truss WD, Weber F, Pamboukian SV, Tripathi A, Peter S. Early implementation of video capsule enteroscopy in patients with left ventricular assist devices and obscure gastrointestinal bleeding. ASAIO J. 2016;62(1):40–5.
56. Daas AY, Small MB, Pinkas H, Brady PG. Safety of conventional and wireless capsule endoscopy in patients supported with nonpulsatile axial flow Heart-Mate II left ventricular assist device. Gastrointest Endosc. 2008;68(2):379–82.
57. Harris LA, Hansel SL, Rajan E, Srivathsan K, Rea R, Crowell MD, et al. Capsule endoscopy in patients with implantable electromedical devices is safe. Gastroenterol Res Pract. 2013;2013:959234.
58. Wever-Pinzon O, Selzman CH, Drakos SG, Saidi A, Stoddard GJ, Gilbert EM, et al. Pulsatility and the risk of nonsurgical bleeding in patients supported with the continuous-flow left ventricular assist device HeartMate II. Circ Heart Fail. 2013;6(3):517–26.
59. Imamura T, Kinugawa K, Uriel N. Therapeutic strategy for gastrointestinal bleeding in patients with left ventricular assist device. Circ J. 2018;82(12):2931–8.
60. Rennyson SL, Shah KB, Tang DG, Kasirajan V, Pedram S, Cahoon W, et al. Octreotide for left ventricular assist device-related gastrointestinal hemorrhage: can we stop the bleeding? ASAIO J. 2013;59(4):450–1.
61. Loyaga-Rendon RY, Hashim T, Tallaj JA, Acharya D, Holman W, Kirklin J, et al. Octreotide in the management of recurrent gastrointestinal bleed in patients supported by continuous flow left ventricular assist devices. ASAIO J. 2015;61(1):107–9.
62. Ray R, Kale PP, Ha R, Banerjee D. Treatment of left ventricular assist device-associated arteriovenous malformations with thalidomide. ASAIO J. 2014;60(4):482–3.
63. Schettle SD, Pruthi RK, Pereira NL. Continuous-flow left ventricular assist devices and gastrointestinal bleeding: potential role of danazol. J Heart Lung Transplant. 2014;33(5):549–50.
64. Imamura T, Nguyen A, Rodgers D, Kim G, Raikhelkar J, Sarswat N, et al. Omega-3 therapy is associated with reduced gastrointestinal bleeding in patients with continuous-flow left ventricular assist device. Circ Heart Fail. 2018;11(10):e005082.
65. Suarez J, Patel CB, Felker GM, Becker R, Hernandez AF, Rogers JG. Mechanisms of bleeding and approach to patients with axial-flow left ventricular assist devices. Circ Heart Fail. 2011;4(6):779–84.
66. Boudoulas KD, Pederzolli A, Saini U, Gumina RJ, Mazzaferri EL, Davis M, et al. Comparison of Impella and intra-aortic balloon pump in high-risk percutaneous coronary intervention: vascular complications and incidence of bleeding. Acute Card Care. 2012;14(4):120–4.
67. Généreux P, Cohen DJ, Mack M, Rodes-Cabau J, Yadav M, Xu K, Parvataneni R, Hahn R, Kodali SK, Webb JG, Leon MB. (2014). Incidence, predictors, and prognostic impact of late bleeding complications after transcatheter aortic valve replacement. J Am Coll Cardiol. 64(24):2605–615. https://doi.org/10.1016/j.jacc.2014.08.052.

Chapter 15
Patients on NSAIDs/Anticoagulation

Asra Batool and Rosa T. Bui

Mechanism of NSAIDs

Most NSAIDs are nonselective inhibitors of cyclooxygenase-1 (COX-1) and cyclo-oxygenase-2 (COX-2) enzymes. While aspirin acetylates COX-1 and COX-2 irreversibly, NSAIDs do so reversibly. COX-1 is constitutively expressed and produces mucosal protective prostaglandins to the gastric and duodenal mucosa. In addition, COX-1 contributes to platelet aggregation through thromboxane production. COX-2 is inducible and plays a lesser role in protection of mucosal lining from acid and pepsin. On that basis, it has been thought that COX-2 selective inhibitors have a safer GI side effect profile. However, at clinically significant doses, COX-2 inhibition leads to similar adverse gastrointestinal effects. Moreover, animal studies have refuted this "COX-2 hypothesis", suggesting that both COX-1 and COX-2 inhibition are required for ulcer formation. [8, 21, 28] Therefore, it is not the selective COX-2 inhibition alone, but perhaps the absence of dual inhibition of both isoforms that explains the decreased GI side effects with COX-2 selective NSAIDs such as celecoxib.

Most NSAIDs are completely absorbed and have trivial first pass hepatic metabolism. Side effects including renal, cardiovascular and gastrointestinal vary, and are largely dependent on pharmacodynamics and pharmacokinetics [27]. It is also important to note that NSAIDs notoriously interact with commonly used medications such as methotrexate and ACE inhibitors. Figures 15.1 and 15.2 illustrate the inhibition of COX-1 and COX-2 and the downstream effects.

A. Batool (✉) · R. T. Bui
Albany Medical Center, Gastroenterology, Albany, NY, USA
e-mail: batoola@amc.edu; buir@amc.edu

© The Author(s), under exclusive license to Springer Nature
Switzerland AG 2021
M. Tadros, G. Y. Wu (eds.), *Management of Occult GI Bleeding*, Clinical
Gastroenterology, https://doi.org/10.1007/978-3-030-71468-0_15

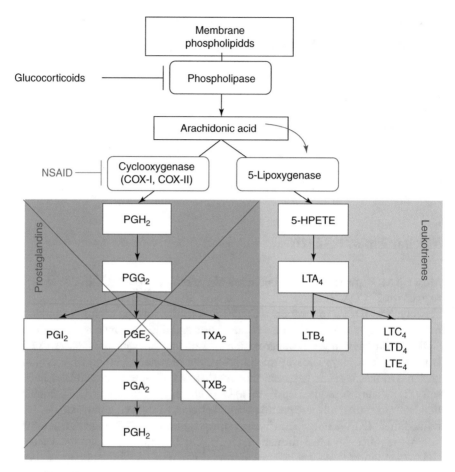

Fig. 15.1 Mechanism of NSAIDs. https://link.springer.com/article/10.1007/s40629-018-0064-0

Pathogenesis of NSAID-Induced Enteropathy and Colopathy

While some studies report 15–30% of patients on chronic NSAIDs develop peptic ulcer disease, other studies observed as high as 80% of long term users eventually develop NSAID-induced enteropathy [2, 6].

Aspirin has a pKa of 3.5 and ibuprofen 4.85. The more positive the pKa value, the weaker the acid and so therefore, aspirin and NSAIDs are not ionized in the gastric lumen but rather can travel across the mucosa. As the mucosa has a neutral pH, NSAIDs then linger in the epithelial cells and can damage the epithelial cells through this mechanism. The second and most critical means of destruction is by inhibiting COX-1 and COX-2, thereby decreasing prostaglandin synthesis. Aspirin dosages as low as 10 mg/day can inhibit gastric prostaglandins [8, 24]. In turn,

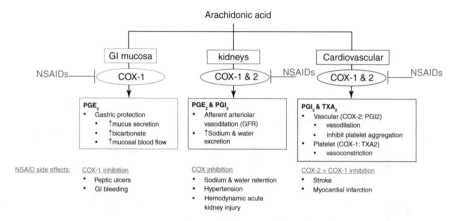

Fig. 15.2 Mechanism of NSAIDs. https://media.springernature.com/original/springer-static/image/art%3A10.1007%2Fs40266-019-00660-1/MediaObjects/40266_2019_660_Fig 1_HTML.png

human gastric mucosa can require up to 8 days to restore its COX-1 activity. Without prostaglandins, the mucosal layer loses its cytoprotective properties and is now susceptible to unimpeded gastric acid secretion, proteolytic enzymes, bile acid and toxins [6]. First, prostaglandins stimulate epithelial cell secretion of mucin and bicarbonate which together form a protective alkaline barrier. Secondly, prostaglandins also enhance mucosal blood flow and oxygen through vasodilation. In addition, prostaglandins promote epithelial cell proliferation and movement towards the luminal side [8]. Other proposed protective mechanisms include interference with nitric oxide such that some studies are now investigating NSAIDs coupled with nitric oxide and aspirin coupled with nitric oxide. In addition to interfering with a variety of gastroduodenal defensive pathways, NSAIDs also promote subsequent bleeding from peptic ulcer disease by inhibiting platelet aggregation and vasoconstriction.

With increased utilization of capsule endoscopy, small bowel enteropathy is more and more frequently identified. Pathogenesis in contrast to gastroduodenal disease, involves intestinal gram-negative "dysbiosis" and bile toxicity as seen in Fig. 15.3, particularly in those with NSAIDs plus a proton pump inhibitor (PPI) [2, 8]. In animal studies, NSAIDs with PPI causes disruption of the microbiome, with overgrowth of gram-negative bacteria in the ileum and subsequent ulceration while those with gram-positive bacteria such as *Bifidobacteria* and *Firmicutes* tend to be without ulcers [8]. Similarly, human studies such as Washio et al. study showed that COX-2 selective NSAIDs in combination with PPI had significantly higher incidence of ulcers, particularly in the jejunum as compared to COX-2 selective NSAIDs and placebo due to small bowel dysbiosis [8]. Interestingly, current prospective studies including GI-REASONS trial and CONDOR trial are also finding that occult GIB is more common in nonselective NSAIDs coupled with PPI compared to celecoxib alone [8].

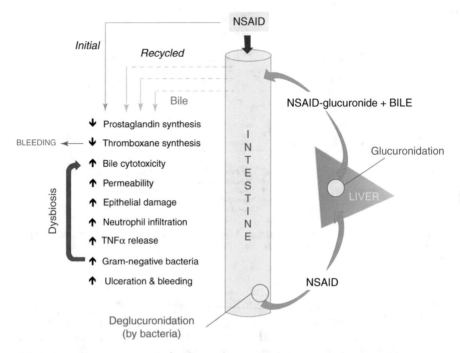

Fig. 15.3 Pathogenesis of NSAID-induced enteropathy. https://link.springer.com/article/10.1007/s10620-015-3963-7

In the lower GI tract, NSAIDs, especially enteric-coated and slow release formulations which permit more exposure of the drug in the colon, increase colonic ulcers, diverticular bleeding and exacerbations of inflammatory bowel disease [12]. In comparison to gastric and small bowel ulcers, colonic ulcers are much less common, less described and found in less than 5% of patients on chronic NSAIDs [9]. There is also a predilection for right-sided and proximal colon. With increasing use of the sustained release formulation, more drug reaches the cecum which then acts as a "reservoir" and becomes directly toxic to the right colon [11, 12, 14, 15]. Histologic exams have reported pill-coated NSAID particles in histiocytes in ulcer and granulation tissue biopsied in the right colon. Distally, proctitis can develop with rectal NSAIDs. Primary mechanisms for NSAID-induced colopathy are decreased blood flow and disruption of epithelial cells as well as decreased prostaglandin production by colonic mucosa [15]. Disruption of epithelial cells leads to exposure to and bacterial translocation and inflammatory reactions. Colopathy can occur within days of NSAID use [11].

Although much of literature focuses on oral NSAIDs, it is important to remember that NSAIDs also come in topical formulations. There have been case reports where topical NSAIDs have also led to occult GI bleeding. Hirose et al. reported a case of an occult GI bleed in an elderly woman using eight sheets of 20 mg of ketoprofen patches every day [5].

Risk Factors for NSAID-Induced Enteropathy

Dosage, duration and individual risk factors and co-morbidities dictate the risk of developing peptic ulcers. Expectedly, both increased dosage and duration augment the risk. An overall average of three months is generally noted but even continuous use during a two-week period can cause mucosal injury. Oral NSAIDs in conjunction with glucocorticoids, warfarin, antiplatelets, topical NSAIDs, and SSRIs potentiate GI bleeding. The following factors increase risk of GI toxicity: previous ulcer disease, age greater than 60, high dose NSAIDs combined with steroids, antiplatelet agents and anticoagulants, chronic NSAID use, untreated H. pylori infection, hemodialysis and SSRIs [8]. In 2009, the ACG stratified risk of NSAID-induced PUD into low, moderate and high as seen in Fig. 15.4 below.

Clinical Presentation and Complications

Melena and hematemesis from NSAID-induced ulcers are well known consequences. Close to 15% of peptic ulcers bleed with a mortality rate of roughly 10%. Patients with peptic ulcers can experience epigastric pain or remain asymptomatic, with many eventually presenting with occult GI bleeding or iron deficiency over time [3]. [51]Chromium-labelled erythrocyte studies in NSAID-induced enteropathy cases estimate occult blood loss from one cc to up to 10 cc a day [1]. When symptomatic, patients usually describe the pain as a hunger sensation with pain worse

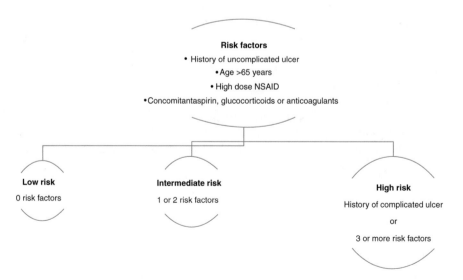

Fig. 15.4 Risk stratification of gastroduodenal toxicity in NSAID use. (Adapted from 2009 American College of Gastroenterology)

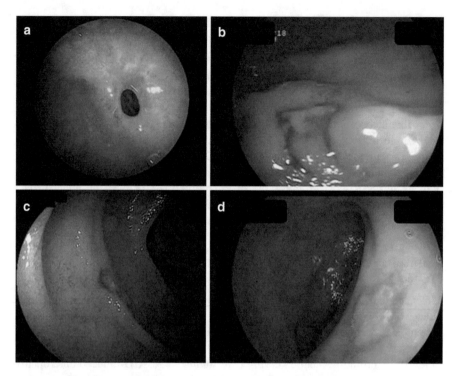

Fig. 15.5 (**a**) Small bowel diaphragm. (**b–d**) Small bowel NSAID-induced ulcers. https://link.springer.com/article/10.1007/s00535-009-0102-2

after eating in gastric ulcers and better with eating in the case of duodenal ulcers. The emergence of early satiety and vomiting suggests obstruction secondary to the ulcer itself or formation of diaphragms. Diaphragms often develop in the ileum but can occur throughout the small bowel, as seen in Fig. 15.5 [6]. Dysphagia may be due to peptic strictures. Worsening abdominal pain may be the initial clue to perforation.

In NSAID-induced colopathy, iron deficiency anemia, change in bowel habits, abdominal pain are reported signs and symptoms [12, 14, 25]. Like the upper GI tract, ulcers leading to occult or overt GI bleed and strictures leading to obstruction can also form in the colon.

Diagnosis

Surrogate markers such as fecal excretion of 111-Indium, fecal calprotectin, and ^{51}Chromium-labelled erythrocyte studies can indicate intestinal inflammation due to NSAIDs [8, 24, 28]. In current practice, endoscopy is the standard for diagnosis. NSAID-induced enteropathy can range from red spots, erosions to round, annular or linear ulcers seen during upper endoscopy [1]. While varied in appearance, these

ulcers are usually superficial and less than one centimeter in diameter. Most duodenal ulcers will form in the duodenal bulb and gastric ulcers in antrum or pyloric
channel. In the colon, ulcers can occur throughout but rarely on the ileocecal valve.

The first diagnostic step in occult GI bleeding is upper endoscopy and/or lower
endoscopy. If unrevealing, capsule endoscopy or small bowel enteroscopy should
be utilized to evaluate the small bowel [1]. Studies have shown the positive predictive value of small bowel enteroscopy exceeds that of a capsule endoscopy when
looking for small bowel ulcers, however more large-scale studies are still needed.
Regardless, capsule endoscopy studies have estimated up to 50–80% of NSAID-
induced enteropathy can occur in the small bowel. Capsule studies have seen small
bowel erosions and ulcers in as little as seven days of 100 mg of enteric-coated
aspirin. Jejunum and ileum are affected equally. Equally important to note, is that
discontinuation of aspirin and other NSAIDs can lead to negative capsule study,
especially as small erosions and superficial ulcers can heal quickly with cessation of
culprit medications [7].

In the colon, NSAID-induced ulcers typically occur in the right colon and transverse and less so in the left colon [10]. They are usually well-circumscribed, circular
or semicircular. Most ulcers heal within four weeks of drug withdrawal [10].
Persistent ulceration, healing and fibrosis lead to diaphragm-like strictures, especially in the right colon [13].

Prevention and Management

Perhaps the best and ideal strategy is to avoid NSAIDs in patients already at
increased risk for peptic ulcer disease. These patients include those with H. pylori,
Zollinger-Ellison syndrome, inflammatory bowel disease, sarcoidosis, CKD, CMV
and HSV infections. However, given the myriad chronic conditions including cardiovascular and rheumatologic diseases, avoidance may be next to infeasible and so
additional strategies can be incorporated in preventing and managing NSAID-
induced enteropathy and colopathy.

Screening for occult bleeding in those taking NSAIDs or anticoagulants through
biomarkers such as FOBT is not recommended [17]. However, testing for and eradi-
cating H. pylori is recommended in those requiring prolonged NSAID use. Proton
pump inhibitor remains the mainstay primary and secondary prevention strategy. In
those who must continue on NSAIDs or aspirin for long term, PPI should be prescribed for as long as they are on those medications. There is no overwhelmingly
convincing data that one PPI is superior than another PPI. As previously mentioned,
while protective of the gastroduodenal tract, PPI in combination with NSAIDs can
lead to small bowel ulcers through intestinal dysbiosis. This however, does not
change the current recommendations in adding a PPI to long term NSAID and aspirin users.

Despite conflicting evidence, some practitioners still gravitate towards selective
or relatively selective COX-2 inhibitors such as celecoxib, etodolac, diclofenac and
meloxicam rather than nonselective NSAIDs in high risk patients. Although not

rigorously studied, high risk patients who must take aspirin and NSAIDs together, can derive benefit from switching to selective COX-2 inhibitor plus PPI versus non-selective NSAID plus PPI. Of note however, selective COX-2 inhibitors do not provide any added benefit in decreasing lower GI bleeding related to NSAIDs [9].

In the lower GI tract, most ulcerations heal but strictures usually do not and may require balloon dilation and even surgical intervention or segmental colectomy if symptomatic [11, 15].

Alternative Therapies

While avoidance of NSAIDs and aspirin seems impossible, one alternative is utilizing topical NSAIDs in cases of pain relief, with the idea that there are less systemic effects. PPIs are preferred in prevention of peptic ulcer disease in NSAID users, but there are several other alternatives, although inferior, which can serve as adjuvant therapy. Misoprostol is a prostaglandin E analog. A study showed a relative risk reduction of 40% in bleeding and complications related to NSAIDs and aspirin when patients were taking 200 mcg four times a day for at least six months compared to placebo. A more recent 2018 randomized, double-blind, placebo-controlled trial conducted by Taha et al. looked at obscure GI bleeding in patients taking aspirin and NSAIDs and found that there was a statistically significant difference in healing of small bowel ulcers and erosions in the misoprostol group compared to the placebo group after eight weeks of therapy [4]. Unfortunately, misoprostol is not well tolerated due to substantial GI side effects including abdominal pain and diarrhea. Nonetheless, it may be worthwhile to consider misoprostol in patients with recurrent peptic ulcer disease on NSAIDs.

Sucralfate is another adjuvant therapy that can be effective in treating particularly duodenal ulcers by forming an adhesive "bandage" at the site to encourage healing. In addition, sucralfate can also impede pepsin activity in gastric secretion.

There are several other new alternatives currently being studied. Rebamipide enhances intracellular prostaglandin synthesis and has been shown to reduce NSAID-induced enteropathy in animals in the STORM trial [8]. Tranexamic acid, dipeptidyl peptidase inhibitors, geranylgeranylacetone which facilitates mucous production, irsogladine a PDE inhibitor which promotes gap junction integrity, nitric oxide releasing NSAIDs are all under investigation. Given evidence that PPI can add insult to NSAID-induced enteropathy through intestinal dysbiosis, studies such as Satoh et al. have also looked at soluble fiber and probiotics as a preventative approach [22].

Anticoagulation: Mechanism and Pathogenesis

The mechanism of warfarin, as seen in Fig. 15.6, is inhibition of vitamin K dependent clotting factors (II, VII, IX, X), protein C and protein S and thereby systemic anticoagulation. Apixiban, rivaroxaban and edoxaban are factor Xa inhibitors which prevent thrombin formation. Dabigatran inhibits thrombin, which in turn impedes fibrin production.

But in addition to its action in the coagulation cascade, DOACs also have a direct effect on intestinal mucosa as most are only partially absorbed. In particular, the tartaric acid in dabigatran is erosive to the gastroduodenal mucosa [18].

Warfarin can be reversed using Vitamin K, fresh frozen plasma or prothrombin complex concentrate. Reversal agents available for dabigatran include hemodialysis and idarucizumab, which is a humanized monoclonal antibody fragment targeted against dabigatran. For the other DOACs, andexanet alfa is a recombinant modified protein mimicking factor Xa and thus binds apixiban, rivaroxiban and edoxoban. Aripazine is a cation and still being studied in reversal of all DOACs.

Overall, DOACs are associated with decreased risk of mortality due to fatal bleeding but associated with higher risk of GI bleeding compared to warfarin [18, 19]. Compared to warfarin, dabigatran and edoxaban at higher dosages and standard dose rivaroxaban are associated with higher gastrointestinal bleeding events. Rivaroxaban is thought to be higher risk for GIB due to its higher peak serum concentrations.

Unlike NSAIDs which tend to affect the upper tract, DOACs tend to affect the lower GI tract. This is seen in the RE-LY trial looking at dabigatran, particularly given its incomplete absorption in the upper GI tract and therefore subsequent erosive effect in the lower tract [19]. In addition to its obvious effect on systemic anticoagulation, current phase 3 trials have identified additional risk factors for bleeding including age greater than 75, history of GIB, diverticulosis, angiodysplasias, renal disease, use of antiplatelets or NSAIDs and a HAS-BLED score of equal to or greater than 3 [19].

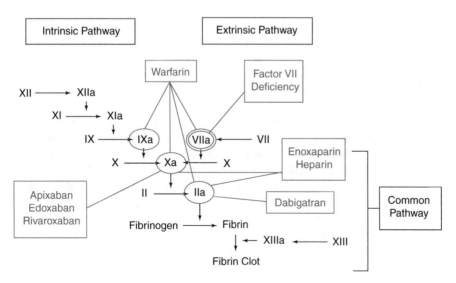

Fig. 15.6 Mechanism of warfarin and DOACs. https://link.springer.com/article/10.1007/s40800-016-0031-y

Etiology of Occult GI Bleeding in the Setting of Anticoagulation

A prospective study by Jaffin et al. suggested that those on anticoagulants with occult bleeding were not due to the anticoagulant itself but pre-existing intestinal and colonic lesions [9, 16]. Many studies such as the COMPASS trial have looked at the higher incidence of GIB with anticoagulation and relation to occult malignancies, whereby initiation of anticoagulation unveils the presence of pre-existing cancer. The study found that anticoagulation therapy significantly increased the incidence of a positive fecal occult blood test (FOBT). However, positive FOBT was not related to increasing PT/PTT [16]. This suggests occult bleeding in anticoagulated patients was due to underlying organic lesions rather than systemic anticoagulation. With that being said, the most common causes of occult bleeding are seen in Fig. 15.8.

Management of Occult GI Bleeding on Anticoagulants

While many practitioners test FOBT to gauge a patient's risk of GI bleeding prior to starting therapeutic anticoagulation, this is not recommended [17]. First off, FOBT has only been validated for colorectal cancer screening and not a means to evaluate GIB risk. Moreover, FOBT is an imperfect test, known for false positives in individuals consuming certain peroxidase-containing foods and false negatives in ascorbic acid-containing food items. Thus, it should not be used to predict bleeding risk prior to starting anticoagulation or used to dictate the discontinuation of anticoagulants.

In contrast, tools such as the HAS-BLED score, HEMORR$_2$HAGES and ATRIA can be used to predict and assess a patient's risk of GIB on anticoagulation. HAS-BLED has been favored as it more reliably predicts clinically significant GIB [20]. HAS-BLED takes into account hypertension, renal and liver dysfunction, bleeding disorder, labile INR, age greater than 65, concurrent alcohol, NSAID or aspirin use.

Certain prevention strategies can be employed however in minimizing GI bleeding from angiodysplasias, pre-existing ulcers, portal hypertensive gastropathy and colopathy and underlying malignancy. For example, adding proton pump inhibitor may mitigate the risk of GIB especially from pre-existing ulcers. Target INR for warfarin should be maintained within range and dosage of DOACs should be renally adjusted. The 2008 ACCF/ACG/AHA consensus statement recommends keeping the INR between 2.0 and 2.5 for patients (excluding high risk patients such as those with mechanical valves) on warfarin plus aspirin and clopidogrel [21]. Combination therapy with other antiplatelets and NSAIDs should be minimized and prescribed for the shortest duration indicated. As seen in Fig. 15.7 above, serum concentration of DOACs can be notoriously increased by azoles and protease inhibitors that inhibit CYP3A4 and therefore should be dose-adjusted accordingly when applicable.

Anticoagulant	Mechanism	Indication	Safety profile	Notable drug interactions	Reversal agent
Warfarin Coumadin Jantoven	Inhibits factor II, VII, IX, X, protein C and S	Nonvalvular afib, aflutter, mechanical prosthetic cardiac valves, VTE, PE		Macrolide antibiotics Amiodarone Carbamazepine Fosphenytoin Cimetidine Fenofibrate Fluconazole	Vitamin K FFP PCC
Dabigatran Pradaxa	Thrombin inhibitor	Nonvalvular afib, VTE, PE, VTE prophylaxis in hip surgery	↑ GI bleeding compared to warfarin (RE-LY trial)	Ketoconazole Tacrolimus Ritonavir Dronedarone Cyclosporine Rifampicin Carbamazepine Phenytoin Barbituates Dexamethasone	Idarucizumab Hemodialysis Nonactivated PCC Activated PCC *Aripazine
Apixaban Eliquis	Factor Xa inhibitor	HIT(off-label) Nonvalvular afib, VTE, PE, VTE prophylaxis in hip surgery		Ketoconazole Ritonavir Dronedarone Rifampicin Carbamazepine Phenytoin Barbituates	Andexanet alfa Nonactivated PCC Activated PCC *Aripazine
Rivaroxiban Xarelto	Factor Xa inhibitor	HIT(off-label) Nonvalvular afib, VTE, PE, VTE prophylaxis in hip surgery	↑ GI bleeding compared to warfarin (ROCKET AF trial)	Ketoconazole Ritonavir Dronedarone Rifampicin Carbamazepine Phenytoin Barbituates	Andexanet alfa Nonactivated PCC Activated PCC *Aripazine
Edoxaban Savaysa	Factor Xa inhibitor	Nonvalvular afib, VTE, PE	↑ GI bleeding compared to warfarin (ENGAGE AF trial)	Ketoconazole Dronedarone Cyclosporine Rifampicin Carbamazepine Phenytoin Barbituates Dexamethasone	Andexanet alfa Nonactivated PCC Activated PCC *Aripazine

Fig. 15.7 Mechanism and reversal agents of warfarin and DOACs. *Aripazine is under investigation

Upper	Both	Lower
Celiac disease	Ulcers	Polyps
Esophagitis/Gastritis	Angiodysplasia	Colitis
Cameron lesions	Malignancy	Portal hypertensive colopathy
Portal hypertensive gastropathy		

Fig. 15.8 Causes of occult GI bleeding

Resumption of Anticoagulants after GIB

In the setting of normal renal function, DOACs are generally out of systemic circulation in approximately 12–24 h. A retrospective study by Sengupta et al. showed that restarting DOACs after GI bleeding was not associated with recurrent GI bleeding [20]. Currently, there are no formal set guidelines on resumption of DOACs. Figure 15.9 below outlines the following recommendations taken from 2016 ASGE guidelines:

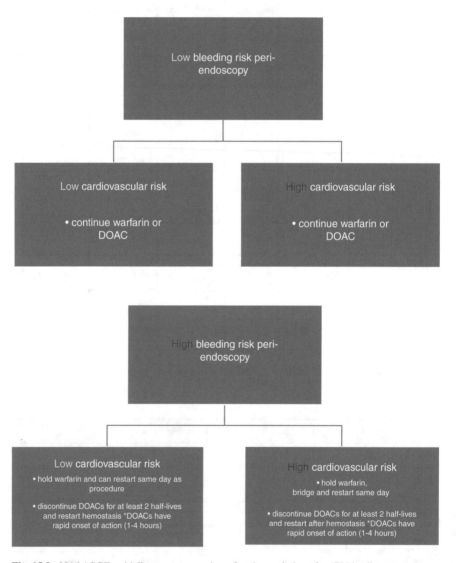

Fig. 15.9 2016 ASGE guidelines on resumption of anticoagulation after GI bleeding

References

1. Tachecí I, Bradna P, Douda T, Baštecká D, Kopáčová M, et al. 2013 DecNSAID-induced enteropathy in rheumatoid arthritis patients with chronic occult gastrointestinal bleeding: a prospective capsule endoscopy study. Image on Internet. 2013 Dec. Cited 30 July 2019]. Available from: https://www.ncbi.nlm.nih.gov/pubmed/24382953
2. Park J, et al. Rebleeding rate and risk factors in nonsteroidal anti-inflammatory drug-induced enteropathy. J Dig Dis. 2018 May;19(5):279–87. https://doi.org/10.1111/1751-2980.12600.
3. Johann HP, Ingvar B, Einar BS. The outcome and role of drugs in patients with unexplained gastrointestinal bleeding. Am J Gastroenterol [Internet]. 2015 Jun [Cited 30 July 2019];50(12):1482–9. Available from: https://www.tanfonline.com/doi/full/10.3109/0036552 1.2015.1057861. https://doi.org/10.3109/00365521.2015.1057861
4. Taha AS, et al. Misoprostol for small bowel ulcers in patients with obscure bleeding taking aspirin and nonsteroidal anti-inflammatory drugs (MASTERS): a randomised, double-blind, placebo-controlled, phase 3 trial. Lancet Gastroenterol Hepatol. 2018 Jul;3(7):469–76.
5. Hirose S, Matsuura K, Kato-Hayashi H, Suzuki A, Ohata K, Kobayashi R, et al. Gastrointestinal bleeding associated with chronic excessive use overdosing with topical ketoprofen patch in elderly patient. Scand J Gastroenterol [Internet]. 2017 Oct [Cited 30 July 2019];53(1):120–3. Available from: https://www.tanfonline.com/doi/full/10.1080/00365521.2017.1390602. https://doi.org/10.1080/00365521.2017.1390602.
6. Deabes A, Gavin M. Obscure occult GI bleeding: an iatrogenic tale?. Dig Dis Sci [Internet]. 2016 Jan [Cited 30 July 2019];61(1):42–5. Available from: https://doi.org/10.1007/s10620-015-3957-5
7. Matsumura T, Makoto A, Sazuka S, Saito M, Takahashi Y, Maruoka D, et al. Negative capsule endoscopy for obscure gastrointestinal bleeding is closely associated with the use of low-dose aspirin. Scand J Gastroenterol [Internet]. 2010 Dec [Cited 30 July 2019];46(5):621–6. Available from: https://www.tandfonline.com/doi/full/10.3109/00365521.2010.545833. https://doi.org/10.3109/00365521.2010.545833.
8. Tai F, Way D, McAlindon ME. NSAIDS and the small bowel. Curr Opin Gastroenterol. 2018;34(3):175–82.
9. Laine L. Lower gastrointestinal events in a double-blind trial of the cyclo-oxygenase-2 selective inhibitor etoricoxib and the traditional nonsteroidal anti-inflammatory drug diclofenac. Gastroenterology. 2008 Nov;135(5):1517–25.
10. Momoko A, et al. Multiple Colon ulcers with typical small intestinal lesions induced by nonsteroidal anti-inflammatory drugs. Intern Med. 2015;54(16):1995–9.
11. Mokhtare M, Valizadeh SM, Emadian O. Lower gastrointestinal bleeding due to non-steroid anti-inflammatory drug-induced Colopathy case report and literature review. Middle East J Dig Dis. 2013;5:107–11.
12. Klein M, Linnemann D, Rosenberg J. Non-steroidal anti-inflammatory drug-induced colopathy. BMJ publishing group. Case Rep. 2011 Feb;2011:2011.
13. Masannat, YA, Harron, M, Harinath, G. Nonsteroidal anti-inflammatory drugs-associated colopathy. ANZ Journal of Surgery [Internet]. 2010 Feb [Cited 30 July 2019];80(1–2):96–9. Available from: https://onlinelibrary.wiley.com/doi/abs/10.1111/j.1445-2197.2009.05180.x. https://doi.org/10.1111/j.1445-2197.2009.05180.x.
14. Byrne MF, et al. Nonsteroidal anti-inflammatory drug-induced diaphragms and ulceration in the colon. Eur J Gastroenterol Hepatol. 2002 Nov;14(11):1265–9.
15. Gopal D, Katon R. Endoscopic balloon dilation of multiple NSAID-induced colonic strictures: case report and review of literature on NSAID-related colopathy. Gastrointest Endosc. 1999 Jul;50(1):120–3.
16. Jaffin BW, et al. Significance of occult gastrointestinal bleeding during anticoagulation therapy. Am J Med. 1987 Aug;83(2):269–72.
17. Urbas R, et al. Utility of Hemoccult testing before therapeutic anticoagulation in venous thromboembolism. South Med J. 2017 May;110(5):375–80.

18. Cheung KS, Leung WK. Gastrointestinal bleeding in patients on novel oral anticoagulants: risk, prevention and management. World J Gastroenterol [Internet]. 2017 Mar [Cited 30 July 2019];23(11):1954–63. Available from: https://www.wjgnet.com/1007-9327/full/v23/i11/1954.htm. https://doi.org/10.3748/wjg.v23.i11.1954.

19. Makam RCP, Hoaglin DC, McManus DD, Wang V, Gore JM, Spencer FA, et al. Efficacy and safety of direct oral anticoagulants approved for cardiovascular indications: systemic review and meta-analysis. PLoS One [Internet]. 2018 May [Cited 30 July 2019];13(5):e0197583. Available from: https://journals.plos.org/plosone/article?id=10.1371/journal.pone.0197583. https://doi.org/10.1371/journal.pone.0197583.

20. Acosta R, Abraham N, Chandrasekhara V, Chathadi K, Early D, Eloubeidi M, et al. The management of antithrombotic agents for patients undergoing GI endoscopy. Gastrointest Endosc [Internet]. 2016 Jan [Cited 30 July 2019];83(1): 3–16. Available from https://www.giejournal.org/article/S0016-5107(15)02950-8/fulltext. https://doi.org/10.1016/j.gie.2015.09.035.

21. Bhatt DL, Scheiman J, Abraham NS, Antman EM, Chang FK, Furberg CD, Johnson DA, Mahaffey KW and Quigley EM. ACCF/ACG/AHA 2008 Expert consensus document on reducing the gastrointestinal risks of antiplatelet therapy and NSAID use. Circulation. [Internet]. 2008 Oct [Cited 30 July 2019];118(18):1894–1909. Available from https://www.ahajournals.org/doi/pdf/10.1161/CIRCULATIONAHA.108.191087.

22. Wallace, J. Prevention of NSAID-enteropathy: a soluble problem? digestive diseases and sciences. [Internet]. 2016a Jan [Cited 30 July 2019];61(1):1–3. Available from: https://link.springer.com/article/10.1007%2Fs10620-015-3963-7.   https://doi.org/10.1007/s10620-015-3963-7.

23. Taha As, McCloskey C, Craigen T, Simpson A, Angerson WJ. Occult vs. overt upper gastrointestinal bleeding – inverse relationship and the use of mucosal damaging and protective drugs. Aliment Pharmacol Ther. [Internet]. 2015 May [Cited 30 July 2019];42(3):1–8. Available from: https://onlinelibrary.wiley.com/doi/full/10.1111/apt.13265.   https://doi.org/10.1111/apt.13265.

24. McCarthy DM. Occult GI bleeding in NSAID users – the base of the iceberg! Clin Gastroenterol Hepatol. [Internet]. 2005 Nov [Cited 30 July 2019];3(11):1071–4. Available from: https://www.cghjournal.org/article/S1542-3565(05)00851-7/fulltext.   https://doi.org/10.1016/S1542-3565(05)00851-7.

25. Schwake L, Schlenker T, Schwake S, Hofmann WJ, Stremmel W. Ulcers of the colon in association with nonsteroidal anti-inflammatory drugs (NSAID) – a rare cause of gastrointestinal bleeding? Report of 3 cases. Zeitschrift für Gastroenterologie [Internet]. 2000 Dec [Cited 30 July 2019];38(12):957–61. Available from https://www.ncbi.nlm.nih.gov/pubmed/11194886. https://doi.org/10.1055/s-2000-10024.

26. Wöhrl S. NSAID hypersensitivity – recommendations for diagnostic work up and patient management. Allergo J Int. 2018;27:114–21. https://doi.org/10.1007/s40629-018-0064-0.

27. Cooper C, Chapurlat R, Al-Daghri N, et al. Safety of Oral non-selective non-steroidal anti-inflammatory drugs in osteoarthritis: what does the literature say? Drugs Aging. 2019;36:15–24. https://doi.org/10.1007/s40266-019-00660-1.

28. Higuchi K, Umegaki E, Watanabe T, et al. Present status and strategy of NSAIDs-induced small bowel injury. J Gastroenterol. 2009;44:879–88. https://doi.org/10.1007/s00535-009-0102-2.

29. Paulus E, Komperda K, Park G, et al. Anticoagulation therapy considerations in factor VII deficiency. Drug Saf – Case Rep. 2016;3:8. https://doi.org/10.1007/s40800-016-0031-y.

Chapter 16
Patients with Genetic Diseases

Krishnakumar Hongalgi, Katherine Donovan, David Miller, and Nikki Allmendinger

Introduction

There are multiple genetic conditions that predispose an individual to occult gastrointestinal bleeding. These genetic mutations lead to disorders of hemostasis, and the vascular, inflammatory, or immune systems and therefore predispose one to occult gastrointestinal bleeding. Most of these conditions present with outward signs that will make it apparent that there is an increased risk of occult bleeding and raise suspicion to the point that there is a low threshold for endoscopic evaluation. Family history is critical in evaluating a patient with occult gastrointestinal bleeding as this information can allow for a more focused approach to the evaluation.

Vascular Causes

Hereditary Hemorrhagic Telangiectasia Syndrome (HHT) HHT or Osler Weber Rendu syndrome is an autosomal dominant disorder with varying expression and penetrance. The prevalence is about 1 in 5000 to 1 in 8000. There are three genes (Tables 16.1 and 16.2) most commonly affected; although over 600 mutations have been identified to be related to HHT. The occult bleeding can originate from epistaxis or gastrocutaneous telangiectasias and can lead to iron deficiency anemia. Gastrointestinal bleeding can be seen in about one third of patients with HHT in the form of occult bleeding or bright red blood per rectum and is one of four criteria to diagnose HHT. Most occult blood loss in HHT will due to unrecognized nasal

K. Hongalgi · K. Donovan · D. Miller · N. Allmendinger (✉)
Albany Medical Center, Albany, NY, USA
e-mail: hongalk@amc.edu; donovak2@amc.edu; allmenn@amc.edu

© The Author(s), under exclusive license to Springer Nature   265
Switzerland AG 2021
M. Tadros, G. Y. Wu (eds.), *Management of Occult GI Bleeding*, Clinical
Gastroenterology, https://doi.org/10.1007/978-3-030-71468-0_16

Table 16.1 Summary of genetic diseases: cause and site of bleeding

	Cause of Bleeding	Location of Lesions
HHT	Vascular abnormalities	Stomach and duodenum
BRBNS	Vascular abnormalities	Anywhere in GI tract
FAP	Abnormal mucosa	Colon
JPS	Abnormal mucosa	Colon, stomach, duodenum
Inflammatory bowel disease	Abnormal mucosa	Anywhere in GI tract
Celiac	Abnormal mucosa	Small bowel

Table 16.2 Summary of genetic diseases: their mutations

	Disease	Chromosome	Gene
Vascular	HHT	9q34.11, 2q24.1, 18q21.1	ENG, ACVLR1, SMAD4
	BRBNS	9p21.2	TEK
	KPS	3q26.32	PIK3CA
Polyposis	FAP	5q21-q22	APC
	JPS	18q21.1	SMAD4
		10q22023	BMPRIA
IBD		16q12.1, 5q33.1, 2q37.1, 1p31.3, 18p11.21	NOD2, IR GM, ATG 16 L1, IL23R, PTPN2
Celiac		6 p21–32	HLA DQA1
Immune	WAS	X chromosome	WAS
	SCID	X chromosome	IL2RG
		11 p12	RAG1, RAG2
	XLA	X chromosome	BTK
	Neurofibromatosis	17 q11.2	NF-1

bleeding. The bleeding occurs due the fragile nature of the telengiectatic vessels. Gastrointestinal loss is more common over the age of 40 years.

The initial presentation of occult blood loss is usually in childhood and usually associated with a known family history of HHT. The presence of epistaxis with characteristic telangiectasias on the lips, oral mucosa and/or fingertips should lower one's threshold for investigating the entire gastrointestinal tract for further vascular anomalies that could be treated in various manners. Telangiectasias are more commonly seen in the stomach and duodenum and less so in the colon in patients with HHT. (Fig. 16.1).

When there is persistent anemia in the setting of HHT, further investigation into a gastrointestinal source should be pursued. This may include but is not limited to upper endoscopy, colonoscopy and wireless capsule endoscopy. Therapeutic interventions available include surgical resection, sclerosing and clipping. Vascular interventional techniques also play a role in managing the occult bleeding in HHT.

Blue Rubber Bleb Nevus Syndrome (BRBNS) BRBNS is a rare condition. It has been associated with somatic mutations of the TEK gene which produces the TIE2 protein (Tables 16.1 and 16.2). Patients with BRBNS are born with a "dominant"

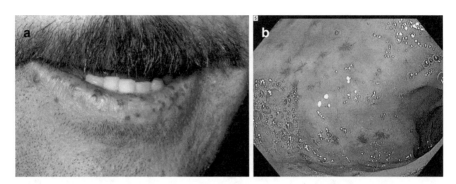

Fig. 16.1 (a) https://commons.wikimedia.org/wiki/File:Case_115.jpg. LIP telangiectasias in HHT; (b) Patient with hereditary hemorrhagic telangiectasia scientific figure on ResearchGate. Available from: https://www.researchgate.net/figure/Multiple-spider-like-mucosal-telangiectases-of-the-gastric-antrum-and-proximal-duodenum_fig 2_317678694 [accessed 25 Apr, 2020]. Multiple spider-like – mucosal telangiectasias in the duodenal bulb

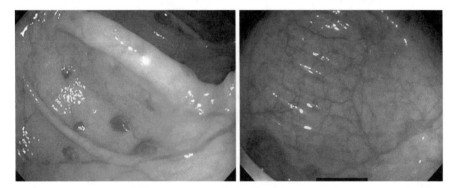

Fig. 16.2 https://www.eventscribe.com/2017/wcogacg2017/ajaxcalls/PosterInfo.asp?efp=S1lVT UxLQVozODMy&PosterID=115945&rnd=8.069134E-02. Isolated colonic lesions in a patient with Blue rubber bled nevus syndrome

lesion and the number of lesions increases with age. The lesions are cutaneous and internal venous malformations. Cutaneous lesions present as small round rubbery lesions on the palms and soles. Gastrointestinal lesions are sessile lesions described as hemangiomas and are seen in about 75% of patients with BRBNS. All parts of the gastrointestinal tract have been documented to be involved although most commonly lesions are identified in the small intestine.

Investigation for sources of gastrointestinal bleeding should include upper endoscopy, colonoscopy, wireless capsule endoscopy and magnetic resonance imaging. Small bowel enterography/enteroscopy can also be considered as a modality for both investigation and possible treatment.

Gastrointestinal lesions in BRBNS lead to chronic bleeding and therefore iron deficiency anemia. In more severe cases the lesions can cause intussusception and intestinal ischemia. (Fig. 16.2)

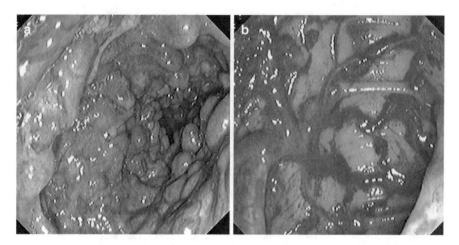

Fig. 16.3 https://www.thieme-connect.com/products/ejournals/pdf/10.1055/s-0042-119038.pdf.
Endoscopic finding of ectasias and congestion of the submucosal and mucosal venous vessels and
hemangiomas affecting the rectum and the left colon

Treatment of BRBNS tends to be conservative and includes lifelong iron supplementation and blood transfusions. Surgical resection is reserved for the most severe
and involved cases due to the risk of recurrence. Interventional vascular treatments
can also be considered. Sirolimus has been successfully used to cause regression of
lesions and therefore decreased bleeding.

Klippel-Trenaunay Syndrome (KTS) KTS is characterized by the triad of capillary malformation, venous malformation, and limb overgrowth with or without lym-
phatic malformation (Fig. 16.3). Most patients with KTS have postzygotic somatic
mutations in the phosphatidylinositol-4, 5-bisphospate 3-kinase, catalytic subunit
alpha (*PIK3CA*) gene on Chromosome 3q26.32 (Tables 16.1 and 16.2). The risk of
coagulopathy generally correlates with the extent of venous disease. Gastrointestinal
venous malformations and varicosities may result in occult or life-threatening gastrointestinal bleeding most commonly originating from the rectum. The lack of significant venous disease of the extremity or skin does not preclude the presence of
pelvic anomalies nor of a coagulopathy. Supportive care, interventional radiologic
procedures and surgical intervention should all be considered in the management of
all the various lesions seen in KPS.

Polyposis Syndromes

Juvenile Polyposis Syndrome (JPS) JPS presents in the first decade of life and is
characterized by painless rectal bleeding. Iron deficiency anemia from occult blood
loss may also be the presenting symptom. Patients can develop 5 to hundreds of

polyps throughout their lifetime. Lesions are most commonly found in the colon, but polyps may also be found in the stomach and small intestine. The lesions are hamartomas and are due to the abnormal collection of tissue elements normally found in the GI tract. These lesions are generally nonmalignant but adenomatous changes can be seen in about 50% of juvenile polyps in the setting of JPS. The lifetime risk of malignancy in an individual with JPS is between 38% and 68%.

The genetic mutations seen in people with JPS are in the SMAD4 (18Q21.1) and BMPRIA (10Q23.2) genes. One of these genes will have a mutation in up to 60% of patients with JPS (Tables 16.1 and 16.2). The relationship between the clinical picture and the genotype is inconsistent. The age of presentation and the number of polyps is variable even with in the same family. The risk of gastric polyps and gastric cancers seems to be higher in those patients with the SMAD4 mutation. JPS patients may also have features associated with HHT and therefore systematic HHT screening is recommended by NASPGHAN for all those with JPS and a SMAD4 mutation. This includes investigation of cerebral and pulmonary AVMs.

If a patient with JPS has an isolated BMPRIA mutation, then no further investigation beyond endoscopy is recommended. Children with this mutation and a severe phenotype with or without extraintestinal manifestation should be screened for PTEN mutations.

If there is a known mutation in a family with JPS, genetic counseling and genetic testing should be pursued between 12 and 15 years of age in an asymptomatic child. If the mutation is not known then screening endoscopy (including EGD and colonoscopy) should be done at the same age. If a child has symptoms and is found to have more than 5 juvenile polyps on colonoscopy then genetic counseling and testing should be pursued. Screening colonoscopies should then be done everyone to five years. Further upper tract surveillance should be pursued in those with unexplained anemia or upper tract symptoms but is not needed in the pediatric population.

Familial Adenomatous Polyposis (FAP) FAP is characterized by the presence of a large number of adenomatous colonic polyps, frequently more than 100 polyps are seen. It occurs in about 3 in 100,000 individuals but only accounts for about 1% of colorectal cancers in the United Stated. In the classic form of the disease there is a 100% chance of developing colorectal cancer. An attenuated version of FAP also exists and his characterized by more than 10 but less than 100 adenomatous polyps and these patients have an 80% chance of developing cancer. The average being 56 years old at diagnosis of cancer. (Fig. 16.4).

Most patients present when they have signs and symptoms of colorectal cancer including gastrointestinal bleeding, abdominal pain and diarrhea. Most patients with FAP are diagnosed between 20 and 40 years old. The mean age of onset of polyps is 16 years old. The more diffuse the polyps, the younger the age of presentation. Cancer is diagnosed, on average, at 39 years old.

FAP is inherited in an autosomal dominant pattern. The mutation is in the adenomatous polyposis coli (APC) gene located on chromosome 5 q21-q22 (Tables 16.1

Fig. 16.4 By Samir at the English language Wikipedia, CC BY-SA 3.0. Endoscopic image of a colon with thousands of polyps

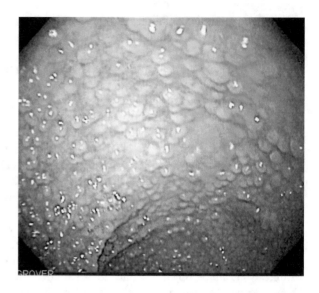

and 16.1). There are more than 1000 mutations in the APC gene identified that can lead to FAP. There is nearly complete penetrance of colonic polyposis but not of the extracolonic manifestations. Twenty-five percent of cases of FAP are due to de novo mutations in the APC gene, therefore these individuals will not have any family history of FAP. Somatic *APC* mutations are found in as many as 80% of sporadic colorectal adenomas and cancers and are not related to the FAP phenotype.

The diagnosis of FAP should be suspected in any individual with 10 or more cumulative adenomatous polyps. FAP should also be suspected in anyone with any number of adenomatous polyps and extraintestinal manifestations. The constellation of inherited colonic adenomatosis polyps together with extracolonic lesions has become known as Gardner syndrome (GS). The benign extracolonic growths include osteomas, epidermal cysts, fibromas, adrenal adenomas and desmoid tumors. Other malignant extraintestinal manifestations include polyps outside the colon (30–100%), thyroid cancer (up to 12%), hepatoblastoma (1–2%), pancreatic cancer (2%). Brain tumors, most commonly medulloblastoma, may also be associated with FAP (1–2%). FAP and CNS involvement is referred to as Turcot's syndrome. The presence of the APC gene mutation should trigger investigation for these extracolonic lesions by history and physical exam.

For FAP, colon cancer screening should begin with colonoscopies starting between 10 and 12 years old in those individuals at risk for FAP. Those at risk include patients with a first degree relative with known FAP or those with more than 10 adenomatous polyps or an individual with any number of polyps with extraintestinal manifestations. Colonoscopies should be done annually while waiting for colectomy. All individuals with typical FAP will need a colectomy in their lifetime.

Inflammatory

Inflammatory Bowel Disease (IBD) IBD encompasses Crohn's disease and ulcerative colitis. Both diseases are caused by unchecked inflammation that effects the gastrointestinal tract as well other parts of the body including joints. IBD is characterized by relapsing and remitting chronic inflammation of the GI tract. The inflammation that occurs in the GI tract leads to chronic anemia due to both blood loss and malabsorption. Blood loss can be obvious or occult. Microcytic anemia with occult positive stool should trigger a concern for IBD. Twin studies have shown the best evidence that there is a genetic role in the development of IBD. There is 50% concordance in monozygotic twins and only less than 10% concordance in dizygotic twins. Like many other diseases, IBD occurs in an individual with genetic predisposition and an environmental trigger. The environmental trigger is usually not obvious.

The understanding of the genetic basis of IBD is just emerging and will continue to grow rapidly. There have been, at least, 163 susceptibility loci identified thus far that confirm increased risk of IBD. NOD2 was the first gene identified to have susceptibility variants that predisposed one to Crohn's disease (Tables 16.1 and 16.2). Given what is known thus far, IBD seems to be a group of polygenic disorders in which there are hundreds of susceptibility loci that confer risk for development of IBD. Continued advances in whole genome sequencing and whole exome sequencing are sure to lead to a better understanding of the genetic contribution to IBD. In the future, genetic information is sure to play a larger clinical role in the diagnosis and treatment of IBD. For now endoscopy is the gold standard for diagnosing inflammatory bowel disease as this allows biopsies and histologic evaluation.

Celiac Disease Although this disease does not generally present with occult bleeding, it can cause malabsorption and therefore iron deficiency anemia. In looking for the cause of anemia, one should always consider celiac disease even when fecal occult blood is negative. Celiac disease is an immune mediated inflammatory process in the small intestine in response to exposure to dietary gluten in genetically susceptible individuals. The genetic susceptibility lies in the human leukocyte antigen (HLA) DR3-DQ2 and/or DR4-DQ8 gene locus on chromosome 6. More than 99% of individuals with celiac disease have HLA DR3-DQ2 and/or DR4-DQ8, compared with approximately 40% of the general population. Homozygotes for DR3-DQ2 are at the highest risk for celiac disease. The presence of either the HLA-DQ2 or DQ8 genotype is required to have celiac disease (Tables 16.1 and 16.2). In addition, other gene mutations at non-HLA loci are also required and the risk of disease varies depending on these other mutations. The presence of gluten in the diet is also required to confirm disease.

The inflammatory response leads to villous atrophy and crypt hyperplasia in the proximal small intestines (Fig. 16.5). The malabsorption that occurs can lead to

Fig. 16.5 Celiac_disease.
https://librepathology.org/
wiki/File:Celiac_
disease_-_high_mag.jpg

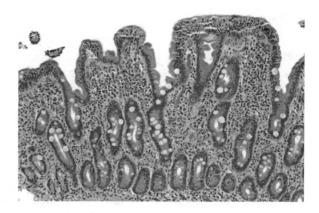

diarrhea, weight loss, and iron/vitamin deficiency. This is all easily reversed with removal of gluten from the diet. The mucosa heals itself with removal of the protein, resumes normal function and the occult blood loss resolves.

Immune Deficencies

Severe Combined Immunodeficiency (SCID) SCID are a heterogeneous group of diseases due to defective development and function of both T and B cells. Both cellular and humoral immunity is compromised. Failure to diagnose and treat early leads to severe infections. GI bleeding is usually secondary to opportunistic infections.

SCID is uncommon; 11 newborn screening programs in the United States identified SCID in 1 in 58,000 infants. Based on molecular defects SCID is broadly classified into typical SCID, leaky SCID, and Omenn syndrome. Patients who are not diagnosed in neonatal period usually present with recurrent severe infections, chronic diarrhea, and failure to thrive. Typical SCID have severe lymphopenia with reduced autologous T cell count of <300/microL. Chest xray may show absent thymic shadow. Genetic defects are either x linked or autosomal recessive involving chromosome 11.

Given the immune defects common gastrointestinal infections can lead to GI bleeding more readily. Campylobacter jejuni is a common bacteria that is more likely to lead to gross or occult bleeding in an individual with SCID. Many common viral infections affecting the GI tract may be more likely to lead to GI bleeding than in an immuncompetent host.

Wiskott-Aldrich Syndrome (WAS) WAS is characterized by susceptibility to infections due to both adaptive and innate immune deficiency, microthrombocytopenia, and eczema (Fig. 16.6). However, there is a wide spectrum of disease severity due to *WAS* gene mutations. The most severe phenotype (classic form) of WAS is

Fig. 16.6 https:// emedicine.medscape.com/ article/137015-overview. Eczematous lesions in Wiskott-Aldrich syndrome. The lesion is essentially indistinguishable from that of atopic dermatitis except for the presence of purpura and petechiae

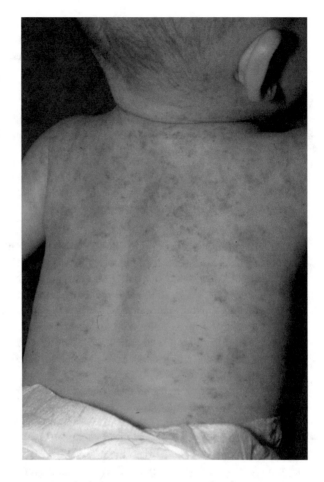

associated with bacterial and viral infections, severe eczema autoimmunity, and/or malignancy. A milder variation is characterized by thrombocytopenia and less severe or sometimes absent infections and eczema, called X-linked thrombocytopenia (XLT), to X-linked neutropenia (XLN) (Tables 16.1 and 16.2).

X-Linked Agammaglobulinemia XLA or Bruton-type agammaglobulinemia is mainly a humoral immunodeficiency seen in male infant's ages 3–18 months characterized by recurrent bacterial respiratory tract infections and increased susceptibility to enteroviral infection. Patient is usually a male with positive family history, typical clinical features such as absence of the tonsils and adenoids. Their serology with show agammaglobulinemia/hypogammaglobinemia and very low to absent CD19+ B cells.

XLA is caused by mutations in the BTK gene (Tables 16.1 and 16.2) which has a major role in promoting pre-B cell expansion. Salmonella and Campylobacter species can cause gastroenteritis. Less commonly chronic rotavirus gastroenteritis and Giardia lamblia gastrointestinal infections can occur. Enteroviral infections can present as dermatomyositis, meningoencephalitis and/or chronic hepatitis.

One third of patients had gastrointestinal manifestations and 11% were diagnosed with IBD or enteritis in a retrospective review study. Monitoring for autoimmune or gastrointestinal disease is recommended. Colorectal cancer has been reported in 3 of 52 patients with XLA. (6%).

The diagnosis may be confirmed with a molecular study identifying a defect in the BTK gene or BTK protein expression. Treatment involves replacement immune globulin therapy and appropriate antibiotic use.

Chronic Granulomatous Disease (CGD)

Chronic granulomatous disease (CGD) is a genetically heterogeneous disorder of phagocyte oxidative metabolism characterized by recurrent, life-threatening bacterial and fungal infections with granuloma formation (Tables 16.1 and 16.2).

GI involvement is a common and recurring problem in CGD with predilection for those with X-linked inheritance. GI involvement should be sought in children usually younger than five years with abdominal pain, growth delay, or hypoalbuminemia. In a case series of 140 patients, 65% of the patients had either granulomatous or ulcerative colonic lesions. IBD is noted to be common in CGD up to one third effected and increases with age.

Noncirrhotic portal hypertension owing to microvasculature damage from repeated liver and systemic injury was noted in a cohort of 194 patients was associated with poor prognosis. In portal hypertension it is important variceal bleeding as a cause of occult bleeding.

In the immune deficiency disorders discussed, the occult blood loss is due to inflammation caused by infections. These infections are due to do the genetic disorders that cause immune deficiency and therefore susceptibility to infections. Treatment of occult bleeding in the setting of immune dysfunction lies in establishing maximum immune function, supportive care such as intravenous fluids and antibiotics when clinically indicated. In patients with CGD and inflammatory bowel disease, anti-tumor necrosis factor medications are not recommended given the increased risk of infections.

Neurofirmatosis

Neurofibromatosis type (NF-1), also known as von Recklinghausen disease, is the most common type of neurofibromatosis. The hallmarks of NF1 are the multiple café-au-lait macules and neurofibromas. Frequently (up to 80%) cognitive

Fig. 16.7 GIST: https://
www.wjgnet.
com/1007-9327/full/v23/
i27/WJG-23-4856-g001.
htm. Endoscopic a view of
a gastric gastrointestinal
stromal tumors

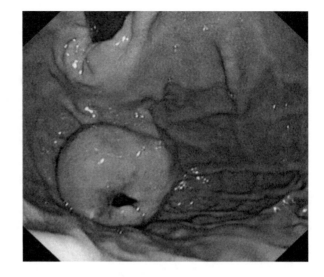

disabilities are also associated with NF-1. Optic pathway gliomas are the most common central nervous system tumor seen in NF-1. NF-1 is due to a mutation in the NF-1 gene on chromosome 17q 11.2 (Tables 16.1 and 16.2).

NF-1 can be associated with gastrointestinal stromal tumors (GIST) that can be located anywhere in the GI tract but are most commonly found in the stomach and small bowel (Fig. 16.7). Most GIST are seen in adults over 40 years old but in the setting of NF-1, these tumors are commonly seen in childhood. Occult gastrointestinal bleeding may be the presenting sign in 28–50% of cases. These lesions can be identified on endoscopy, CT scan and MRI. Endoscopic ultrasound may also be helpful in defining lesions suspicious for GIST. Surgical resection is the treatment of choice with multiple prognostic factors considered to determine further evaluation and management beyond removal of the tumor.

Hermansky-Pudlak Syndrome

Hermansky-Pudlak Syndrome (HPS) is a rare autosomal recessive disorder with a wordwide prevalence of 1 in 500,000 to 1 in 1,000,000 with a prevalence of nearly 1 in 1800 in Puerto Rico (Tables 16.1 and 16.2). It typically presents with oculocutaneous albinism, bleeding diathesis, and different subtypes can lead to pulmonary fibrosis, granulomatous colitis, and kidney failure. At present, 10 subtypes of HPS have been recognized. HPS 1, 2, and 4 present with the most severe symptoms. HPS 3, 5, and 6, present with the most mild symptoms. Severity of HPS 7, 8, and 9 are largely unknown.

The pathogenesis of HPS involves dysregulation of genes involved in production of protein complexes associated with trafficking of lysosomes and lysosome-related organelles. In subtypes of HPS associated with bleeding diathesis, platelet dense bodies, otherwise known as delta granules, are absent or decreased in number, leading to defective secondary platelet aggregation. This manifests as typical symptoms of defects in primary hemostasis, which would present as mucocutaneous bleeding, prolonged bleeding after dental procedures, petechiae, easy bruising, and epistaxis.

Manifestations of the bleeding-diathesis of HPS with respect to gastrointestinal bleeding present as both non-discriminant upper and lower GI tract bleeding due to secondary platelet dysfunction in addition to bleeding from granulomatous colitis.

As the bleeding pathogenesis of HPS is due to a qualitative platelet disorder, platelets levels are expected to be normal or slightly decreased. Treatment of bleeding is largely supportive and should include platelet transfusion and desmopressin, and TNF-a inhibitors have shown to be successful for treatment of bleeding from granulomatous colitis.

Ehlers-Danlos Syndrome Type IV

Ehlers-Danlos Syndrome is an inherited connective tissue disorder characterized by hypermobility and hyperelasticity of the skin. There are thirteen recognized subtypes ranging in severity. One of the most severe subtypes, Ehlers-Danlos Syndrome Type IV (vEDS) is an autosomal dominant condition that refers to the vascular form of the disease. A defect in COL3A1 dictating production of collagen type III, critical for blood vessel and organ integrity, is implicated (Tables 16.1 and 16.2). Classical presentations of vEDS include easy bruising, skin lucency, visible vasculature, and acrogeria. The major cause of death in vEDS patients is arterial dissection and organ failure.

Several gastrointestinal complications have been described in association with vEDS including spontaneous gastrointestinal hemorrhage and hemoperitoneum, paraesophageal hernias, and arterial lesions. Most arterial lesions manifest as aneurysms, dissections, and ruptures of the celiac trunk, splenic, and hepatic arteries. The most common reported complications are bowel perforation, spleen rupture, hernias, rectal prolapse, and altered gut motility.

Vascular Ehlers-Danlos associated intestinal perforation has been widely documented and investigated. Both spontaneous and non-spontaneous perforations secondary to constipation have been reported, spontaneous events being the most common. Perforations can be repaired with resection and diversion, but re-perforation of the bowel frequently occurs. Treatment with total abdominal colectomy (TAC) has been more successful in avoiding subsequent perforating events. It is recommended that vEDS patients be counseled and treated for constipation, a common symptom of EDS, in an attempt to avoid bowel perforation.

References

HHT

1. Guttmacher AE, Marchuk DA, White RI Jr. Hereditary hemorrhagic telangiectasia. N Engl J Med. 1995;333:918.
2. Govani FS, Shovlin CL. Hereditary haemorrhagic telangiectasia: a clinical and scientific review. Eur J Hum Genet. 2009;17:860.
3. Abdalla SA, Letarte M. Hereditary haemorrhagic telangiectasia: current views on genetics and mechanisms of disease. J Med Genet. 2006;43:97.

BRBNS

4. Soblet J, Kangas J, Nätynki M, et al. Blue rubber bleb nevus (BRBN) syndrome is caused by somatic TEK (TIE2) mutations. J Invest Dermatol. 2017;137:207.

KTS

5. Wassef M, Blei F, Adams D, et al. Vascular anomalies classification: recommendations from the International Society for the Study of vascular anomalies. Pediatrics. 2015;136:e203.

WAS

6. Imai K, Morio T, Zhu Y, et al. Clinical course of patients with WASP gene mutations. Blood 2004; 103:456; Ochs HD, Thrasher AJ. The Wiskott-Aldrich syndrome. J Allergy Clin Immunol. 2006;117:725.

Polyposis Syndromes

7. Cohen S, Hyer W, Mas E, et al. Management of Juvenile Polyposis Syndrome in children and adolescents: a position paper from ESPGHAN polyposis working group. JPGN. 2019;68:453.

IBD

8. Abraham C, Cho JH. Inflammatory bowel disease. N Engl J Med 2009; 361:2066; Kaser A, Zeissig S, Blumberg RS. Inflammatory bowel disease. Annu Rev Immunol. 2010;28:573.

9. Ye BD, McGovern DP. Genetic variation in IBD: progress, clues to pathogenesis and possible clinical utility. Expert Rev Clin Immunol. 2016;12:1091.
10. Loddo I, Romano. Inflammatory bowel disease: genetics, epigenetics, and pathogenesis. Frontimmunol. 2015;6:551.

Celiac

11. Fasano A, Berti I, Gerarduzzi T, et al. Prevalence of celiac disease in at-risk and not-at-risk groups in the United States: a large multicenter study. Arch Intern Med. 2003;163:286.
12. Kagnoff MF. Celiac disease. A gastrointestinal disease with environmental, genetic, and immunologic components. Gastroenterol Clin N Am. 1992;21:405.
13. Schuppan D. Current concepts of celiac disease pathogenesis. Gastroenterology. 2000;119:234.

Immunodeficiency

14. Aguilar C, Malphettes M, Donadieu J, Chandesris O, Coignard-Biehler H, Catherinot E, Pellier I, Stephan JL, Le Moing V, Barlogis V, et al. Prevention of infections during primary immunodeficiency. Clin Infect Dis. 2014;59(10):1462–70. Epub 2014 Aug 14
15. Imai K, Morio T, Zhu Y, et al. Clinical course of patients with WASP gene mutations. Blood. 2004;103:456.
16. Ochs HD, Thrasher AJ. The Wiskott-Aldrich syndrome. J Allergy Clin Immunol. 2006;117:725.

CGD

17. Marciano BE, Rosenzweig SD, Kleiner DE, et al. Gastrointestinal involvement in chronic granulomatous disease. Pediatrics. 2004;114:462.
18. Winkelstein JA, Marino MC, Johnston RB Jr, et al. Chronic granulomatous disease. Report on a national registry of 368 patients. Medicine (Baltimore). 2000;79:155.
19. Jones LB, McGrogan P, Flood TJ, et al. Special article: chronic granulomatous disease in the United Kingdom and Ireland: a comprehensive national patient-based registry. Clin Exp Immunol. 2008;152:211.
20. Towbin AJ, Chaves I. Chronic granulomatous disease. Pediatr Radiol. 2010;40:657.

Agammagluninemia

21. Hermaszewski RA, Webster AD. Primary hypogammaglobulinaemia: a survey of clinical manifestations and complications. Q J Med. 1993;86:31.
22. Halliday E, Winkelstein J, Webster AD. Enteroviral infections in primary immunodeficiency (PID): a survey of morbidity and mortality. J Infect. 2003;46:1.

SCID

23. Kwan A, Abraham RS, Currier R, et al. Newborn screening for severe combined immunodeficiency in 11 screening programs in the United States. JAMA. 2014;312:729.
24. Bousfiha A, Jeddane L, Picard C, et al. The 2017 IUIS phenotypic classification for primary Immunodeficiencies. J Clin Immunol. 2018;38:129.
25. Picard C, Bobby Gaspar H, Al-Herz W, et al. International Union of Immunological Societies: 2017 primary immunodeficiency diseases committee report on inborn errors of immunity. J Clin Immunol. 2018;38:96.

NF

26. North K. Neurofibromatosis type 1. Am J Med Genet. 2000;97:119.
27. Lorenzo J, Barton B, Arnold SS, North KN. Developmental trajectories of young children with neurofibromatosis type 1: a longitudinal study from 21 to 40 months of age. J Pediatr. 2015;166:1006.
28. Miettinen M, Sobin LH, Lasota J. Gastrointestinal stromal tumors of the stomach: a clinicopathologic, immunohistochemical, and molecular genetic study of 1765 cases with long-term follow-up. Am J Surg Pathol. 2005;29:52.
29. Miettinen M, Makhlouf H, Sobin LH, Lasota J. Gastrointestinal stromal tumors of the jejunum and ileum: a clinicopathologic, immunohistochemical, and molecular genetic study of 906 cases before imatinib with long-term follow-up. Am J Surg Pathol. 2006;30:477.

Hermansky-Pudlak

30. Online Mendelian Inheritance in Man, OMIM®. Johns Hopkins University, Baltimore, MD. 203300: {203300}. 27 July 2016. World Wide Web URL: https://omim.org/entry/203300.
31. Hermansky-Pudlak Syndrome: National Library of Medicine (US). Genetics home reference [Internet]. Bethesda, MD: The Library. 15 Apr 2020. Hermansky-Pudlak syndrome. Reviewed May 2014; cited 25 Apr 2020. Available from: https://ghr.nlm.nih.gov/condition/hermansky-pudlak-syndrome.
32. Mora AJ, Wolfsohn DM. The management of gastrointestinal disease in Hermansky-Pudlak syndrome. J Clin Gastroenterol. 2011;45(8):700–2. https://doi.org/10.1097/MCG.0b013e3181fd2742.
33. Ozdemir N, Celik E, Baslar Z, Celkan T. A rare cause of thrombocyte dysfunction: Hermansky-Pudlak syndrome. Turk Pediatri Ars. 2014;49(2):163–6. https://doi.org/10.5152/tpa.2014.1071.

vEDS

34. Germain D. P. (2007). Ehlers-Danlos syndrome type IV. Orphanet J Rare Dis, 2, 32; Fikree A, Chelimsky G, Collins H, Kovacic K, Aziz Q. Gastrointestinal involvement in the Ehlers-Danlos syndromes. Am J Med Genet C. 2017;175(1):181–7. https://doi.org/10.1002/ajmg.c.31546.

35. Frank M, Adham S, Zinzindohoué F, Jeunemaitre X. Natural history of gastrointestinal manifestations in vascular Ehlers-Danlos syndrome: a 17-year retrospective review. J Gastroenterol Hepatol. 2018;34(5):857–63. https://doi.org/10.1111/jgh.14522.
36. Park KY, Gill KG, Kohler JE. Intestinal perforation in children as an important differential diagnosis of vascular Ehlers-Danlos syndrome. Am J Case Rep. 2019;20:1057–62. https://doi.org/10.12659/ajcr.917245.
37. Byers PH, Belmont J, Black J, et al. Diagnosis, natural history, and management in vascular Ehlers-Danlos syndrome. Am J Med Genet C. 2017;175(1):40–7. https://doi.org/10.1002/ajmg.c.31553.

Index

ted in the United States
ker & Taylor Publisher Services